T0199983

Psychopharmacology Algorithms

Clinical Guidance from the Psychopharmacology Algorithm Project at the Harvard South Shore Psychiatry Residency Program

Psychopharmacology Algorithms

Clinical Guidance from the Psychopharmacology Algorithm Project at the Harvard South Shore Psychiatry Residency Program

David N. Osser, MD
Associate Professor of Psychiatry
Harvard Medical School at the VA Boston Healthcare System
Brockton, Massachusetts

Wolters Kluwer

Philadelphia · Baltimore · New York · London
Buenos Aires · Hong Kong · Sydney · Tokyo

Acquisitions Editor: Chris Teja
Product Development Editor: Ariel S. Winter
Marketing Manager: Phyllis Hitner
Production Project Manager: Kirstin Johnson
Design Coordinator: Holly McLaughlin
Manufacturing Coordinator: Beth Welsh
Editorial Coordinator: Dave Murphy
Prepress Vendor: S4Carlisle Publishing Services

9

Printed in the United States of America

Library of Congress Cataloging-in-Publication Data

Names: Osser, David N. (David Neal), editor.
Title: Psychopharmacology algorithms: clinical guidance from the
    Psychopharmacology Algorithm Project at the Harvard South Shore
    Psychiatry Residency Program / [edited by] David N. Osser.
Description: Philadelphia: Wolters Kluwer Health, [2021] | Includes
    bibliographical references and index. | Summary: "Algorithms are useful
    in the field of psychopharmacology as they can serve as guidelines for
    avoiding the biases and cognitive lapses that are common when treating
    conditions that rely on uncertain data. In spite of this, evidence-based
    practices in psychopharmacology often require years to become widely
    adopted. The Psychopharmacology Algorithm Project at Harvard's South
    Shore Medical Program is an effort to speed up the adoption of
    evidence-based research into the day-to-day treatment of patients"—
    Provided by publisher.
Identifiers: LCCN 2020018487 | ISBN 9781975151195 (paperback)
Subjects: MESH: Psychopharmacology Algorithm Project at the Harvard South
    Shore Psychiatry Residency Program. | Mental Disorders—drug therapy |
    Psychotropic Drugs—administration & dosage | Algorithms | Practice
    Guidelines as Topic | Evidence-Based Medicine
Classification: LCC RC483 | NLM WM 402 | DDC 616.89/18—dc23
LC record available at https://lccn.loc.gov/2020018487

shop.lww.com

CONTRIBUTORS

Harmony Raylen Abejuela, MD
Clinical Fellow in Psychiatry
Harvard Medical School
Boston Children's Hospital
Boston, Massachusetts

Arash Ansari, MD
Instructor in Psychiatry
Department of Psychiatry
Harvard Medical School
Attending Psychiatrist
Faulkner Hospital
Boston, Massachusetts

Laura A. Bajor, DO
Clinical Fellow in Psychiatry
Harvard Medical School
Harvard South Shore Psychiatry
Residency Training Program
Brockton, Massachusetts

Ashley M. Beaulieu, DO
Clinical Fellow in Psychiatry
Department of Psychiatry
Harvard Medical School
VA Boston Healthcare System
Brockton, Massachusetts

Lance R. Dunlop, MD
Acting Medical Director
Cambria County Mental Health/Mental
Retardation Clinic
Johnstown, Pennsylvania

Christoforos Iraklis Giakoumatos, MD
Clinical Fellow in Psychiatry
Harvard Medical School
VA Boston Healthcare System
Brockton, Massachusetts

Leonard S. Lai, MD
Clinical Instructor
Department of Psychiatry
Harvard Medical School
Attending Psychiatrist
Faulkner Hospital
Boston, Massachusetts

James J. Levitt, MD
Assistant Professor of Psychiatry
Harvard Medical School
VA Boston Healthcare System
Brockton, Massachusetts

Theo Manschreck, MD
Clinical Professor of Psychiatry
Harvard Medical School at the
VA Boston
Healthcare System
Brockton, Massachusetts
Corrigan Mental Health Center
Fall River, Massachusetts
Harvard Commonwealth Center of
Excellence in Clinical Neuroscience and
Psychopharmacological Research
Beth Israel Deaconess Medical Center
Boston, Massachusetts

Othman Mohammad, MD
Clinical Fellow in Psychiatry
Harvard Medical School
Boston Children's Hospital
Boston, Massachusetts

David N. Osser, MD
Associate Professor of Psychiatry
Harvard Medical School at the VA Boston
Healthcare System
Brockton, Massachusetts

Robert D. Patterson, MD
Lecturer in Psychiatry
Harvard Medical School
McLean Hospital
Belmont, Massachusetts

Kenneth C. Potts, MD
Assistant Professor of Psychiatry
Harvard Medical School
Associate Chief of Psychiatry
Faulkner Hospital
Boston, Massachusetts

Mohsen Jalali Roudsari, MD
Laboratory for Clinical and Experimental
Psychopathology
Corrigan Mental Health Center
Fall River, Massachusetts
Harvard Commonwealth Center of
Excellence in Clinical Neuroscience and
Psychopharmacological Research
Beth Israel Deaconess Medical Center
Boston, Massachusetts

Paul M. Schoenfeld, MD
Instructor in Psychiatry
Department of Psychiatry
Harvard Medical School
Attending Psychiatrist
Faulkner Hospital
Boston, Massachusetts

Dana Wang, MD
Rivia Medical PLLC
New York, NY

Edward Tabasky, MD
Department of Psychiatry
NYS Psychiatric Institute
Columbia University College of
Physicians and Surgeons
New York, New York

Michael Tang, DO
Clinical Fellow in Psychiatry
Harvard Medical School
VA Boston Healthcare System
Brockton, Massachusetts

Ana Nectara Ticlea, MD
Clinical Fellow in Psychiatry
Harvard Medical School
Harvard South Shore Psychiatry
Residency Training Program
Brockton, Massachusetts

INTRODUCTION
AND HOW TO USE THIS BOOK*

This book contains reprints of nine peer-reviewed algorithms that were published between 2010 and 2020. I have carefully re-read each one. In a very few instances, sentences were found that did not convey the authors' intended point correctly. With permission of the publishers, these sentences were improved. Each paper is followed by a freshly-written Update which includes any changes from the original algorithm recommendations and a review of new information that adds or modifies the level of support for previous recommendations.

I am not sure if you should read the article first, and then the Update or vice-versa. You may want to try both sequences with different chapters. Maybe by reading the Update first you will be prepared for what has changed when you encounter it in the original paper. However, there are relatively few changes in most algorithms, and the main discussions and arguments supporting the reasoning for the recommendations are in the main paper. In either case, after reading both, the reader should be clear on how the algorithm should be sequenced (and the supporting evidence) as of the time of completion of the writing which was January, 2020.

The first chapter is a reprint of a paper giving a perspective on why we need psychopharmacology algorithms and the evidence-base for their utility.

The last two chapters are reprints of other papers (of which I was a co-author) that provide supplementary information and add support to the users of the algorithms. There is a long book chapter on Inpatient Psychopharmacology which reviews many issues pertinent to inpatient work with medications but also is applicable in outpatient settings as well. Though published in 2009, it seems surprisingly current and very few corrections were needed even though this was not a peer-reviewed publication. The final chapter describes a teaching program in psychopharmacology for the residents at the Harvard South Shore Psychiatry Residency Training Program (HSSRTP) that utilizes algorithms as one of the methods of teaching the subject. The algorithms in this book could be used in a similar manner by teachers. The courses that we give now at HSSRTP have changed somewhat in the 15-20 years since this publication. However, we still teach basic psychopharmacology (medications, their pharmacology, their uses, their side effects) in the early years of residency and use the algorithms in this book in the teaching with more advanced residents. Each of the algorithm teaching sessions includes a study of an important paper that helped influence some part of the algorithm, looking critically at methodology, statistics

*I thank Robert D. Patterson, M.D. for his contributions to this introductory chapter.

used, biases that could have affected the results, and the relationship with other studies of the same issues.

PATIENT ASSESSMENT PRIOR TO CONSULTING ALGORITHMS

The first step before prescribing psychiatric medication for a patient is to undertake a thorough psychiatric assessment. This involves reviewing past treatments and their effectiveness, considering the medical problems of the patient and noting the treatments for them that they are currently receiving (or perhaps should be receiving, as the case may be), conducting a psychiatric interview that considers the chief complaint(s), history of present illnesses, past and developmental histories, psychosocial and relationship histories, and mental status examination. It concludes with a formulation of the apparent causes of the person's problems and a diagnostic impression based on the criteria in the Diagnostic and Statistical Manual of Mental Disorders, 5th edition (DSM-5). One must evaluate the whole patient in order to understand the context of the specific disorders that might be targets for pharmacotherapy.[1] Anything less than this adds to the risks of errors in the choice of medications. This evaluation may need to be spread over several meetings before reaching final (but still tentative) initial conclusions. Ninety minutes is a time frame frequently required to evaluate a new patient in this manner, including the time for reviewing the previous record and writing the assessment. It might require longer or shorter times. Often, in the current managed care environment or in public sector care, clinicians are not allowed this much time (if employed) or may elect to take less time (in private practice) because of financial pressures. Clinical experience may convince practitioners that they can do an adequate psychiatric assessment in less time than just indicated and chose the correct medication for the correct diagnoses. Patients are usually not fooled, however: they very often can recognize when someone has taken a very short time to evaluate problems that the patient knows to be quite complex. They may be dubious when they are quickly sent home with a prescription. Subsequent very brief visits may strengthen the patient's impression of receiving "fast food" style care. This kind of practice is undermining the public's confidence in our profession.[2]

Use of the DSM-5 criteria for diagnosis is required in order to use these algorithms. This in not because we believe it is a perfect system for diagnosis but because the studies on which these algorithms rely are all based on evidence derived from psychopharmacology treatment studies of patients who met these criteria. Any use of these algorithms in patients diagnosed idiosyncratically or by some improvisational method that attempts to shortcut the DSM-5 diagnostic process may produce suboptimal results and may not be worthy of being called evidence-supported practice.

In many of the earlier studies cited, the patients met criteria for DSM-IV or DSM-III diagnoses. When there have been important differences between the older and newer DSM criteria the authors have done their best to help determine the relevance of these studies to current criteria. Some diagnostic criteria have changed relatively little and the current criteria are still largely adequate for applying the findings from studies using previous criteria. Schizophrenia is an example of this situation. However, generalized anxiety disorder (GAD) criteria, for example, have changed considerably and the algorithm for GAD takes this into account.

Many patients fall short of meeting DSM-5 criteria for one or more diagnoses which otherwise seem appropriate. These are difficult situations, but it may be reasonable to consider the algorithm's recommendations though with less confidence because the patients on which the recommendations are based are not fully comparable.

You may notice that there is no algorithm for schizoaffective disorder, though we have one for schizophrenia and for mania with psychosis. This is because there is no adequate or significant quantity of evidence out there from which an algorithm can be derived. See the algorithm for schizophrenia for a full discussion of that issue with appropriate references and suggestions for how to treat patients who meet the DSM-5 criteria for schizoaffective disorder.

HOW TO HANDLE COMORBIDITY

Some have said: "All my patients are complex and have lots of comorbidity, so the algorithms are useless to me." Sometimes, this is an excuse to not be informed about the best evidence for treating each diagnosis separately. In response, I suggest the following: when there is comorbidity, delineate the various diagnoses that are present. Then, determine (in collaboration with the patient) the one that seems to be contributing the most to the patient's distress or dysfunction, and treat that first with evidence-derived treatments as in these algorithms. For example, if the patient has rapid cycling bipolar disorder plus other problems, getting the bipolar disorder under control may be the top priority, and if that is accomplished some or all of the other problems may become milder or subclinical in severity. Another example would be a patient actively using substances. Getting the patient into remission from their use disorders will, in many cases, deserve priority. Even cannabis use disorder, which can exacerbate bipolar disorder and post-traumatic stress disorder,[3] may need to be addressed before one can expect medications normally effective for those comorbidities to have the usual benefit.

There is some information about management of important comorbidities in each algorithm paper, showing how the presence of these comorbidities modifies the basic algorithm for that diagnosis. When there is no useful evidence on how to manage the primary disorder with comorbidities that may be present, it seems reasonable to treat the primary diagnosis in accordance with the algorithm unless a good reason to not do so is apparent. Then, if there is some success in managing the primary problem, address the next most important diagnosis that is still causing distress or disability. If there is a lack of success with the first diagnosis, reassess the differential diagnoses again and perhaps on this reconsideration it will appear that there is another diagnosis that is most important. Continue with one diagnosis at a time, and usually one change of treatment at a time, until all the major diagnoses are managed optimally. With complex patients, this can be a project that can take many months of fairly intensive care, but it can be gratifying for the clinician and patient to see a process of gradual improvement of one diagnosis after another that is affecting their quality of life.

Other factors may affect the order of treatment of the different diagnoses, including the patient's willingness to accept the risks of side effects of the medications for the diagnosis, patient willingness to accept the diagnosis itself (due to stigma or other considerations), and drug interactions or other medical considerations that may require certain diagnoses to be managed first.

Remember that a change in treatment can include addition or subtraction of a medication – both can have significant positive and adverse effects, so it is best not to do two changes at once if possible. Even discontinuation of nicotine can have major adverse neuropsychiatric effects.[4]

WHAT ABOUT PSYCHOTHERAPY AND OTHER NON-MEDICATION TREATMENTS?

These algorithms are designed to help choose the most evidence-supported medication if the practitioner decides to use medication. They do not generally offer guidance for when to select medication as a first-line treatment over psychotherapy, or when to add medication to psychotherapy if psychotherapy is chosen first-line. The focus of the algorithms is to provide help with deciding which medication should be chosen first, second and third.

WHAT DETERMINES THE ORDER OF RECOMMENDED MEDICATIONS IN THE ALGORITHMS?

The order of selection of medications in the algorithms is derived from consideration of efficacy (results in randomized, placebo-controlled trials), effectiveness (outcome in less-well-controlled or observational studies, case series, and other reports), ability to maintain initial efficacy or effectiveness, and side effect burden that is acceptable to patients over the short term and (importantly) long term. These are important considerations, with greater or lesser importance depending on the level of treatment-resistance of the target problem. For example, a medication that is very well tolerated but does not have the largest effect size might be chosen for the first treatment for a disorder instead of one that has a large effect size but more side effects. Patients who have already failed several trials might need to try a medication which has more severe side effects but greater evidence of effectiveness. Whenever possible, algorithms in this book offer a selection of medications at each node that are judged by the authors to be of approximately equal efficacy and tolerability. The specifics vary and the choice will be made by the prescriber and patient agreeing on the medication that seems the best fit for their needs given what side effects they would be most willing to risk. Sometimes there will be first-line options at a particular node but also some second line options that are reasonable to consider if the side effects of the first-line choices are all unacceptable to the patient or clinician.

Occasionally cost is a consideration, but only if deciding between two or more choices of approximately equal efficacy and safety. In that case we suggest choosing the less expensive option.

THE WEBSITE FOR THESE ALGORITHMS

The recommendations in the algorithms in this book may also be accessed online at the website www.psychopharm.mobi. There one can find flowcharts of each algorithm, and each node has a box that is linked to a short text which is an abbreviated version of the texts in the algorithm papers. There are a few references in each box, and these are linked to PubMed so if you click on them, the article abstract will appear. The website is best employed to quickly obtain a reminder of the recommendations with which the reader is already familiar from having read the full text with the nuanced analysis of the evidence base leading to the recommendations. Sometimes there will be only subtle preferences for some options over others and this can only be appreciated by having read the full texts: the web version can seem unduly rigid or be misleading without having read the full explanation. An advantage of the versions on the web is that they are updated when there are important new developments, so they are always the latest versions. Also, as new algorithms are developed they will appear on the website.

EVIDENCE-BASED MEDICINE: AN ART

The practice of evidence-based medicine is an art - because it requires making decisions based on voluminous, uncertain and very hard-to-quantify data.[5] These algorithms help provide users with the important evidence and what it might mean for practice. However, the art involves the ability to determine how well the evidence applies to any given patient. Competent practitioners may "deviate" from the what the evidence suggests when that evidence does not seem generalizable to their patient because of comorbidities or complexities not addressed by the evidence. The algorithms in this book endeavor to address many of these complexities so as to make them as useful as possible to the largest number of patients, but there will be many gaps. Patients may not be willing to take the most effective treatments. Some of the art of medicine is in the ability to persuade patients to take the most evidence-based treatment. Part of this persuasiveness comes from the patient having confidence that the prescriber has listened well, understands the total patient and appears ready to be available in a timely manner with practical solutions to side effects that might occur.[6]

Clinicians who are also academicians and specialize in certain diagnoses may not find these algorithms that useful. They already know the evidence as well or better than the authors of these papers. They see in consultation or treat directly many treatment-resistant patients and apply their knowledge to the best of their considerable ability. However, the generalist practitioner who treats many kinds of patients may not be able to devote the huge amount of time required to critically evaluate the evidence base for all the diagnoses they encounter. For them, it may seem reasonable to have one place to go where they can find thoughtful analyses of the evidence distilled into algorithmic heuristics. However, there does have to be some trust involved that the experts writing these algorithms (and the peer reviewers who contributed) have produced reliable and actionable advice.

Clinical experience is also important in decision making, but there will be more to say about that in the next chapter.

WHAT ALGORITHMS ARE NEXT?

We have published one new algorithm in 2020 since this book went to production, so it could not be included in the book: An Algorithm for Core Symptoms of Autism Spectrum Disorder in Adults.[7] There are two new algorithms that are being drafted and hopefully are coming soon: Psychopharmacology for Behavioral Symptoms in Dementia., and Adults with Attention-Deficit Hyperactivity Disorder. A revision of the 2011 Posttraumatic Stress Disorder algorithm also has a manuscript in draft form.

It is the author's intention to update this book with future editions.

DISCLOSURE OF COMPETING INTERESTS

The author of this book has received no compensation from drug companies. Royalties are earned from another book: Ansari A and Osser DN. Psychopharmacology: A concise Overview for Students and Clinicians, 2nd Edition 2015, published by CreateSpace. A third edition will appear in 2020 with Oxford University Press. These books do not contain algorithms.

IMPORTANT NOTE

The information presented in this book is meant to be a summary or overview of prescribing suggestions for different diagnostic situations. The content should be used by prescribing clinicians as a consultation, but the recommendations should not be followed rigidly. There should be thoughtful and thorough evaluation of the appropriateness of the suggestions herein before prescribing. The author is not rendering professional services through this book. Although every effort has been made to present the material accurately, no representations are made as to the accuracy or completeness of the contents. There may be typographical or other errors including misinterpretations of the evidence base or failure to take into account uncited studies. Before prescribing anything, the package insert of the medication should be reviewed and the medication should be administered in accordance with the relevant information. Patients should not make any changes in their treatment based on the contents of this book without consulting with their prescribing provider.

REFERENCES

1. Baldessarini RJ. Status and prospects for psychopharmacology. In: *Chemotherapy in Psychiatry* 3ed. New York: Springer; 2013:251-63.
2. Zulman DM, Haverfield MC, Shaw JG, et al. Practices to Foster Physician Presence and Connection With Patients in the Clinical Encounter. *JAMA* 2020;323:70-81.
3. Mammen G, Rueda S, Roerecke M, Bonato S, Lev-Ran S, Rehm J. Association of Cannabis With Long-Term Clinical Symptoms in Anxiety and Mood Disorders: A Systematic Review of Prospective Studies. *J Clin Psychiatry* 2018;79.
4. Anthenelli RM, Benowitz NL, West R, et al. Neuropsychiatric safety and efficacy of varenicline, bupropion, and nicotine patch in smokers with and without psychiatric disorders (EAGLES): a double-blind, randomised, placebo-controlled clinical trial. *Lancet* 2016;387:2507-20.
5. Worsham C, Jena AB. Decision making: The art of evidence-based medicine. In: *Harvard Business Review*. Cambridge, MA: Harvard Business School; 2019.
6. Salzman C, Glick I, Keshavan MS. The 7 sins of psychopharmacology. *J Clin Psychopharmacol* 2010;30:653-5.
7. Gannon S, Osser DN. The psychopharmacology algorithm project at the Harvard South Shore Program: An algorithm for core symptoms of autism spectrum disorder in adults. *Psychiatry Res* 2020;287:112900.

ACKNOWLEDGMENTS

The author wishes to thank his many collaborators that contributed to the development and publication of these algorithms, those who provided support and encouragement in these endeavors, and those who aided in bringing them to the awareness of clinicians and others who have found them useful.

First of all, there are the coauthors of the articles, who are also listed on the title page of each algorithm reprint. These 20 authors (many of them were residents in training at the Harvard South Shore Psychiatry Residency Training Program) spent, in many cases, hundreds of hours on nights and weekends searching for articles, reading them, communicating with coauthors in discussions of their importance, and preparing draft after draft of the algorithm articles before submission and in response to reviewers' critiques. Without their hard work and energy, these articles would never have been written.

I also thank the blinded reviewers of each article. Though I do not know who they were, these individuals were clearly experts on the subject matter of the articles and made substantive and sophisticated criticisms that required resolution and achievement of consensus before the articles could be accepted for publication. These reviews added significant validity to the final versions of each algorithm in that they reduced any initial biases detected and broadened the number of persons in agreement with the interpretations of the literature in the final published version.

My supporters over the years deserve heartfelt thanks. Algorithms are controversial, and some physicians do not welcome the appearance of medication treatment algorithms in psychiatry no matter how evidence-supported and peer-reviewed they may be. I have more to say about this in the introductory chapter. The following mentors and supporters from the United States and in corners of the world have offered strong moral and practical support at different points (or continuously) over the years: (listed alphabetically) Ross Baldessarini, MD; Mark Bauer, MD; Rogelio Bayog, MD; Mesut Çetin, MD (Turkey); B. Eliot Cole, MD; Joseph Coyle, MD; Anne Dantzler, MD; John Davis, MD; Lynn DeLisi, MD; Serdar Dursun, MD (Canada); Jan Fawcett, MD; Eugene Fierman, MD; Ira Glick, MD; Shelly Greenfield, MD; Susan Gulesian, MD; Flavio Guzman, MD (Argentina); Philip Janicak, MD; Kenneth Jobson, MD; Gary Kaplan, MD; Xiang-Yang Li, MD; Steven Locke, MD; Mansfield Mela, MD (Canada); Herbert Meltzer, MD; Dean Najarian, RPh, BCPP; Jessica Oesterheld, MD; Jonathan Osser (my brother); Chester Pearlman, MD; Ronald Pies, MD; John Renner, MD; Raluca Savu, MD; Richard I. Shader, MD (my first and perhaps most significant mentor in psychopharmacology); Miles Shore, MD; Tian-Mei Si, MD (China); Robert Sigadel, MD; Stephen Soreff, MD;

Dan Stein, MD (South Africa); Cheng-Hua Tien, MD (China); Ming Tsuang, MD; Xin Yu, MD (China); and Carlos Zarate, MD.

Next, there is perhaps my most significant supporter, collaborator, overall mentor, friend, and the psychiatrist who did the most by far to encourage me to keep producing these algorithms and who made extraordinary efforts (that I never could have done on my own) over decades to circulate the algorithms in computerized versions and over the Internet using progressively improved interfaces: Robert D. Patterson, MD. Surely, without his input, these academic products would never have been completed much less achieved the level of recognition, such as it is, that they may have achieved. He is the director of the Information Technology component of this work and is the creator of our website www.psychopharm.mobi.

And finally, I want to thank from the bottom of my heart my beloved and beautiful wife of 38 years, Stephanie, and our children Roselin and Daniel, who put up with my many, many hours devoted to this calling when I could have been spending more quality time with them.

I hope I have not left out anyone that should be on this list and if so please accept my apology.

David N. Osser, MD
Needham, Massachusetts
January 2020

CONTENTS

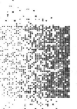

On the Value of Evidence-Based Psychopharmacology Algorithms

David N. Osser, MD[1] and Robert D. Patterson, MD[2]

Lucian Leape raised awareness of the high error rate in medicine (1). These errors may be due to "slips" (unintentional mistakes) or may result from not obtaining key facts about the patient's history or from not knowing or applying the best evidence for optimal care of the patient. The remedy for the latter is said to be the practice of Evidence-Based Medicine (EBM) – which has been defined by Sackett and colleagues as "…integrating clinical expertise with the best available external clinical evidence from systematic research" (2).

However, EBM is easier said than done. For psychopharmacology, it requires a laborious process of activity and thinking. First one must make a criteria-based Diagnostic and Statistical Manual diagnosis, identifying subtypes, specifiers, and comorbidity that may affect what treatment will be preferred. This is necessary because almost all of the psychopharmacology evidence is derived from studies of patients that are carefully diagnosed by these criteria. The treatment history must then be explored in detail for adequacy and outcomes of trials in order to avoid repeating ineffective or harmful approaches used in the past. Finally, it is necessary to search for, find, read, and interpret the pertinent literature. This idealized approach to clinical practice is impractical because it takes far too much time and requires use of cognitive processes that may be unfamiliar to some clinicians.

These barriers have limited the usefulness of EBM in the day-to-day practice of medicine and psychopharmacology.

Instead of using EBM, clinicians often resort to quicker but more error-prone processes of decision-making (3). Reflexive decisions are decisions made without consciously considering any alternative, usually because you are in a hurry. Under this heading there are bias-driven judgments, which are decisions motivated by overconfidence based on some bias. Also there is the availability heuristic, which is grabbing the first idea that comes to mind (4,5). Another cause of errors is the affective heuristic which is the tendency of affect-laden practice experiences (either positive or negative) to be far more influential than considerations based on the scientific evidence. For example, if you once had a patient who had a Stevens-Johnson syndrome from lamotrigine, you may be reluctant to prescribe that medication again even if it is a preferred option for preventing recurrence of bipolar depression. If statistics are presented on the low frequency of this syndrome, you will not believe them.

[1]Associate Professor of Psychiatry, Harvard Medical School at the VA Boston Healthcare System, Brockton Division, 940 Belmont Street, Brockton, MA 02301, USA
E-mail: david.osser@va.gov
[2]Lecturer in Psychiatry, Harvard Medical School, McLean Hospital, 115 Mill Street, Belmont, MA 02478, USA,
E-mail: bpatterson5961@gmail.com
Bulletin of Clinical Psychopharmacology 2013;23(1):XX-X

These quick, intuitive decisions are sometimes excused (or praised) as being part of the art of medicine. Faith in this art is part of the culture of medicine, with deep historical roots. For thousands of years, the apprentice model dominated training in medical practice. The art is initially conveyed by more experienced mentors, and then augmented by personal experience as the emerging practitioner makes his/her own mistakes. As Groopman has noted, we do not want airline pilots to learn from their mistakes – we want them to make the right decisions every time. However, the healthcare system continues to be built on a foundation of mistakes followed by "corrective action plans" (3).

Busy physicians typically do a limited review of the patient's history and mental status, focusing on certain symptoms or historical details that seem likely to explain the patient's chief complaint, after which the treatment plan just "falls into place" (6). Practice is centered on faith in a collection of "rules of thumb" that can be applied rapidly and confidently. However, Michael O'Donnell, M.D., former editor of the British Medical Journal, quipped that this kind of clinical experience ran result in "… making the same mistakes over and over with increasing confidence over an impressive number of years" (7).

There is a neurobiology of how people react to information and experience. Risk-taking tendency, for example, is a strongly heritable personality trait (0.58 heritability in twins (8)). Thus, while some psychiatrists will rarely use clozapine even when clearly indicated because of fear of its risks, others may have minimal fear and even overlook necessary monitoring. This is not the only reason that clozapine is under-prescribed, however: it has been found that when scientifically validated, well-evidenced treatment approaches take more time than what physicians do now and believe works well, they will not provide the time-consuming treatment (9).

Other problems with using clinical experience as the primary basis for practice are the generally small Ns of the experience, and sampling differences: i.e., the patient to be treated now may not in fact be at all similar to the dimly-recollected previous patients.

Drug companies are also shaping decision-making, sometimes against EBM, taking advantage of "novelty preference bias," "familiarity effect" and "overoptimism bias" (10). Their representatives provide education that may be neither objective nor comprehensive but is quick, easy, and often accompanied by free samples. The pharmaceutical firms (usually in collaboration with academic psychiatry) produce most of the psychopharmacological studies and influence their design, interpretation, and publication in ways that tend to encourage excessive valuation of new expensive products (11,12). These studies are typically done for short lengths of time in otherwise healthy and uncomplicated patients who are not representative of the more difficult patients seen in typical practice who may be suicidal, use substances, and have much medical comorbidity. This has undermined confidence in the applicability of much of the evidence-base (13), and at the least requires that EBM practitioners become sophisticated in their ability to detect the flaws and biases of studies so that they will not draw false conclusions from them.

This brings us to the proposed solution to these problems in teaching and learning psychopharmacology: psychopharmacology algorithms that are informed by the evidence and that distill and synthesize the available research and organize it into a coherent blueprint for practice. The algorithms should be developed and updated frequently by consensus among respected EBM experts who have distanced themselves from drug-company support. They should clearly indicate best or preferred practice for cases of progressive complexity, and from initial treatment through very treatment-resistant scenarios. They should provide a scaffolding structure for organizing the data relevant to specific kinds of patients. Thus, if a new study is published, or a new medication becomes available, information about these developments can be combined with and compared with the other knowledge on the shelf for that decision point. The clinician can decide if the new information should change practice for a typical patient at that node of the algorithm – or wait for the expert consensus update. Experts have argued that healthcare desperately needs such syntheses, and the production of them needs to be recognized as a methodology and field in its own right (14,15).

What are some of the qualities of these algorithms/guidelines that would indicate that they are valid enough for clinical use? The Institute of Medicine has proposed a comprehensive set of standards (16). Few existing guidelines meet all the criteria, which include authors (a) having few to no conflicts of interest, (b) providing explanations of the reasoning behind each recommendation, (c) obtaining rigorous external review before publication, and (d) updating frequently. To these it there should be added that evidence of short and long term safety are considerations that are just as important as efficacy evidence in motivating the sequencing of medication recommendations (17). Further, there should be acknowledgement of other published algorithms with different conclusion and an analysis of the basis for the differences with attempts to resolve them (17). The impact of comorbidity, medical and psychiatric, including the effect if the patient is a woman of child-bearing potential, should be assessed and recommendations offered.

Finally, it should be emphasized that algorithms, no matter how well-constructed, should not be followed rigidly as if they represent absolute truth. They are aids to judgment, and practitioners should be free to determine whether or not they are suitable for application to an individual patient. Despite this caveat, it is worth noting that evidence from other fields (e.g. - engineering) suggests that when algorithm-based decisions and individual expert judgment have been compared, the results have favored algorithm adherence (18, 19). Occasionally, the expert makes a "brilliant" judgment when deviating from the algorithm that proves correct, but more often when the expert deviates, the result is an error. A good algorithm or guideline will offer and discuss some of the alternatives that could be considered at each node and why they are not favored first-line but could be reasonable under some circumstances.

What is the evidence that following psychopharmacology algorithms improves outcome? While standardized care driven by evidence-supported algorithms is a model that has produced good outcomes with other illnesses such as diabetes, pneumonia, and heart disease (20), there have not been very many studies in psychiatry and the results have been modest. Bauer examined tests of guidelines up to the year 2000 and found that 6 of 13 studies reported improved outcomes associated with guideline adherence (21). More recent psychopharmacology algorithm studies in depression were reviewed by Adli and colleagues (22) who found that patients treated with the algorithm initially benefitted more than the control group but further separation from "treatment as usual" did not necessarily occur over time (23). The early benefits could have been due to more intensive patient involvement with the project coordinator in the algorithm group. Studies in schizophrenia have found small advantages from following an algorithms (Texas Algorithm Project and German Society for Psychiatry guideline), including reduced side effects and less polypharmacy with antipsychotics (24,25). The differences were not robust perhaps because all controlled studies to date have compared use of an entire algorithm versus treatment as usual. In an algorithm there are multiple recommendations. Clinicians in the treatment-as-usual arms also usually do most of them. Of the recommendations that clinicians do not follow so often, the alternatives chosen will sometimes produce a significant difference in outcome and some may not. In the schizophrenia studies, physicians rarely complied with the algorithm recommendation to use clozapine after two adequate trials of antipsychotics. The control groups also did not use much clozapine. This may account for the lack of strong outcome differences: the algorithm-following physicians did not choose to follow the recommendation with the greatest likelihood of producing a better overall outcome for their patients!

The Texas and German algorithm groups did find that regular intensive educational discussions about the guidelines (which requires support by hospital and clinic leadership) can overcome some of these barriers. Discussions with patients to convince them of the value of the algorithm recommendations may be another critical factor.

A recent objection to EBM in general and the algorithms/guidelines derived from the evidence has come from the new emphasis on the potential for "personalized medicine (PM)" (26). Since evidence is gathered from studies of heterogeneous patient populations (e.g. – major depression) it can only give an average or typical response rate in such a group. However, this conflict between EBM and PM appears to be based on a false dichotomy. When specific biological markers or other tests enable the delineation of subgroups with specific treatment, this will be added to the diagnostic process that precedes the application of the algorithm, and the personalized treatment will be applied to those eligible for it. Then, the others in the population will be appropriate candidates for the general recommendations.

An unsolved problem with the clinical use of even the best algorithms is that some clinicians may feel pressed to make hasty consultations with the algorithm's summary flowchart rather than reading the full text and appreciating all the nuances of the reasoning. The result can be grossly inaccurate appreciation of what is recommended and significant patient care errors. On the other hand, caveat emptor (let the buyer beware) is an appropriate aphorism to warn those too eager to utilize algorithms. Some of the algorithms that have been presented in a variety of publications are oversimplified, subject to significant biases, or may give bad advice due to reasoning errors.

The Psychopharmacology Algorithm Project at the Harvard South Shore Program based at the VA Boston Healthcare System, Brockton Division, has been publishing and revising psychopharmacology algorithms for over 20 years. The more recent ones seem to meet many but not all of the IOM guidelines for quality (27-33). Most are available on the project's web site www.psychopharm.mobi. Their strongest feature is that the facts cited, analysis of the literature, and reasoning are examined in a blinded peer review process by up to 5 content experts selected by the journal editors. If the reasoning, based on the evidence interpretations provided, was plausible to all reviewers, then it was retained. When there were differences of opinion, adjustments were made or further exploration of pertinent evidence was done until consensus was achieved or a stronger argument in support of the authors' interpretation was composed.

Algorithms will be of more practical value when their most important advice – advice that differs from usual practice and may give better results – can be provided to the prescribing clinician at the point of care as part of a computerized medical record and order-entry system. Computerized expert systems are not yet common in psychiatric practice, though they are in many other complex endeavors such as flying airplanes, piloting boats, driving cars to reach a specific destination, complying with tax laws, and analyzing case law to come up with the best legal arguments. Patient outcomes could improve if algorithm-based computer applications to aid the practice of psychopharmacology were to be developed and then utilized by clinicians.

REFERENCES

1. Leape LL. Error in medicine. JAMA. 1994;272(23):1851-7.
2. Sackett DL, Rosenberg WM, Gray JA, Haynes RB, Richardson WS. Evidence based medicine: what it is and what it isn't. BMJ. 1996;312(7023):71-2.
3. Groopman J. How Doctors Think. Boston: Houghton Mifflin Company; 2007.
4. Tversky A, Kahneman D. Judgment under Uncertainty: Heuristics and Biases. Science. 1974;185(4157):1124-31.
5. Kassirer JP, Kopelman RI. Derailed by the availability heuristic. Hosp Pract (Off Ed). 1987;22(6):59-60, 5-9.
6. Patel VL, Arocha JF, Kaufman DR. A primer on aspects of cognition for medical informatics. J Am Med Inform Assoc. 2001;8(4):324-43.
7. O'Donnell M. A Sceptic's Medical Dictionary. London: BMJ Publishing Group; 1997.
8. Ebstein RP, Zohar AH, Benjamin J, Belmaker RH. An update on molecular genetic studies of human personality traits. Appl Bioinformatics. 2002;1(2):57-68.
9. Buchman TG, Patel VL, Dushoff J, Ehrlich PR, Feldman M, Feldman M, et al. Enhancing the use of clinical guidelines: a social norms perspective. J Am Coll Surg. 2006;202(5):826-36.
10. Makhinson M. Biases in medication prescribing: the case of second-generation antipsychotics. J Psychiatr Pract. 2010;16(1):15-21.
11. Osser DN. Cleaning up evidence-based psychopharmacology. Psychopharm Review. 2008;43(3):19-26.
12. Sen S, Prabhu M. Reporting bias in industry-supported medication trials presented at the American Psychiatric Association meeting. J Clin Psychopharmacol. 2012;32(3):435.
13. Levine R, Fink M. The case against evidence-based principles in psychiatry. Med Hypotheses. 2006;67(2):401-10.
14. Dickersin K. Health-care policy. To reform U.S. health care, start with systematic reviews. Science. 2010;329(5991):516-7.
15. Davidoff F, Miglus J. Delivering clinical evidence where it's needed: building an information system worthy of the profession. JAMA. 2011;305(18):1906-7.
16. Ransohoff DF, Pignone M, Sox HC. How to decide whether a clinical practice guideline is trustworthy. JAMA. 2013;309(2):139-40.
17. Osser DN, Patterson RD. Algorithms for psychopharmacology. In: Shader RI, ed. Manual of Psychiatric Therapeutics, Third Edition. Boston: Little, Brown and Co.; 2003:479-84.

18. Dawes RM. The robust beauty of improper linear models in decision making. In: Kahneman D, Slovic P, Tversky A, eds. Judgment Under Uncertainty: Heuristics and Biases. New York: Cambridge University Press; 1983:391-407.

19. Dawes RM, Faust D, Meehl PE. Clinical versus actuarial judgment. Science. 1989;243(4899):1668-74.

20. Mullaney TJ. Doctors wielding data. Business Week. 2005;94:98.

21. Bauer MS. A review of quantitative studies of adherence to mental health clinical practice guidelines. Harv Rev Psychiatry. 2002;10(3):138-53.

22. Adli M, Bauer M, Rush AJ. Algorithms and collaborative-care systems for depression: are they effective and why? A systematic review. Biol Psychiatry. 2006;59(11):1029-38.

23. Trivedi MH, Rush AJ, Crismon ML, Kashner TM, Toprac MG, Carmody TJ, et al. Clinical results for patients with major depressive disorder in the Texas Medication Algorithm Project. Arch Gen Psychiatry. 2004;61(7):669-80.

24. Miller AL, Crismon ML, Rush AJ, Chiles J, Kashner TM, Toprac M, et al. The Texas medication algorithm project: clinical results for schizophrenia. Schizophr Bull. 2004;30(3):627-47.

25. Weinmann S, Hoerger S, Erath M, Kilian R, Gaebel W, Becker T. Implementation of a schizophrenia practice guideline: clinical results. J Clin Psychiatry. 2008;69(8):1299-306.

26. de Leon J. Evidence-based medicine versus personalized medicine: are they enemies? J Clin Psychopharmacol. 2012;32(2):153-64.

27. Ansari A, Osser DN. The psychopharmacology algorithm project at the Harvard South Shore Program: an update on bipolar depression. Harv Rev Psychiatry. 2010;18(1):36-55.

28. Bajor LA, Ticlea AN, Osser DN. The Psychopharmacology Algorithm Project at the Harvard South Shore Program: an update on posttraumatic stress disorder. Harv Rev Psychiatry. 2011;19(5):240-58.

29. Hamoda HM, Osser DN. The Psychopharmacology Algorithm Project at the Harvard South Shore Program: an update on psychotic depression. Harv Rev Psychiatry. 2008;16(4):235- 47.

30. Osser DN, Dunlop LR. The Psychopharmacology Algorithm Project at the Harvard South Shore Program: an update on generalized social anxiety disorder. Psychopharm Review. 2010;45(12):91-8.

31. Tang M, Osser DN. The Psychopharmacology Algorithm Project at the Harvard South Shore Program: 2012 update on psychotic depression. Journal of Mood Disorders. 2012;2(4):167-79.

32. Osser DN, Jalali-Roudsari M, Manschreck T. The Psychopharmacology Algorithm Project at the Harvard South Shore Program: an update on schizopnrenia. Harv Rev Psychiatry. 2013;21(1):18-41.

33. Mohammad OM, Osser DN. The Psychopharmacology Algorithm Project at the Harvard South Shore Program: an algorithm for acute mania. 2013:Submitted.

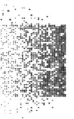

The Psychopharmacology Algorithm Project at the Harvard South Shore Program: An Update on Bipolar Depression

Dana Wang, MD[1] and David N. Osser, MD[2]

Abstract

Background: *The Psychopharmacology Algorithm Project at the Harvard South Shore Program (PAPHSS) published algorithms for bipolar depression in 1999 and 2010. Developments over the past 9 years suggest that another update is needed.*

Methods: *The 2010 algorithm and associated references were reevaluated. A literature search was conducted on PubMed for recent studies and review articles to see what changes in the recommendations were justified. Exceptions to the main algorithm for special patient populations, including those with attention-deficit hyperactivity disorder (ADHD), posttraumatic stress disorder (PTSD), substance use disorders, anxiety disorders, and women of childbearing potential, and those with common medical comorbidities were considered.*

Results: *Electroconvulsive therapy (ECT) is still the first-line option for patients in need of urgent treatment. Five medications are recommended for early usage in acute bipolar depression, singly or in combinations when monotherapy fails, the order to be determined by considerations such as side effect vulnerability and patient preference. The five are lamotrigine, lurasidone, lithium, quetiapine, and cariprazine. After trials of these, possible options include antidepressants (bupropion and selective serotonin reuptake inhibitors are preferred) or valproate (very small evidence-base). In bipolar II depression, the support for antidepressants is a little stronger but depression with mixed features and rapid cycling would usually lead to further postponement of antidepressants. Olanzapine+fluoxetine, though Food and Drug Administration (FDA) approved for bipolar depression, is not considered until beyond this point, due to metabolic side effects. The algorithm concludes with a table of other possible treatments that have some evidence.*

Conclusions: *This revision incorporates the latest FDA-approved treatments (lurasidone and cariprazine) and important new studies and organizes the evidence systematically.*

Keywords: algorithms, bipolar depression, cariprazine, lurasidone, psychopharmacology

---

[1]Rivia Medical PLLC, New York, NY, USA

[2]Department of Psychiatry, Harvard Medical School, VA Boston Healthcare System, Brockton Division, Brockton, MA, USA

Correspondence: David Osser, 150 Winding River Road, Needham, MA 02492.

Email: davidosser0846@gmail.com

DOI: 10.1111/bdi.12860

INTRODUCTION

Bipolar depression (BP-DEP) is the predominant mood state for patients with bipolar disorder and is associated with significantly more long-term impairment in psychosocial functioning and quality-of-life compared with unipolar depression.[1] Unipolar depression and bipolar depression differ in response to pharmacotherapeutic agents.[2] BP-DEP can present in bipolar I or bipolar II disorders, with mixed features or rapid cycling. There is a lifetime prevalence of up to 20% for comorbidity with posttraumatic stress disorder (PTSD), 47% for substance use disorders,[3,4] and 75% for anxiety disorders.[5] These comorbidities complicate diagnosis and selection of pharmacotherapy.

There is a paucity of evidence-supported treatment choices.Only four medications have received United States Food and Drug Administration (FDA) approval for acute BP-DEP. The olanzapine-fluoxetine combination (OFC) was the first approved, in 2003. Quetiapine was approved in 2006. In 2013, lurasidone was approved as a monotherapy and as an adjunct to ongoing lithium or valproate for bipolar I depression. The fourth, cariprazine, was approved in 2019. Lamotrigine is approved for prevention of relapse in bipolar I disorder (mainly against BP-DEP), though studies did not provide sufficient support for approval for acute episodes. Lithium has FDA approval for acute mania and for prevention of bipolar mood episodes, but not for acute BP-DEP. There is a variety of options without solid evidence of efficacy or FDA-labeling for BP-DEP, including traditional antidepressants. Clinical experience and other heuristics contribute to decisions to prefer less-evidenced strategies.[6] In this paper, a treatment approach is presented that considers the most up-to-date evidence and shows how to best apply it in a variety of clinical scenarios ranging from initial treatment to the most treatment-resistant cases while taking into account some of the comorbidities frequently encountered.

This is an update of the 2010 algorithm of the Psychopharmacology Algorithm Project at the Harvard South Shore Program (PAPHSS).[7] It includes new recommendations for bipolar depression with comorbid attention-deficit hyperactivity disorder (ADHD), PTSD, substance use disorders, anxiety disorders, and women of childbearing potential or pregnant, and some medical conditions.

MATERIALS AND METHODS

The methods used in developing new and revised PAPHSS algorithms have been described previously.[7-11] In brief, the authors reviewed the 2010 BP-DEP algorithm, conducted literature searches using PubMed with keywords pertaining to available psychopharmacological agents with a focus on new randomized controlled trials (RCTs), and consulted recent guidelines, reviews, and meta-analyses. The authors consider short- and long-term efficacy, effectiveness, tolerability, and safety of the different treatment options, and then formulate an opinion-based qualitative distillation of this literature focused on what changes seem appropriate to make in the previous peer-reviewed and published version. Basic principles include a preference for using the fewest medications whenever possible and emphasizing acute effectiveness but also with particularly strong focus on long-term safety and tolerability, given that bipolar disorder may be life-long. The evidence that a regimen can prevent future illness episodes is also important.

After informal review by other experts, PAPHSS algorithm drafts are submitted for publication in peer-reviewed journals. The review process provides additional validation of the appropriateness and plausibility of the authors' interpretation of the literature.

The algorithm is meant as a heuristic to aid judgment but should not be applied rigidly: practitioners must be free to determine whether the recommendations seem reasonable taking into account the unique aspects of each patient.

DIAGNOSIS OF BIPOLAR DEPRESSION

By definition, patients diagnosed with BP-DEP meet criteria for a major depressive episode and have a history of manic or hypomanic episodes. Hypomania is difficult to diagnose retrospectively and vigorous pursuit of the diagnosis may be required. A "pre-bipolar" depression[12] should be suspected in patients with: a family history of bipolar disorder or suicide, a relatively young age at onset, a history of quick remissions and frequent recurrences, current or past postpartum psychosis or major mood disturbance, past poor response to antidepressants, and history of antidepressant-emergent agitation, irritability, or suicidality. In addition, depression with "atypical" features (hypersomnia, hyperphagia with weight gain, leaden paralysis, and rejection sensitivity) also warrants close monitoring for emergence of hypomania or mania.[13] Those with a seasonal pattern of mood fluctuation can also be at risk for bipolar disorder.[14]

THE ALGORITHM

The flowchart

A summary and overview of the algorithm appears in Figure 1. The questions, evidence analysis, and reasoning that support the recommendations at each node are presented below. The following discussion focuses on a sequence of options most pertinent to BP-DEP patients that are relatively uncomplicated by comorbidities. Later, exceptions to these recommendations in special patient populations will be considered in Table 2.

Node 1: Is electroconvulsive therapy urgently indicated?

Electroconvulsive therapy (ECT) is a highly effective treatment for BP-DEP.[15] ECT can be urgently indicated in patients with severe suicidality, catatonia, insufficient oral intake, and medical conditions that limit the use of psychotropic medications. In BP-DEP, ECT produced a 65%-80% short-term response rate (≥50% symptomatic improvement) and 53% remission rate.[16-18] An RCT of ECT in treatment-resistant BP-DEP, defined as two trials with adequate dose and duration of antidepressants or lithium, quetiapine, lamotrigine, or olanzapine, found a 74% response rate compared with 35% with an algorithm-based pharmacological approach.[19] Medication treatment failure is not a reliable predictor for ECT response, coadministration of psychotropic medication does not alter efficacy, and patients with longer depressive episodes may be more likely to respond.[20] BP-DEP may need fewer treatments to respond to ECT than those with unipolar depression.[16,21] ECT may be viewed as a treatment of "first resort" given the morbidity associated with prolonging depressive

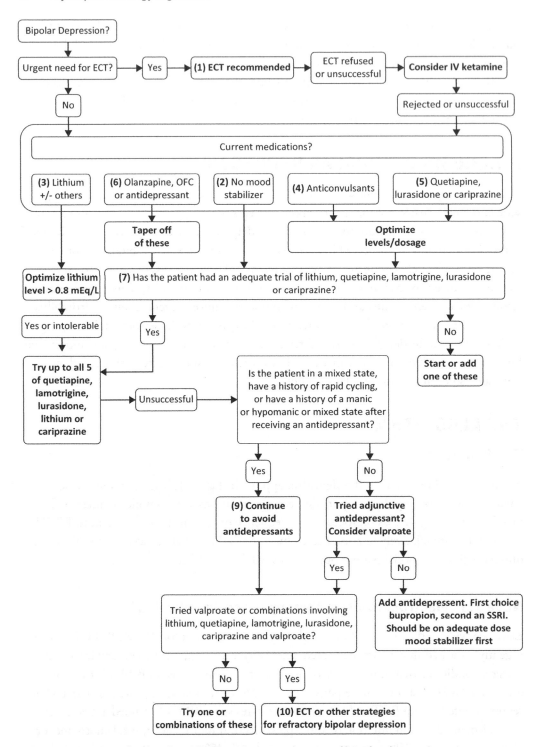

Figure 1. Flowchart for the algorithm for pharmacotherapy of bipolar depression

Abbreviations: ECT, electroconvulsive therapy; IV, intravenous; OFC, olanzapine and fluoxetine combined; SSRI, selective serotonin reuptake inhibitor

illness with medication trials with a low probability of effectiveness. Use of ECT as a maintenance treatment of BP-DEP, however, remains poorly evaluated.

The N-methyl-D-aspartate antagonist ketamine has been tested in treatment-resistant BP-DEP with single intravenous infusions (0.5 mg/kg over 40 minutes) added to a mood stabilizer, with positive response in 50%-80% of subjects that lasted 7-10 days, with a decrease in suicidality.[22-24] Repeated dosing on 6 of the following 12 days was well tolerated except for transient dissociative symptoms, but eight of nine subjects relapsed into depression within 19 days after the last dose of ketamine.[25]

A role for ketamine is possible for hospitalized, treatment-resistant patients who refuse or do not tolerate ECT.[26,27] It can produce rapid improvement and patients may then accept other treatments for maintenance. Little is known about the effectiveness or safety of ketamine given repeatedly over prolonged periods. Nasal spray preparations of ketamine (esketamine) and similar agents[28] have so far received little evaluation in bipolar depression.

Node 2: The patient is not currently on a mood stabilizer

If ECT is refused, not available, or not indicated, there are five algorithm pathways (Nodes 2-6) depending on which medicines a patient is taking at the time of evaluation. Node 2 is the pathway if the patient is currently not taking any mood-stabilizing medication. Five treatment options are recommended for priority consideration here, all of which have some proven effectiveness in BP-DEP: lithium, quetiapine, lamotrigine, lurasidone, and cariprazine. Each is discussed below, with information about their effectiveness and adverse effect risks. It seems reasonable to select any of these as a first choice in Node 2, depending on clinician and patient preferences and considering expected vulnerability to harmful effects. OFC is also discussed although it is not among the first-line choices in this algorithm.

Node 2 is a core node in the algorithm and has the longest text. Other node discussions may refer the reader back to analyses presented in Node 2.

Lithium

Lithium has not been demonstrated to have efficacy in acute BP-DEP and it does not have FDA approval for this indication. Early studies provided positive data, mostly from long-term observational studies.[29,30] However, the only large rigorously controlled study was Astra-Zeneca's EMBOLDEN I, which was a randomized, double-blind comparison of quetiapine, lithium, and placebo in 802 BP-DEP patients (62.5% bipolar I).[31] Lithium was not better than placebo ($P = .13$) but quetiapine was significantly better ($P < .001$). The mean serum lithium concentration was only 0.61 mEq/L, which is rather low. In post-hoc analysis, however, even a subgroup of 34 patients with lithium levels >0.8 mEq/L, while doing slightly better than the lower lithium level group, had a non-significant improvement.

A placebo-controlled study in 117 outpatients by Nemeroff et al is often cited as evidence supporting lithium as a monotherapy for BP-DEP.[32] In this trial, BP-DEP patients treated with lithium were collected into two groups, one with serum lithium levels ≤0.8 mEq/L vs >0.8. Lithium was then augmented for 10 weeks with placebo, imipramine, or paroxetine. There was no difference in efficacy among the three groups regardless of lithium level, but the high lithium level group (plus placebo) did quite well. It would have been informative if the authors had provided a direct comparison of the results with high vs low levels of lithium (with suitable controls) but this secondary analysis was not included in the paper. Higher levels of lithium ≥ 0.6 mEq/L were associated with better prevention of BP-DEP recurrences than lower levels in a comparison study with quetiapine.[33]

Comprehensive reviews of lithium treatment have consistently shown lithium to have a significant antisuicidal effect and to decrease long-term mortality.[34-37] This is important due to the high rate of suicide attempts of up to 32.4% in bipolar I and 36.3% in bipolar II.[38,39] Even though its antisuicidal property is not rapidly apparent, the benefits accrue over time.[40] Stopping lithium increases the risk of suicide by ninefold.[41]

Another benefit of lithium is its proposed unique neuroprotective effects.[42-46] Bipolar disorder patients on long-term lithium have better-preserved white matter structural integrity.[47] Lithium treated bipolar patients were spared the loss of cortical thickness and hippocampal volume that occurred in non-lithium-treated bipolar patients, and brain preservation was similar to matched healthy controls.[45,48,49] Aside from possibly improving the clinical course of bipolar disorder, the neuroprotective effect seems to confer additional benefits in delaying the onset of Alzheimer's disease, and it may favorably alter the course of Parkinson's disease.[50]

Lithium is also associated with reduced risk of stroke in bipolar patients compared to other treatments, perhaps because of reduction in atherosclerosis.[51]

The benefits of lithium treatment seem to exist for patients across the life span,[52,53] but recent data suggest that the long-term benefit is greatest when started early in the course of the illness. Lithium monotherapy prevents both mania (risk ratio 0.52) and depression relapses (risk ratio 0.78),[54] and is also more likely than the other treatments used for bipolar disorder to be maintained as a monotherapy over time.[55-57] In an RCT comparing quetiapine vs lithium for 1 year of maintenance effects, lithium was superior, especially in the second half of the year.[58] Finally, a new "real-world effectiveness" nationwide Finnish cohort study found lithium to be associated with the lowest rate of psychiatric and medical hospitalizations in bipolar disorder patients.[59] Lithium works less well in rapid cyclers but so do all other mood-stabilizing medications.[60-62]

Lithium has many adverse effects, both common and infrequent, that contribute to its avoidance by many clinicians and refusal by some patients. Many patients do not tolerate even relatively minor side effects such as tremor, nausea, loose stools, hair loss, and blunted high moods.[63] Training, clinical experience, tenacious effort in patient education, and consulting the literature on side effect management[64,65] can all assist the prescriber in overcoming some of these problems. Weight gain with lithium is a common concern, but it is significantly less than with quetiapine, valproate, and olanzapine.[66] Another area of significant concern with the use of lithium is the possibility that abrupt lithium discontinuation may worsen the natural course of bipolar disorder, leading to increased or earlier manic and depressive relapses.[67] In a group of patients who were stable for years, 50% relapsed within 8 months after abrupt lithium discontinuation, vs within 37 months with gradual discontinuation.[68] Consequently, if lithium treatment is initiated, it should be done with the expectation that it would be continued as a long-term maintenance agent and that it would be tapered off gradually if and when it needed to be discontinued.[35,69] Initial and ongoing discussions with the patient about this issue are important.

Regarding lithium's risk for end-stage kidney disease, the number needed to harm (NNH) has been estimated to be 300, but this may be an overestimate because of biases in the study design.[70] A recent large observation study actually found no increase in end-stage kidney disease on lithium compared with controls and no difference from patients on valproate.[71] However, chronic kidney disease (not end-stage) was more frequent with over 20 years of lithium use.[71,72] Lithium patients should have regular kidney function monitoring.[73]

Thyroid function should be monitored routinely as well, using thyroid-stimulating hormone (TSH) for initial screening. Lithium interferes with thyroid function by several possible mechanisms, and if untreated up to 50% of patients may develop goiters, especially women.[74] Some vulnerable patients may develop rapid cycling as a consequence.[75]

Quetiapine

Quetiapine is an FDA-approved medicine for acute BP-DEP, based on evidence from two large manufacturer-supported studies BOLDEN I (the BipOLar DEpressioN study group) and II. Both trials showed clear, but not dose-dependent, separation from placebo for patients being treated daily with either 300 or 600 mg of quetiapine.[76,77] In BOLDEN I, 58% of patients treated with quetiapine responded (>50% reduction of initial depression ratings) compared to 36% with placebo, and separation was apparent by 1 week. The bipolar II subjects did not respond as well as bipolar I patients, but rapid cyclers in both groups responded to quetiapine more than placebo.[76] In the BOLDEN II replication study, bipolar II subjects may have responded better than in the preceding trial. Clinical improvement was also greater with quetiapine than placebo in both bipolar I and II disorder subjects in ratings of quality-of-life[78] and anxiety.[79]

The EMBOLDEN (Efficacy of Monotherapy Seroquel in BipOLar DEpressioN) I (mentioned earlier) and II trials are placebo-controlled studies that compared quetiapine vs lithium (level 0.6-1.2 mEq/L) and quetiapine vs paroxetine (20 mg/d). Both trials found that quetiapine produced greater response than placebo or the active comparators.[31,80] Treatment-emergent mania/hypomania was infrequent with quetiapine and somewhat more prevalent in the paroxetine group than with placebo.[80]

Several adverse effects were associated with quetiapine treatment in these studies. Serum triglyceride levels increased with quetiapine but decreased with placebo and lithium. Subjects with clinically important weight changes were ≥7% with quetiapine vs 2% with lithium.[31,66] Unpublished trials of quetiapine in the 1990s found high rates of clinically significant weight gain.[81,82] Quetiapine has also been reported to reduce insulin sensitivity in youths aged 9-18, more than risperidone or placebo.[83]

Quetiapine can also prolong the electrocardiographic QTc repolarization interval. In 2011, the FDA added a warning about this to the quetiapine package insert, similar to the one for citalopram.

There is one placebo-controlled maintenance trial of quetiapine as a monotherapy for bipolar disorder, based on an enrichment and discontinuation design.[84] BP-DEP subjects improved with open-label quetiapine were then randomized to continue quetiapine or switch, over 2 weeks, to lithium or placebo for up to 2 years. Both lithium and quetiapine were similarly superior to placebo. The study has been criticized for using a sample that was enriched with quetiapine responders and for a possible negative impact of quetiapine discontinuation. Nevertheless, lithium showed similar increased time to new episodes of both depression and mania, and thus performed better than might have been expected.[84,85] The FDA did not approve quetiapine monotherapy as a maintenance treatment for bipolar disorder.

Lamotrigine

Lamotrigine monotherapy has emerged as a possible first choice medication for BP-DEP because of its lower risk of adverse effects (other than rashes) compared with alternatives including lithium and quetiapine. It is not associated with weight gain and may actually decrease weight.[86] It is also less likely to cause unwanted neurocognitive effects and sedation.[87] Most of the rashes associated with lamotrigine are benign, but dermatologic and mucosal necrosis (Stevens-Johnson syndrome) have been associated with early use of lamotrigine in about 1/1000 cases, especially with rapidly escalating doses and in association with valproate co-treatment.[88,89]

The evidence supporting lamotrigine efficacy for acute BP-DEP, however, appears to be mixed, at best. One double-blind, placebo-controlled study of lamotrigine (at 50 or 200 mg/d) in bipolar I depression (n = 195) found favorable results.[90] At 50 mg, 41% of patients improved compared to 26% with placebo; at 200 mg, 51%of patients showed improvement. A small, placebo-controlled, crossover study of patients with refractory (mostly rapid cycling) BP-DEP also found a similar response rate with lamotrigine.[91] Results from multiple open-label or less well-controlled studies also suggest that lamotrigine may be effective for acute BP-DEP in both bipolar I and II disorders, though benefits are delayed by the need for slow increases of dosing to effective levels (typically 200-300 mg/d).[92-96]

These positive findings have been countered by four large, negative, placebo-controlled RCTs supported and designed by the manufacturer for the treatment of acutely depressed bipolar I and II patients.[97] None of the four studies found a statistical difference between lamotrigine and placebo. Lamotrigine did not receive FDA approval for acute BP-DEP. Nevertheless, a meta-analysis[98] of these five studies found a modest overall benefit with a 27% drug-placebo difference in effect size. In the more severely ill patients (initial 17-item Hamilton Rating Scale for Depression score of 24 or more), however, lamotrigine had a greater separation from placebo (47%) because placebo effect was lower in these subjects. Lamotrigine was not better than placebo if the baseline Hamilton was lower than 24 (7% difference).

A case series of 40 consecutive subjects with bipolar I disorder found that the optimal plasma level of lamotrigine for the maintenance treatment for BP-DEP was about 4 µg/mL.[99]

The efficacy of lamotrigine as maintenance treatment in delaying recurrences of BP-DEP (but not [hypo]manic episodes) is fairly robust. Two large, 18-month trials[100,101] showed efficacy, enabling lamotrigine to obtain FDA approval for maintenance use. It had no efficacy for preventing mania, but at least did not increase the risk of mania compared with placebo. Another study[101] compared lithium and lamotrigine for maintenance against depressive relapse. It favored lamotrigine, but may have been influenced by enrichment with patients who initially responded to lamotrigine for acute BP-DEP and were then randomized to continue lamotrigine or switch to lithium.

Lamotrigine has shown no efficacy in treating acute mania,[15] which makes it less desirable than lithium, quetiapine, or cariprazine for many patients with acute BP-DEP in that there may be no coverage for [hypo]manic phases of the illness. Thus, for any patient whose hypomanias have been more than mild and others who have had full mania, a second medication to address mania will be needed. On the other hand, the relatively benign adverse effect profile of lamotrigine might make it a first choice for some patients, especially if previous hypomanias have been mild or infrequent and not necessarily in urgent need of coverage, as in type II bipolar disorder.

Lurasidone

In the only trials of lurasidone monotherapy vs placebo to date,[102] patients were randomized to 20-60 or 80-120 mg/d. After 6 weeks, similar improvement was found in the low and high dosage groups, with the number needed to treat (NNT) being 6 and 7, respectively, but adverse reactions of nausea, vomiting, sedation, and extrapyramidal symptoms (EPS) were greater with the higher doses though there was no difference in the rate of discontinuation. Lurasidone appears to have fewer problems with weight gain than lithium and QTc prolongation compared with quetiapine.[103,104] Akathisia and nausea[105] are the most distressing side effects for patients taking lurasidone.

The efficacy of lurasidone and quetiapine in BP-DEP appears to be similar with different outcome measures.[106,107] However, the lurasidone monotherapy study mentions the use of a "quality control process" for some of the data that are not described. The cited "Concordant Rater Systems" has a website that cites a reference[108] describing procedures to enhance rater assessment stability including eliminating raters with the 15% highest or lowest ratings of patient symptoms. With different approaches to optimizing signal enhancement from the rater data, one may wonder whether the reported efficacy of lurasidone is as similar to quetiapine as it appears.

Lurasidone trials conducted so far have included bipolar I patients with BP-DEP. Post-hoc analysis found efficacy for treating BP-DEP with mixed features.[109]

Lurasidone has not been studied as a treatment for acute mania nor as a long-term treatment to prevent recurrences of [hypo]mania. Contrary to expectation (most antipsychotics are also antimanic), case reports have suggested that lurasidone may precipitate [hypo]mania, perhaps especially in relatively low doses used in BP-DEP (eg, 40 mg).[110]

Cariprazine

Cariprazine is a new second-generation antipsychotics (SGA) that received FDA approval for bipolar mania with and without mixed features[111-113] in 2015. In June 2019, cariprazine received FDA approval for acute bipolar depression in doses of 1.5 or 3 mg daily. There are three published studies and a fourth one will be published soon.[114] All but the first reported positive results. In the most recent published report, there was a comparison of 1.5 and 3 mg with placebo in bipolar I depressed (but not suicidal) patients without psychosis who had not failed on other bipolar depression medications.[115] Both doses produced improvement vs placebo by the primary outcome measure of rating scale score change, but the secondary measure of global impression of improvement only found efficacy on 3 mg and the NNT was 8.3 (12 for the 1.5 mg dose).

Citrome performed a data synthesis of all four studies and, usefully, compared the cariprazine results with the results with other medications approved for acute bipolar depression.[114] The overall NNT for improvement (50% reduction in rating scale scores) was 10 for cariprazine. This may be compared to an NNT of 5 for the lurasidone studies and 6 for the quetiapine studies. The NNH for weight gain was 16 with quetiapine, 58 for lurasidone, and 50 for cariprazine. Weight gain could be greater over the long term: these were all 6-week studies. There were also no significant lipid or glucose changes with cariprazine. The major side effects of cariprazine were nausea, akathisia, restlessness, and EPS, and these were dose related. Considering the evidence on benefits and these harms, the lower approved dose (1.5 mg) seemed best for most patients. In the 2019 study, patients were begun on 1.5 mg and increased to 3 mg after 2 weeks if there was no response.

Cariprazine joins quetiapine as the second SGA that is FDA-approved for both mania and depression, but it has significant advantages in metabolic side effects over quetiapine. However, it may be less effective for depression, and the approved doses for mania (3 to 6 mg) are significantly higher than the optimal dose for depression. Thus, at the optimal dose of 1.5 mg for depression, there may not be protection against mania. However, the same may be said for quetiapine, which is effective for depression at 300 mg, but doses for mania are usually higher.

Other SGAs for bipolar depression

Some other atypical antipsychotics tested in BP-DEP have not shown efficacy. Examples include adjunctive use of ziprasidone[116] and aripiprazole monotherapy in two large RCTs.[117] In the 8-week aripiprazole studies, there was separation from placebo in some of the earlier weeks, but by week 8, there was no difference (NNT = 44). Dosage at endpoint reached a mean of 16.5 mg. Some have speculated that lower doses (eg, starting at 2-5 mg and titrating up to 5-10 mg) might have produced a comparable and more sustained antidepressant effect (perhaps due to less akathisia), and this deserves study. In the only maintenance study of aripiprazole in bipolar disorder (following successful treatment of acute mania at higher doses), there was no difference from placebo in preventing depressions or mixed states with depressive symptoms over 6 months follow-up.[118] It seems that BP-DEP treatment priority should be given to the SGAs with stronger supporting evidence.

Olanzapine-fluoxetine combination and olanzapine monotherapy

Another FDA-approved treatment for acute BP-DEP is OFC. A large (n = 788) RCT comparing placebo, olanzapine monotherapy, and OFC in depressed patients with bipolar I disorder demonstrated a statistically significant and clinically meaningful response with OFC. Olanzapine alone was statistically better than placebo, but the difference did not appear clinically significant and seemed to be due mostly to improvement in sleep and appetite, rather than in the core symptoms of depression.[119] Another study compared OFC to lamotrigine with no placebo arm.[120] It found similar remission rates with both active treatments, with somewhat more rapid improvement in BP-DEP with OFC, whereas lamotrigine was better tolerated overall and did not worsen parameters of metabolic syndrome.

Olanzapine monotherapy was tested in another trial in Japan.[121] Again, the benefits for BP-DEP were statistically significant, but the effect size appeared clinically insignificant with most improvement in appetite and sleep. Long-term follow-up in two East Asian samples found reduced risk of recurrences of both depression and [hypo]mania but with an increased risk of weight gain.[122,123]

Despite its effectiveness in acute BP-DEP, OFC is not recommended in the early nodes of this algorithm. The severe metabolic effects of olanzapine contribute to long-term risk for morbidity and mortality.[124] Even a single dose of olanzapine was found to alter glucose and lipid metabolism and increase insulin resistance.[125] Olanzapine monotherapy is not recommended at all in this algorithm.

The effectiveness of OFC does not seem to generalize to other combinations of SGAs and antidepressants. In a recent meta-analysis of six controlled studies of other combinations, no clinically significant benefit was found. Over 1-year follow-up, there was an increased risk of [hypo]manic mood switching with antidepressants vs placebo combined with SGAs.[126]

Are there any other options for early use in bipolar depression?

Valproate might be effective in BP-DEP, but this impression is based on four small studies with a total of only 142 subjects and some significant problems (eg, one had a drop-out rate of 53% on valproate).[127,128] As a maintenance treatment to prevent BP-DEP episodes, according to a 2014 meta-analysis of 33 RCTs, valproate did not demonstrate efficacy, whereas lithium and lamotrigine did have significant preventative effect.[129] The large 2010 BALANCE study contributed to the evidence-base for valproate's inferiority as a treatment for bipolar disorder, compared with lithium, and the combination was only slightly more effective than lithium alone.[130-132] Valproate also has important adverse effects especially weight gain and is a severe teratogen.[133] Therefore, valproate might be considered later as an option for BP-DEP, but is not recommended among first-line treatments.

Neither carbamazepine (CBZ) nor oxcarbazepine have sufficient evidence to support efficacy in BP-DEP.[134]

No antidepressant is FDA-approved explicitly for the treatment of BP-DEP except for fluoxetine when combined with olanzapine, as discussed. Antidepressant monotherapy in bipolar I disorder is discouraged in expert consensus evaluations of the literature, especially when mixed features are present, and even when added to a mood stabilizer.[2,135] More recently, data from the Systematic Treatment Enhancement Program for Bipolar Disorder (STEP-BD) study confirmed that rapid cyclers continued on antidepressants (despite concurrent mood stabilizer treatment) had much worse maintenance outcomes.[136] They had triple the rate of depressive episodes per year compared with subjects whose antidepressants were discontinued. These were patients who seemed initially to have a good response to the added antidepressant. The STEP-BD study also found that antidepressants seem to cause a unique syndrome of dysphoria, irritability, and insomnia that is not part of the natural course of most bipolar patients.[137] Patients treated with an antidepressant for acute depression were 10 times more likely to develop this "antidepressant-associated chronic irritable dysphoria" (ACID) syndrome.

Their efficacy with bipolar II depression is less clear, though risks of dangerous mood switching are lower than with bipolar I depression. Evidence is accumulating that antidepressants including sertraline and venlafaxine may be effective and relatively safe (with respect to cycling) from short-term studies without placebo controls in patients with non-mixed bipolar II depressions.[138,139] Sertraline was recently compared to lithium alone or sertraline plus lithium in 142 subjects in a 16-week randomized study of the acute treatment of bipolar II depression.[140] The response and mood switch rates did not differ, but more patients dropped out on the combination treatment, and it did not work faster than the others. However, the switchers on lithium had a mean serum lithium level of only 0.41 mEq/L compared to non-switchers who had a mean level of 0.62 mEq/L.

There is a long-term (1 year), controlled study of maintenance treatment with fluoxetine in patients with bipolar II depression who had responded acutely to open-label fluoxetine monotherapy.[141] Eighty-one patients were randomized to fluoxetine, lithium, or placebo. The time to relapse was significantly longer with fluoxetine. An editorial pointed out that the study suffered from 75% attrition over the course of the protocol, and the sample was 100% enriched with responders to fluoxetine.[142] Also, patients on fluoxetine were three times more likely to present with some hypomanic symptoms at follow-up visits. As noted earlier, STEP-BD found no improvement from adding antidepressants to ongoing mood stabilizers compared with avoiding doing so.[143]

In summary, more study is required before there can be a firm recommendation that antidepressants should be among early options for managing bipolar II depression. Antidepressants do have generally milder side effects compared with SGAs, lithium, and lamotrigine (considering the rash risk). If antidepressants are considered, clinicians should be careful to diagnose bipolar II strictly according to the DSM-IV or -5 criteria,[144] as was done in these studies. A key criterion differentiating bipolar I mania from the hypomania in bipolar II that clinicians may overlook is that manic episodes are associated with "marked impairment in social or occupational functioning." Often, impairment from the [hypo]mania that on superficial evaluation did not appear "marked" may later be recognized as such, and the diagnosis will become bipolar I and antidepressants will drop from early consideration.

In summary for Node 2

Lithium, quetiapine, lamotrigine, lurasidone, and cariprazine are the five preferred options for acute BP-DEP. Clinicians should choose a suitable first choice medication from among these, depending on the patient's tolerance of particular adverse effects, need for an agent that will prevent switching to mania, and other factors.

Nodes 3-6: Overview

Nodes 3-6 start algorithm branches for depressed patients currently taking some medication for BP-DEP and address whether to optimize dose, add or change treatment for the next step (See Figure 1).

Node 3: Is the patient currently on lithium?

As discussed in Node 2, lithium monotherapy may have limited effectiveness for acute BP-DEP especially if the trough level is <0.8 mEq/L. Therefore, clinicians should consider increasing the dose, if tolerated, to reach a serum lithium level >0.8 mEq/L.[32] If the patient already has a level above 0.8, go to Node 7 where quetiapine, lamotrigine, lurasidone, and cariprazine are considered for the next step.

Node 4: Is the patient taking carbamazepine, lamotrigine, or valproate?

One should first optimize the dose of these anticonvulsants: lamotrigine to 200-400 mg/d (optimal level may be about 4 μg/mL, as noted earlier[99]); valproate or CBZ to usually employed levels (for mania, 50-125 or 4-12 μg/mL, respectively).[8] If doses are already optimized, then add or change to lithium, quetiapine, lurasidone, lamotrigine, or cariprazine considering the factors discussed in Node 2. Depending on the medication chosen, adding or switching will depend on whether the patient needs coverage for mania, as discussed in Node 2.

Some clinicians like to add an antidepressant to depressed patients on valproate, but in the STEP-BD study, as noted earlier, this was not better than adding placebo.[143] If CBZ is retained, addition of lurasidone is contraindicated according to the package insert due to particularly strong induction of the metabolism of lurasidone by CBZ, which can result in 85% reduction in serum concentrations of lurasidone. Cariprazine is also a P450 3A4 substrate and metabolism would be induced by CBZ.

Node 5: Is the patient taking quetiapine, lurasidone, or cariprazine monotherapy?

The daily dose of quetiapine used in the BP-DEP registration trials was 300-600 mg and for lurasidone it was 40-120 mg. This dose should be continued for up to 6 weeks especially if partial response occurs and improvement is continuing. If response remains unsatisfactory, then evidence supports adding lithium to lurasidone.[107] There are no studies, however, combining lithium and quetiapine for acute BP-DEP. A maintenance study, however, found quetiapine better than placebo when combined with lithium or valproate.[145] Therefore, addition of lithium to quetiapine is a reasonable choice. Based on this one study, valproate addition might be reasonable as well, but it is not one of the top choices for reasons explained earlier at Node 2.

Another option would be to combine lamotrigine and quetiapine. In the CE-QUEL (Comparative Evaluation of Quetiapine Plus Lamotrigine) double-blind study, 202 patients receiving quetiapine were randomized to addition of lamotrigine up to

200 mg/d, 500 µg/d of folic acid, or placebo.[146] With quetiapine plus lamotrigine, there was improvement in depressive symptoms at 12 and 52 weeks and fewer recurrences of depression. Surprisingly, folate yielded a somewhat less favorable response than with quetiapine alone.

There are no studies as yet combining cariprazine with other medications for BP-DEP.

Alternatively, if the patient has not had an adequate trial of monotherapy with any of the other four recommended options, then one could switch to one of them, as discussed in Node 2.

Node 6: Is the patient taking an antidepressant, or olanzapine alone or with fluoxetine?

These are treatments that are not favored for early use in BP-DEP for the reasons discussed in Node 2. The STEP-BD results showing the harms of continuing patients on antidepressants, including more frequent cycling into depressions and switches into ACID (irritable dysphoric states), argue against this common practice.[136,137] Therefore, if the patient is on one of them now and is depressed, the recommendation is the same as in Node 2. One may discontinue the existing medication with gradual dose reduction over at least 2 weeks to limit any risk of mood destabilization. At the same time, start lithium, quetiapine, lamotrigine, lurasidone, or cariprazine depending on the patient's expected side effect tolerance and the other considerations discussed in Node 2.

Node 7: Is the patient still depressed after an adequate trial of the first treatment selected at Node 2 or after changes recommended in Nodes 3-6?

Options to consider for this second medication trial are any of the five drugs discussed that are first-line but not yet tried. As shown in Figure 1, the algorithm recommends staying at Node 7 in the event of unsatisfactory response, continuing to try up to all five of the recommended first-line treatments (if acceptable to clinician and patient) before continuing to Node 8. Adding or changing treatments are possibilities. The next medication could be *added* even if it is ineffective for [hypo]mania (eg, lamotrigine), provided that the first medication has a mania-preventing effect (eg, lithium). One could *switch* to the next medication if the choice is likely to be effective for mania (eg, lithium, quetiapine, or cariprazine) but probably not lurasidone which is unstudied in mania.

Quetiapine is effective as an acute monotherapy for BP-DEP, and it has maintenance efficacy as an adjunct to another mood stabilizer,[147,148] but it adds metabolic and other adverse effect risks that can be a problem over the long term. Lamotrigine has one (n=124) positive study as an add-on to lithium in bipolar I and II depression[149]: 52% of subjects met criteria for response, compared to 32% with placebo (NNT=5), but 8% switched to [hypo]mania with lamotrigine as did 3% of those given placebo. As noted at Node 2, maintenance efficacy in BP-DEP is reasonably well established for lamotrigine and it is well tolerated by most patients. Lurasidone was found effective and well tolerated as monotherapy and as an adjunct to lithium and other mood stabilizers.[107]

What about adding an antidepressant to the first-line BP-DEP medication?

Antidepressants are a popular choice at Node 7 and earlier, for many clinicians. However, they have inconsistent evidence for efficacy in BP-DEP and they induce recurrent depressions and other negative states as discussed earlier.[143] Also, in a meta-analysis of six placebo-controlled RCTs of adding an antidepressant (selective serotonin reuptake inhibitors [SSRIs], bupropion, or agomelatine) to lithium or other mood stabilizers (mentioned earlier), there was little additional improvement (standardized mean difference 0.165) and no differences in response or remission rates.[126] Furthermore, there was a significantly increased risk of switch to [hypo]mania within a year of follow-up (OR 1.8) suggesting a destabilizing effect on the course of some bipolar disorder patients. See Node 8 for further discussion of the benefits and risks of antidepressants. We still do not recommend OFC here, because of the long-term metabolic side effects of the olanzapine component.

Node 8: Consider an antidepressant in non-rapid cycling BP-DEP or possibly valproate

One arrives at Node 8 after the patient has been tried on up to five BP-DEP medicines (and combinations) without a history of rapid cycling (four or more mood episodes per year) or mixed episodes. Also, there should be no history of [hypo]mania after receiving an antidepressant. For rapid cyclers or patients with BP-DEP with mixed features, go to Node 9.

Use of an antidepressant

The International Society for Bipolar Disorders (ISBP) Task Force of 68 experts reviewed the literature and prepared a report on the use of antidepressants in bipolar disorder in 2013.[2] Twelve recommendations were made, based on consensus of at least 80% of the experts.

Three recommendations pertinent to this step in the algorithm arose from their report. Our comments are in italics:

- Avoid antidepressants in all patients with current or past mixed states. Discontinue any antidepressants in use during a mixed state. [*There are no new studies offering further evidence on this topic.*]
- In bipolar II depression, antidepressant monotherapy can be used but not if there are mixed features (defined as two or more hypomanic symptoms). Observe closely for any manic/mixed symptoms developing. [*There are no studies since 2013 evaluating*

bipolar II mixed cases treated with antidepressants, so this recommendation seems still pertinent.]

- Avoid antidepressants in all patients with recent or past rapid cycling. *[Two recent studies evaluated bipolar II depressed patients with rapid cycling and found no greater mood switching and no reduction in effectiveness compared with non-rapid cyclers.[140,150] However, these studies did not have placebo controls so it is not known if the antidepressants were effective. As noted, rapid cyclers had much worse outcomes with depression in the STEP-BD study.[136]]*

Thus, it might be reasonable to consider adding an antidepressant to a mood stabilizer at Node 8, and even to consider antidepressant monotherapy for a bipolar II depressed patient—but not for patients with previous or current mixed features. For rapid cycling bipolar II patients, cautious antidepressant monotherapy can be considered but clinicians should stay alert for depression recurrences. In choosing an antidepressant, safety may be the primary consideration: bupropion and SSRIs seem to have less risk of inducing cycling than venlafaxine in bipolar I patients.[151] In bipolar II patients, however, venlafaxine monotherapy was not a problem in one study.[150] Fluoxetine is best avoided because of the long half-life of its active metabolite, norfluoxetine, which might prolong an emerging manic episode.

Valproate

Despite having very limited evidence of efficacy in acute BP-DEP as discussed in Node 2, valproate can be considered as an option here. Its dosage should be adjusted to the higher end of the usual serum level, 70-90 μg/mL, according to some expert opinion.[131]

Node 9: Continuing to avoid antidepressant in high-risk patients

Patients who reached this point of the algorithm have been tried on lithium, quetiapine, lurasidone, lamotrigine, and cariprazine unless one or more were deemed unacceptable due to intolerability or side effect risks. In addition, they have risk factors for the use of an antidepressant including mixed features, rapid cycling, and history of [hypo]mania or a mixed state after receiving an antidepressant. Options include, trying valproate (also offered in Node 8) or combinations of the five recommended BP-DEP medicines not yet tried. This may also be the point to consider OFC.

Node 10: Highly refractory bipolar depression

Many evidence-supported treatments have been tried by this point and yet the patient's response remains unsatisfactory. The diagnosis of BP-DEP should be reviewed again, as it also should after each previous trial that produced an unsatisfactory response. Table 1 lists several more options and cites pertinent evidence. ECT is discussed first because of its strong effectiveness, and the others are in no particular order. This is not meant to be an exhaustive list.

Table 1	Options to consider for treatment-resistant bipolar depression	
Treatment	*Comments*
Reconsider ECT	ECT may produce a 50% response rate at this point and thus may be by far the best option.[153,154] See Node 1
Other device-based interventions	Transcutaneous magnetic stimulation, vagus nerve stimulation, and deep brain stimulation have possible value but have not been adequately studied in BP-DEP. Transcranial direct stimulation is a promising new option with efficacy.[155] Adjunctive bright light therapy for an hour given at Noon was much more effective than dim red light for BP-DEP in a recent small study.[156] Patients were on antimanic agents, and rapid cyclers and mixed syndrome patients were excluded
Stimulants, modafinil, or armodafinil	Methylphenidate has many case reports and may be mildly effective based on uncontrolled data. Lisdexamfetamine in a recent RCT in 25 subjects had no efficacy on the total depression scores but depressed mood and fatigue/sleepiness were improved.[157] Modafinil was tested in a placebo-controlled RCT (n = 85) with overall positive effect on depression though primarily due to improvement in energy symptoms. There were no manic switches.[158] Armodafinil has had three large placebo-controlled RCTs as an adjunct. One was positive (NNT = 9) and two were negative. The manufacturer decided not to file for an FDA indication.[159]
Pramipexole	Pramipexole, a D3 agonist, has had two small positive short-term placebo-controlled trials as an adjunct (n = 21, n = 22).[160,161] Note that, rapid cyclers were excluded, and it was poorly tolerated. However, it can have persisting benefit.[162,163]
Clozapine	There are no controlled studies in BP-DEP, but open-label reports show possible benefit in some cases.[164,165] One report documented 4 years of stable improvement in a patient with refractory psychotic bipolar disorder treated with clozapine[166] and another suggested reduced rates of hospitalization for BP-DEP episodes with addition of clozapine.[167]
Add omega-3 fatty acids (O3FAs)	In six RCTs, O3FAs were not effective in BP-DEP.[168] However, another (n = 75) found improvement in mildly to moderately depressed patients.[169] A meta-analysis of adjunctive O3FAs (n=291) found evidence of efficacy in acute BP-DEP with a low-moderate effect size of 0.34.[170] O3FAs may be particularly well tolerated.
Add aripiprazole	This SGA, which is FDA-approved as an adjunct for non-bipolar depression, has had multiple open-label and uncontrolled studies showing some effectiveness in bipolar depressed patients.[171-177] However, unlike quetiapine and lurasidone, it has failed to show efficacy as monotherapy in two large controlled studies,[117] although post-hoc analysis showed some improvement in severely depressed patients.[178] It has been suggested that the average doses (15-18 mg/d) might have been too high in these negative studies.[117] In the most recent positive report, doses up to 5 mg were used.[173]
Add sleep deprivation combined with light therapy	A group in Italy has reported two consecutive large prospective open trials of 24-h sleep deprivation with light therapy added to lithium in inpatients with BP-DEP, 83% of whom had histories of medication resistance.[179] There were significant benefits for depression and suicidality. The findings were replicated by other investigators in an open-label controlled trial comparing with medication alone, and the results were sustained over 7 wk.[180] This "chronotherapy" approach deserves more investigation
Add triiodothyronine (T3)	A retrospective chart review of 125 treatment-resistant, depressed patients with bipolar II and 34 with bipolar NOS disorders found that they had failed trials of an average of 14 previous treatments.[181] With addition of "supraphysiological" doses of T3 averaging 90 µg daily, 33% remitted and 84% improved. There may be investigator bias in addition to other problems with chart review studies

Abbreviations: BP-DEP, bipolar depression; ECT, electroconvulsive therapy; FDA, food and drug administration; O3FAs, omega-3-fatty acids; RCT, randomized controlled trial; SGA, second-generation antipsychotic; T3, triiodothyronine

EXCEPTIONS: COMORBIDITY AND OTHER FEATURES IN BP-DEP AND HOW THEY AFFECT THE ALGORITHM

Table 2 lists common comorbidities and other circumstances with suggestions on how the algorithm might change for these patients based on evidence considerations.

Table 2 | Comorbidity and other features in bipolar depression: How they affect the algorithm		
Comorbid Conditions	*Evidence Considerations*	*Recommendations*
Posttraumatic Stress Disorder (PTSD)	Co-occurring BP-DEP and PTSD are associated with increased suicide risk, rapid cycling, substance use disorder, and greater depressive symptoms.[182,183] PTSD has a higher prevalence in BP-DEP compared with general population, with overall 20% lifetime prevalence rate.[3] Lithium might reduce vulnerability to PTSD.[184]	Common symptoms require differentiation (irritability, insomnia, decreased concentration). PTSD-related insomnia and anxiety could be treated with prazosin.[185] Quetiapine could be reasonable (be aware of weight gain). Lamotrigine has some efficacy in PTSD.[186]
Attention-Deficit/ Hyperactivity Disorder (ADHD)	Stimulants added for ADHD symptoms with effective ongoing mood stabilizer seem safe, but use without a mood stabilizer is associated with 6-7 fold increased risk of inducing [hypo]mania.[187] Atomoxetine and armodafinil have been insufficiently studied in this comorbidity.[188,189]	Patients should be on a mood stabilizer before adding any stimulant to address ADHD symptoms or excessive day time fatigue
DSM 5 Anxiety Disorders	Up to 75% of bipolar disorder patients have at least one comorbid anxiety disorder at some point. These are associated with more frequent mood episodes and poorer treatment outcome.[5]	Anxiolytic agents such as buspirone, gabapentin, and benzodiazepines may be helpful. Valproate sometimes is helpful in treatment-resistant panic disorder. However, quetiapine had no efficacy for BP-DEP nor comorbid generalized anxiety disorder in one RCT.[190]
Women of childbearing potential and pregnant women	Valproate is by far the most teratogenic agent used for bipolar disorder.[191] Valproate (but not lamotrigine) may also lower intelligence scores in young children exposed to it in utero.[192] Carbamazepine is associated with increased spina bifida, cardiac anomalies, and vitamin K deficiencies late in pregnancy.[191]	Avoid valproate in any woman with the potential to become pregnant: should the patient become pregnant it may already be too late to remove it before harm is done. High dose folate (4-5 mg daily) has been recommended[201] but probably has no protective effect.[133] Carbamazepine is almost as harmful and should be avoided. Lithium is preferred over valproate and carbamazepine.

Table 2	Comorbidity and other features in bipolar depression: How they affect the algorithm (*continued*)		
Comorbid Conditions	*Evidence Considerations*	*Recommendations*
	Data on lamotrigine suggest low risk of fetal harm as monotherapy, but cleft palate is a concern.[193-197] Lithium has lower malformation risks than valproate and carbamazepine. Cardiac malformations occurred in 2.4% of infants exposed to lithium (0.6% for ventricular outflow obstruction) vs 1.2% of unexposed babies (0.2% ventricular outflow), an adjusted risk ratio of 1.65. The risk rises with higher doses, but is still lower than previously thought.[198] ECT treatment during pregnancy causes fetal heart rate reduction, uterine contraction, and premature labor in up to 1/3 of the subjects. ECT was found to have an overall fetal mortality rate of 7%.[199] Although the safety of antipsychotics in pregnancy has not been clearly established (due to many limitations in the studies), they seem to be relatively safe.[200] The SGAs that cause weight gain appear to increase risk of gestational metabolic complications including diabetes and babies large for gestational age. Olanzapine may be associated with low and high birth weight and a small risk of malformation including hip dysplasia, meningocoele, ankyloblepharon, and neural tube defects.[201] Patients stopping medication during pregnancy had a relapse rate of 80% for depression, 16% for mania relapse, and 3.9% for mixed episode in postpartum.[202]	For some patients, lithium should be the first choice[203] The SGAs with efficacy in BP-DEP are generally first choice, though data are very limited in pregnancy.[204] Lamotrigine may be considered. ECT treatment during pregnancy warrants more caution than previously thought. It can be used for severe depression, catatonia, medication resistant illness, extremely high risk for suicide, psychotic agitation, severe physical decline due to malnutrition, dehydration, or other life threatening conditions.[199] Prescribe as few drugs as possible—ideally, one. But, when pregnancy occurs during treatment, it is usually best to continue the previous regimen to avoid exposure to even more agents, except if the patient was on valproate or carbamazepine (probably switch). Adjust doses as pregnancy progresses. Blood volume expands 30% in third trimester. Plasma level monitoring is helpful. Anticholinergic drugs should not be prescribed to pregnant women except for acute, short-term need. Depot antipsychotics should not be routinely used in pregnancy: infants may show extrapyramidal symptoms for several months

(*continued*)

Table 2	Comorbidity and other features in bipolar depression: How they affect the algorithm (*continued*)	
Comorbid Conditions	*Evidence Considerations*	*Recommendations*
Substance Use Disorders (SUDs)	Reported lifetime prevalence of BP-DEP and any substance use disorder is as high as 47%, especially in bipolar I disorder (60%). Active SUDs are associated with poorer outcome with medication treatments but there are very limited data in this patient population due to exclusion criteria.[4] Valproate in one small study showed significant reduction in alcohol drinking in patients with BP-DEP.[205] Citicoline added to standard treatment of comorbid cocaine dependence in manic patients showed improvement in substance abuse.[206] Naltrexone and acamprosate have been shown to have modest ability to reduce alcohol drinking behaviors.[207,208]	Remission of SUDs is a high treatment priority
Cardiac disease or use of QTc-prolonging drugs	Quetiapine has had 5 studies measuring QTc prolongation but the manufacturer has refused to release the QTc data.[209] However, in 2011 the FDA mandated a new QTc warning in the quetiapine package insert with requirements for monitoring. Based on clinical trials thus far, lurasidone has been shown to have minimal alteration of QTc.[104]	If risk of QTc prolongation is a significant concern, quetiapine would be relatively undesirable. Consider lurasidone. Review the patient's medications for other QTc-prolonging agents and monitor for risk factors for Torsade's, such as bradycardia and electrolyte abnormalities
Other medical comorbidities	Medical comorbidities are common	Hepatitis and liver cirrhosis: avoid valproate and carbamazepine when possible. Among SGAs, quetiapine and olanzapine have higher risk of transaminase elevations Renal filtration impairment: avoid lithium. Lamotrigine is also renally excreted. Obesity, hyperlipidemia, metabolic syndrome: consider lamotrigine, carbamazepine, or lurasidone

Abbreviations: ADHD, attention-deficit hyperactivity disorder; BP-DEP, bipolar disorder; ECT, electroconvulsive therapy; IM, intramuscular; PTSD, posttraumatic stress disorder; SGA, second-generation antipsychotics; SUDs, substance use disorders.

COMPARISON WITH OTHER BP-DEP GUIDELINES AND ALGORITHMS

A "meta-consensus" of other guidelines found significant disagreements.[152] Though the recommendations herein are generally in accord with most recently published guidelines, there are some differences, in part because the current algorithm places such strong emphasis on long-term side effect considerations. For example, other guidelines propose OFC as a first-line treatment, but in this algorithm it is not recommended until after most other evidenced options. Table 3 summarizes key recommendations in other guidelines published since 2013.

Table 3	Other guidelines and algorithms for the treatment of acute bipolar depression		
Guideline/Algorithm	*Year*	*Key Points*
The psychopharmacology algorithm project at the Harvard South Shore Program: an update on bipolar depression[7]	2010	Last version of the present algorithm. Lithium, quetiapine, and lamotrigine were first-line options, with a slight preference for lithium. Adding an antidepressant could be considered after above options in low-risk patients
Canadian Network for Mood and Anxiety Treatments (CANMAT) and International Society for Bipolar Disorders (ISBP) collaborative update of CANMAT guidelines for the management of patients with bipolar disorder: update 2013[135]	2013	Bipolar I: first-line lithium, lamotrigine, quetiapine monotherapy, olanzapine plus SSRI, or combinations with lithium, valproate plus antidepressant. Bipolar II: first-line quetiapine only; second-line lithium, lamotrigine, atypical antipsychotic plus antidepressants, and others
National Institute for Health and Care Excellence: Clinical Guidelines[210]	2014	First-line medications were quetiapine, olanzapine, OFC, lamotrigine, valproate, and lithium
Royal Australian and New Zealand College of Psychiatrists clinical practice guidelines for mood disorders.[211]	2015	Quetiapine, lurasidone, olanzapine were first-line monotherapy options, followed by lithium, valproate, and lamotrigine as second-line monotherapy choices.
Evidence-based guidelines for treating bipolar disorder: Revised third edition recommendations from the British Association for Psychopharmacology[212]	2016	Firstline medications included quetiapine, lurasidone, olanzapine, and OFC. Lamotrigine was second line. Escitalopram, fluoxetine, lithium, and paroxetine were third-line recommendations
The international College of Neuro-Psychopharmacology (CINP) Treatment Guidelines for Bipolar Disorder in Adults (CINP-BD-2017)[213]	2016	Lurasidone and quetiapine were recommended as first line. Escitalopram, fluoxetine, olanzapine, and OFC were the second-line recommendations. Lithium was fourth line given the level of evidence.

Abbreviation: OFC, olanzapine and fluoxetine combined; SSRI, selective serotonin reuptake inhibitor.

CONCLUDING COMMENT

Notwithstanding the development of this and other algorithms and guidelines, the treatment of BP-DEP remains a challenge for both clinicians and patients. A considerable degree of uncertainty remains about which of the treatments constitute first-, second-, or third-line therapies. Practitioners will need to remain ever alert to emerging evidence and evolving changes in practice in order to provide safe and effective management of their BP-DEP patients.

ACKNOWLEDGMENT

The authors thank Ross J. Baldessarini, MD for his thorough and thoughtful review of a draft of this paper.

CONFLIC T OF INTERESTS

This manuscript represents original material, has not been previously published, and is not under consideration for publication elsewhere. All authors have read and approved the final submitted version of this manuscript. All authors do not have any financial conflict of interest to declare.

DATA AVAILABILITY STATEMENT

Data sharing is not applicable to this article as no new data were created or analyzed in this study.

ORCID

https://orcid.org/0000-0002-9477-241X

REFERENCES

1. Judd LL, Schettler PJ, Solomon DA, et al. Psychosocial disability and work role function compared across the long-term course of bipolar I, bipolar II and unipolar major depressive disorders. *J Affect Disord*. 2008;108:49-58.
2. Pacchiarotti I, Bond DJ, Baldessarini RJ, et al. The International Society for Bipolar Disorders (ISBD) task force report on antidepressant use in bipolar disorders. *Am J Psychiatry*. 2013;170:1249-1262.
3. Hernandez JM, Cordova MJ, Ruzek J, et al. Presentation and prevalence of PTSD in a bipolar disorder population: a STEP-BD examination. *J Affect Disord*. 2013;150:450-455.
4. Pettinati HM, O'Brien CP, Dundon WD. Current status of co-occurring mood and substance use disorders: a new therapeutic target. *Am J Psychiatry*. 2013;170:23-30.
5. Provencher MD, Guimond AJ, Hawke LD. Comorbid anxiety in bipolar spectrum disorders: a neglected research and treatment issue? *J Affect Disord*. 2012;137:161-164.
6. Osser DN, Patterson RD. On the value of evidence-based psychopharmacology algorithms. *Bulletin of Clinical Psychopharmacology*. 2013;23:1-5.

7. Ansari A, Osser DN. The psychopharmacology algorithm project at the Harvard South Shore Program: an update on bipolar depression. *Harv Rev Psychiatry*. 2010;18:36-55.

8. Mohammad O, Osser DN. The psychopharmacology algorithm project at the Harvard South Shore Program: an algorithm for acute mania. *Harv Rev Psychiatry*. 2014;22:274-294.

9. Osser DN, Roudsari MJ, Manschreck T. The psychopharmacology algorithm project at the Harvard South Shore Program: an update on schizophrenia. *Harv Rev Psychiatry*. 2013;21:18-40.

10. Abejuela HR, Osser DN. The psychopharmacology algorithm project at the Harvard South Shore Program: an algorithm for generalized anxiety disorder. *Harv Rev Psychiatry*. 2016;24:243-256.

11. Giakoumatos CI, Osser D. The psychopharmacology algorithm project at the Harvard South Shore Program: an update on unipolar nonpsychotic depression. *Harv Rev Psychiatry*. 2019;27:33-52.

12. O'Donovan C, Garnham JS, Hajek T, Alda M. Antidepressant monotherapy in pre-bipolar depression; predictive value and inherent risk. *J Affect Disord*. 2008;107:293-298.

13. Bowden CL. Strategies to reduce misdiagnosis of bipolar depression. *Psychiatr Serv*. 2001;52:51-55.

14. Byrne EM, Raheja UK, Stephens SH, et al. Seasonality shows evidence for polygenic architecture and genetic correlation with schizophrenia and bipolar disorder. *J Clin Psychiatry*. 2015;76(02): 128–134.

15. Goodwin FK, Jamison KR. Manic-depressive illness, bipolar disorders and recurrent depression (2nd edn). New York: Oxford University Press;2007.

16. Daly JJ, Prudic J, Devanand DP, et al. ECT in bipolar and unipolar depression: differences in speed of response. *Bipolar Disord*. 2001;3:95-104.

17. Medda P, Perugi G, Zanello S, Ciuffa M, Cassano GB. Response to ECT in bipolar I, bipolar II and unipolar depression. *J Affect Disord*. 2009;118:55-59.

18. Dierckx B, Heijnen WT, van den Broek WW, Birkenhager TK. Efficacy of electroconvulsive therapy in bipolar versus unipolar major depression: a meta-analysis. *Bipolar Disord*. 2012;14:146-150.

19. Schoeyen HK, Kessler U, Andreassen OA, et al. Treatment-resistant bipolar depression: a randomized controlled trial of electroconvulsive therapy versus algorithm-based pharmacological treatment. *Am J Psychiatry*. 2015;172:41-51.

20. Kho KH, Zwinderman AH, Blansjaar BA. Predictors for the efficacy of electroconvulsive therapy: chart review of a naturalistic study. *J Clin Psychiatry*. 2005;66:894-899.

21. Loo CK, Mahon M, Katalinic N, Lyndon B, Hadzi-Pavlovic D. Predictors of response to ultrabrief right unilateral electroconvulsive therapy. *J Affect Disord*. 2011;130:192-197.

22. Diazgranados N, Ibrahim L, Brutsche NE, et al. A randomized add- on trial of an N-methyl-D-aspartate antagonist in treatment-resistant bipolar depression. *Arch Gen Psychiatry*. 2010;67:793-802.

23. Zarate CA, Brutsche NE, Ibrahim L, et al. Replication of ketamine's antidepressant efficacy in bipolar depression: a randomized controlled add-on trial. *Biol Psychiatry*. 2012;71:939-946.

24. Ballard ED, Ionescu DF, Vande Voort JL, et al. Improvement in suicidal ideation after ketamine infusion: relationship to reductions in depression and anxiety. *J Psychiatr Res*. 2014;58:161-166.

25. aan het Rot M, Collins KA, Murrough JW, et al. Safety and efficacy of repeated-dose intravenous ketamine for treatment-resistant depression. *Biol Psychiatry*. 2010;67:139-145.

26. Sanacora G, Frye MA, McDonald W, et al. A consensus statement on the use of ketamine in the treatment of mood disorders. *JAMA Psychiatry*. 2017;74:399-405.

27. Zorumski CF, Conway CR. Use of ketamine in clinical practice: a time for optimism and caution. *JAMA Psychiatry*. 2017;74:405-406.

28. Lara DR, Bisol LW, Munari LR. Antide pressant, mood stabilizing and procognitive effects of very low dose sublingual ketamine in refractory unipolar and bipolar depression. *Int J Neuropsychopharmacol*. 2013;16:2111-2117.

29. Baldessarini RJ, Tondo L. Does lithium treatment still work? Evidence of stable responses over three decades. *Arch Gen Psychiatry*. 2000;57:187-190.

30. Frances AJ, Kahn DA, Carpenter D, Docherty JP, Donovan SL. The expert consensus guidelines for treating depression in bipolar disorder. *J Clin Psychiatry*. 1998;59(Suppl4):73-79.

31. Young AH, McElroy SL, Bauer M, et al. A double-blind, placebo-hcontrolled study of quetiapine and lithium monotherapy in adults in the acute phase of bipolar depression (EMBOLDEN I). *J Clin Psychiatry*. 2010;71:150-162.

32. Nemeroff CB, Evans DL, Gyulai L, et al. Double-blind, placebo-controlled comparison of imipramine and paroxetine in the treatment of bipolar depression. *Am J Psychiatry*. 2001;158:906-912.

33. Nolen WA, Weisler RH. The association of the effect of lithiumin the maintenance treatment of bipolar disorder with lithium plasma levels: a post hoc analysis of a double-blind study comparing switching to lithium or placebo in patients who responded to quetiapine (Trial 144). *Bipolar Disord*. 2013;15:100-109.

34. Baldessarini RJ, Tondo L, Faedda GL, Suppes TR, Floris G, Rudas N. Effects of the rate of discontinuing lithium maintenance treatment in bipolar disorders. *J Clin Psychiatry*. 1996;57:441-448.

35. Baldessarini RJ, Tondo L, Hennen J. Effects of lithium treatment and its discontinuation on suicidal behavior in bipolar manic-depressive disorders. *J Clin Psychiatry*. 1999;60(Suppl 2):77-84; discussion 111–6.

36. Cipriani A, Pretty H, Hawton K, Geddes JR. Lithium in the prevention of suicidal behavior and all-cause mortality in patients with mood disorders: a systematic review of randomized trials. *Am J Psychiatry*. 2005;162:1805-1819.

37. Smith KA, Cipriani A. Lithium and suicide in mood disorders: updated meta-review of the scientific literature. *Bipolar Disord*. 2017;19:575-586.

38. Novick DM, Swartz HA, Frank E. Suicide attempts in bipolar I and bipolar II disorder: a review and meta-analysis of the evidence. *Bipolar Disord*. 2010;12:1-9.

39. Tondo L, Pompili M, Forte A, Baldessarini RJ. Suicide attempts in bipolar disorders: comprehensive review of 101 reports. *Acta Psychiatr Scand*. 2016;133:174-186.

40. Young AH. Review: lithium reduces the risk of suicide compared with placebo in people with depression and bipolar disorder. *Evid Based Ment Health*. 2013;16:112.

41. Tondo L, Hennen J, Baldessarini RJ. Lower suicide risk with long-term lithium treatment in major affective illness: a meta-analysis. *Acta Psychiatr Scand*. 2001;104:163-172.

42. Bearden CE, Thompson PM, Dalwani M, et al. Greater cortical gray matter density in lithium-treated patients with bipolar disorder. *Biol Psychiatry*. 2007;62:7-16.

43. Nunes PV, Forlenza OV, Gattaz WF. Lithium and risk for Alzheimer's disease in elderly patients with bipolar disorder. *Br J Psychiatry*. 2007;190:359-360.

44. Fornai F, Longone P, Cafaro L, et al. Lithium delays progression of amyotrophic lateral sclerosis. *Proc Natl Acad Sci USA*. 2008;105:2052-2057.

45. Giakoumatos CI, Nanda P, Mathew IT, et al. Effects of lithium on cortical thickness and hippocampal subfield volumes in psychotic bipolar disorder. *J Psychiatr Res*. 2015;61:180-187.

46. Wingo AP, Harvey PD, Baldessarini RJ. Neurocognitive impairment in bipolar disorder patients: functional implications. *Bipolar Disord*.2009;11:113-125.

47. Gildengers AG, Butters MA, Aizenstein HJ, et al. Longer lithium exposure is associated with better white matter integrity in older adults with bipolar disorder. *Bipolar Disord*. 2015;17(3):248–256.

48. Moore GJ, Cortese BM, Glitz DA, et al. A longitudinal study of the effects of lithium treatment on prefrontal and subgenual prefrontal gray matter volume in treatment-responsive bipolar disorder patients. *J Clin Psychiatry*. 2009;70:699-705.

49. Lyoo IK, Dager SR, Kim JE, et al. Lithium-induced gray matter volume increase as a neural correlate of treatment response in bipolar disorder: a longitudinal brain imaging study. *Neuropsychopharmacology*. 2010;35:1743-1750.

50. Forlenza OV, De-Paula VJ, Diniz BS. Neuroprotective effects of lithium: implications for the treatment of Alzheimer's disease and related neurodegenerative disorders. *ACS Chem Neurosci*. 2014;5:443-450.

51. Lan C-C, Liu C-C, Lin C-H, et al. A reduced risk of stroke with lithium exposure in bipolar disorder: a population-based retrospective cohort study. *Bipolar Disord*. 2015;17:705-714.

52. Lepkifker E, Iancu I, Horesh N, Strous RD, Kotler M. Lithium therapy for unipolar and bipolar depression among the middle-aged and older adult patient subpopulation. *Depress Anxiety.* 2007;24(8):571-576.

53. Patel NC, Delbello MP, Bryan HS, et al. Open-label lithium for the treatment of adolescents with bipolar depression. *J Am Acad Child Adolesc Psychiatry.* 2006;45:289-297.

54. Severus E, Taylor MJ, Sauer C, et al. Lithium for prevention of mood episodes in bipolar disorders: systematic review and meta- analysis. *Int J Bipolar Disord.* 2014;2:15.

55. Baldessarini RJ, Leahy L, Arcona S, Gause D, Zhang W, Hennen J. Patterns of psychotropic drug prescription for U.S. patients with diagnoses of bipolar disorders. *Psychiatr Serv.* 2007;58:85-91.

56. Kessing LV, Hellmund G, Geddes JR, Goodwin GM, Andersen PK. Valproate v. lithium in the treatment of bipolar disorder in clinical practice: observational nationwide register-based cohort study. *Br J Psychiatry.* 2011;199:57-63.

57. Hayes JF, Marston L, Walters K, Geddes JR, King M, Osborn DP. Lithium vs. valproate vs. olanzapine vs. quetiapine as maintenance monotherapy for bipolar disorder: a population-based UK cohort study using electronic health records. *World Psychiatry.* 2016;15:53-58.

58. Berk M, Daglas R, Dandash O, et al. Quetiapine v. lithium in the maintenance phase following a first episode of mania: randomised controlled trial. *Br J Psychiatry.* 2017;210:413-421.

59. Lähteenvuo M, Tanskanen A, Taipale H, et al. Real-world effectiveness of pharmacologic treatments for the prevention of rehospitalization in a finnish nationwide cohort of patients with bipolar disorder. *JAMA Psychiatry.* 2018;75:347-355.

60. Kessing LV, Vradi E, Andersen PK. Starting lithium prophylaxis early v. late in bipolar disorder. *Br J Psychiatry.* 2014;205:214-220.

61. Kemp DE, Gao K, Fein EB, et al. Lamotrigine as add-on treatment to lithium and divalproex: lessons learned from a double-blind, placebo-controlled trial in rapid-cycling bipolar disorder. *Bipolar Disord.* 2012;14:780-789.

62. Tondo L, Hennen J, Baldessarini RJ. Rapid-cycling bipolar disorder: effects of long-term treatments. *Acta Psychiatr Scand.* 2003;108:4-14.

63. Cipriani A, Barbui C, Salanti G, et al. Comparative efficacy and acceptability of antimanic drugs in acute mania: a multiple-treatments meta-analysis. *Lancet.* 2011;378:1306-1315.

64. Jefferson JW, Greist AH, Ackerman DL. Lithium encyclopaedia for clinical Practice. Washington, DC: APA Press;1987.

65. Goldberg JF, Ernst CL. Managing the side effects of psychotropic medications (2nd edn) Washington, DC: American Psychiatric Publishing; 2019.

66. Hayes JF, Marston L, Walters K, Geddes JR, King M, Osborn DP. Adverse renal, endocrine, hepatic, and metabolic events during maintenance mood stabilizer treatment for bipolar disorder: a population-based cohort study. *PLoS Medicine.* 2016;13:e1002058.

67. Cavanagh J, Smyth R, Goodwin GM. Relapse into mania or depression following lithium discontinuation: a 7-year follow-up. *Acta Psychiatr Scand.* 2004;109:91-95.

68. Suppes T, Baldessarini RJ, Faedda GL, Tondo L, Tohen M. Discontinuation of maintenance treatment in bipolar disorder: risks and implications. *Harv Rev Psychiatry.*1993;1:131-144.

69. Goodwin GM. Recurrence of mania after lithium withdrawal. Implications for the use of lithium in the treatment of bipolar affective disorder. *Br J Psychiatry.* 1994;164:149-152.

70. Aiff H, Attman P-O, Aurell M, et al. Effects of 10 to 30 years of lithium treatment on kidney function. *J Psychopharmacol.* 2015;29(5):608-614.

71. Kessing LV, Gerds TA, Feldt-Rasmussen B, Andersen PK, Licht RW. Use of lithium and anticonvulsants and the rate of chronic kidney disease: a nationwide population-based study. *JAMA Psychiatry.* 2015;72:1182-1191.

72. Tondo L, Abramowicz M, Alda M, et al. Long-term lithium treatment in bipolar disorder: effects on glomerular filtration rate and other metabolic parameters. *Int J Bipolar Disord.* 2017;5:27.

73. Aiff H, Attman PO, Aurell M, Bendz H, Schon S, Svedlund J. End-stage renal disease associated with prophylactic lithium treatment. *Eur Neuropsychopharmacol.* 2014;24:540-544.

74. Surks MI, Sievert R. Drugs and thyroid function. *N Engl J Med.* 1995;333:1688-1694.

75. Kupka RW, Luckenbaugh DA, Post RM, Leverich GS, Nolen WA. Rapid and non-rapid cycling bipolar disorder: a meta-analysis of clinical studies. *J Clin Psychiatry.* 2003;64:1483-1494.

76. Calabrese JR, Keck PE, Macfadden W, et al. A randomized, double-blind, placebo-controlled trial of quetiapine in the treatment of bipolar I or II depression. *Am J Psychiatry.* 2005;162:1351-1360.

77. Thase ME, Macfadden W, Weisler RH, et al. Efficacy of quetiapine monotherapy in bipolar I and II depression: a double-blind, placebo- controlled study (the BOLDER II study). *J Clin Psychopharmacol.* 2006;26:600-609.

78. Endicott J, Rajagopalan K, Minkwitz M, Macfadden W. A randomized, double-blind, placebo-controlled study of quetiapine in the treatment of bipolar I and II depression: improvements in quality of life. *Int Clin Psychopharmacol.* 2007;22:29-37.

79. Hirschfeld RM, Weisler RH, Raines SR, Macfadden W. Quetiapine in the treatment of anxiety in patients with bipolar I or II depression: a secondary analysis from a randomized, double-blind, placebo-controlled study. *J Clin Psychiatry.* 2006;67:355-362.

80. McElroy SL, Weisler RH, Chang W, et al. A double-blind, placebo- controlled study of quetiapine and paroxetine as monotherapy in adults with bipolar depression (EMBOLDEN II). *J Clin Psychiatry.* 2010;71:163-174.

81. Vedantam S. A silenced drug study creates an uproar. Washington Post. 2009.

82. Wilson D. Drug maker's email released in Seroquel lawsuit. NY Times. 2009.

83. Ngai YF, Sabatini P, Nguyen D, et al. Quetiapine treatment in youth is associated with decreased insulin secretion. *J Clin Psychopharmacol.* 2014;34:359-364.

84. Weisler RH, Nolen WA, Neijber A, Hellqvist A, Paulsson B. Continuation of quetiapine versus switching to placebo or lithium for maintenance treatment of bipolar I disorder (Trial 144: a randomized controlled study). *J Clin Psychiatry.* 2011;72:1452-1464.

85. Goodwin FK, Whitham EA, Ghaemi SN. Maintenance treatment study designs in bipolar disorder: do they demonstrate that atypical neuroleptics (antipsychotics) are mood stabilizers? *CNS Drugs.* 2011;25:819-827.

86. Bowden CL, Calabrese JR, Ketter TA, Sachs GS, White RL, Thompson TR. Impact of lamotrigine and lithium on weight in obese and nonobese patients with bipolar I disorder. *Am J Psychiatry.* 2006;163:1199-1201.

87. Gualtieri CT, Johnson LG. Comparative neurocognitive effects of 5 psychotropic anticonvulsants and lithium. MedGenMed. 2006;8:46.

88. Calabrese JR, Sullivan JR, Bowden CL, et al. Rash in multicenter trials of lamotrigine in mood disorders: clinical relevance and management. *J Clin Psychiatry.* 2002;63:1012-1019.

89. Mockenhaupt M, Messenheimer J, Tennis P, Schlingmann J. Risk of Stevens-Johnson syndrome and toxic epidermal necrolysis in new users of antiepileptics. *Neurology.* 2005;64:1134-1138.

90. Calabrese JR, Bowden CL, Sachs GS, Ascher JA, Monaghan E, Rudd GD. A double-blind placebo-controlled study of lamotrigine monotherapy in outpatients with bipolar I depression.Lamictal 602 Study Group. *J Clin Psychiatry.* 1999;60:79-88.

91. Frye MA, Ketter TA, Kimbrell TA, et al. A placebo-controlled study of lamotrigine and gabapentin monotherapy in refractory mood disorders. *J Clin Psychopharmacol.*2000;20:607-614.

92. Kusumakar V, Yatham LN. An open study of lamotrigine in refractory bipolar depression. *Psychiatry Res.* 1997;72:145-148.

93. Calabrese JR, Bowden CL, McElroy SL, et al. Spectrum of activity of lamotrigine in treatment-refractory bipolar disorder. *Am J Psychiatry.* 1999;156:1019-1023.

94. Robillard M, Conn DK. Lamotrigine use in geriatric patients with bipolar depression. *Can J Psychiatry.* 2002;47:767-770.

95. Chang K, Saxena K, Howe M. An open-label study of lamotrigine adjunct or monotherapy for the treatment of adolescents with bipolar depression. *J Am Acad Child Adolesc Psychiatry.* 2006;45:298-304.

96. Savas HA, Selek S, Bulbul F, Kaya MC, Savas E. Successful treatment with lamotrigine in bipolar depression: a study from Turkey. *Aust N Z J Psychiatry*. 2006;40:498-500.

97. Calabrese JR, Huffman RF, White RL, et al. Lamotrigine in the acute treatment of bipolar depression: results of five double-blind, placebo-controlled clinical trials. *Bipolar Disord*. 2008;10:323-333.

98. Geddes JR, Burgess S, Hawton K, Jamison K, Goodwin GM. Long- term lithium therapy for bipolar disorder: systematic review and meta-analysis of randomized controlled trials. *Am J Psychiatry*. 2004;161:217-222.

99. Kesebir S, Akdeniz F, Demir A, Bilici M. A comparison before and after lamotrigine use in long term continuation treatment: effect of blood level. *Journal of Mood Disorders*. 2013;3:47-51.

100. Bowden CL, Calabrese JR, Sachs G, et al. A placebo-controlled 18- month trial of lamotrigine and lithium maintenance treatment in recently manic or hypomanic patients with bipolar I disorder. *Arch Gen Psychiatry*. 2003;60:392-400.

101. Calabrese JR, Bowden CL, Sachs G, et al. A placebo-controlled 18-month trial of lamotrigine and lithium maintenance treatment in recently depressed patients with bipolar I disorder. *J Clin Psychiatry*. 2003;64:1013-1024.

102. Loebel A, Cucchiaro J, Silva R, et al. Lurasidone monotherapy in the treatment of bipolar I depression: a randomized, double-blind, placebo-controlled study. *Am J Psychiatry*. 2014;171:160-168.

103. Belmaker RH. Lurasidone and bipolar disorder. *Am J Psychiatry*. 2014;171:131-133.

104. Leucht S, Cipriani A, Spineli L, et al. Comparative efficacy and tolerability of 15 antipsychotic drugs in schizophrenia: a multiple- treatments meta-analysis. *Lancet*. 2013;382:951-962.

105. Ketter TA, Miller S, Dell'Osso B, Calabrese JR, Frye MA, Citrome L. Balancing benefits and harms of treatments for acute bipolar depression. *J Affect Disord*. 2014;169(Suppl 1):S24-S33.

106. De Fruyt J, Deschepper E, Audenaert K, et al. Second generation antipsychotics in the treatment of bipolar depression: a systematic review and meta-analysis. *J Psychopharmacol*.2012;26:603-617.

107. Loebel A, Cucchiaro J, Silva R, et al. Lurasidone as adjunctive therapy with lithium or valproate for the treatment of bipolar I depression: a randomized, double-blind, placebo-controlled study. *Am J Psychiatry*. 2014;171:169-177.

108. Sachs GS. Use of quality metrics as eligibility criteria to improve signal detection. *Biol Psychiatry*. 2014;75(9S):S31.

109. McIntyre RS, Cucchiaro J, Pikalov A, Kroger H, Loebel A. Lurasidone in the treatment of bipolar depression with mixed (sub-syndromal hypomanic) features: post hoc analysis of a randomized placebo-controlled trial. *J Clin Psychiatry*. 2015;76(04):398–405.

110. Doan LA, Williams SR, Takayesu A, Lu B. Case series reports on lurasidone-associated mania. *J Clin Psychopharmacol*. 2017;37:264-266.

111. Calabrese JR, Keck, Jr PE, Starace A, et al. Efficacy and safety of low- and high-dose cariprazine in acute and mixed mania associated with bipolar I disorder: a double-blind, placebo-controlled study. *J Clin Psychiatry*. 2015;76:284-292.

112. Sachs GS, Greenberg WM, Starace A, et al. Cariprazine in the treatment of acute mania in bipolar I disorder: a double-blind, placebo-controlled, phase III trial. *J Affect Disord*.2015;174:296-302.

113. Durgam S, Starace A, Li D, et al. The efficacy and tolerability of cariprazine in acute mania associated with bipolar I disorder: a phase II trial. *Bipolar Disord*.2015;17:63-75.

114. Citrome L. Cariprazine for bipolar depression: What is the number needed to treat, number needed to harm and likelihood to be helped or harmed? *Int J Clin Pract*. 2019;73:e13397.

115. Earley W, Burgess MV, Rekeda L, et al. Cariprazine treatment of bipolar depression: a randomized double-blind placebo-controlled phase 3 study. *Am J Psychiatry*. 2019;176:439-448.

116. Sachs GS, Ice KS, Chappell PB, et al. Efficacy and safety of adjunctive oral ziprasidone for acute treatment of depression in patients with bipolar I disorder: a randomized, double-blind, placebo-controlled trial. *J Clin Psychiatry*. 2011;72:1413-1422.

117. Thase ME, Jonas A, Khan A, et al. Aripiprazole monotherapy in nonpsychotic bipolar I depression: results of 2 randomized, placebo-controlled studies. *J Clin Psychopharmacol*. 2008;28:13-20.

118. Keck PE, Calabrese JR, McQuade RD, et al. A randomized, double-blind, placebo-controlled 26-week trial of aripiprazole in recently manic patients with bipolar I disorder. *J Clin Psychiatry.* 2006;67:626-637.

119. Tohen M, Vieta E, Calabrese J, et al. Efficacy of olanzapine and olanzapine-fluoxetine combination in the treatment of bipolar I depression. *Arch Gen Psychiatry.* 2003;60:1079-1088.

120. Brown EB, McElroy SL, Keck PE, et al. A 7-week, randomized, double-blind trial of olanzapine/fluoxetine combination versus lamotrigine in the treatment of bipolar I depression. *J Clin Psychiatry.* 2006;67:1025-1033.

121. Tohen M, McDonnell DP, Case M, et al. Randomised, double-blind, placebo-controlled study of olanzapine in patients with bipolar I depression. *Br J Psychiatry.* 2012;201:376-382.

122. Katagiri H, Tohen M, McDonnell DP, et al. Safety and efficacy of olanzapine in the long-term treatment of Japanese patients with bipolar I disorder, depression: an integrated analysis. *Psychiatry Clin Neurosci.* 2014;68:498-505.

123. Wang M, Tong JH, Huang DS, Zhu G, Liang GM, Du H. Efficacy of olanzapine monotherapy for treatment of bipolar I depression: a randomized, double-blind, placebo controlled study. *Psychopharmacology.* 2014;231:2811-2818.

124. Ostacher MJ, Tandon R, Suppes T. Florida best practice psycho-therapeutic medication guidelines for adults with bipolar disorder: a novel, practical, patient-centered guide for clinicians. *J Clin Psychiatry.* 2016;77:920-926.

125. Hahn MK, Wolever TMS, Arenovich T, et al. Acute effects of single-dose olanzapine on metabolic, endocrine, and inflammatory markers in healthy controls. *J Clin Psychopharmacol.* 2013;33:740-746.

126. McGirr A, Vohringer PA, Ghaemi SN, Lam RW, Yatham LN. Safety and efficacy of adjunctive second-generation antidepressant therapy with a mood stabiliser or an atypical antipsychotic in acute bipolar depression: a systematic review and meta-analysis of randomised placebo-controlled trials. *Lancet Psychiatry.* 2016;3:1138-1146.

127. Bond DJ, Lam RW, Yatham LN. Divalproex sodium versus placebo in the treatment of acute bipolar depression: a systematic review and meta-analysis. *J Affect Disord.*2010;124:228-234.

128. Wang PW, Nowakowska C, Chandler RA, et al. Divalproex extended-release in acute bipolar II depression. *J Affect Disord.* 2010;124:170-173.

129. Miura T, Noma H, Furukawa TA, et al. Comparative efficacy and tolerability of pharmacological treatments in the maintenance treatment of bipolar disorder: a systematic review and network meta-analysis. *Lancet Psychiatry.* 2014;1:351-359.

130. Geddes JR, Goodwin GM, Rendell J, et al. Lithium plus valproate combination therapy versus monotherapy for relapse prevention in bipolar I disorder (BALANCE): a randomised open-label trial. *Lancet.* 2010;375:385-395.

131. Ghaemi SN, Goodwin FK. Divalproex vs. lithium in the treatment of bipolar disorder: a naturalistic 1.7-year comparison. *J Affect Disord.* 2001;65:281-287.

132. Gyulai L, Bowden CL, McElroy SL, et al. Maintenance efficacy of divalproex in the prevention of bipolar depression. *Neuropsychopharmacology.* 2003;28:1374-1382.

133. Patel N, Viguera AC, Baldessarini RJ. Mood-stabilizing anticonvulsants, spina bifida, and folate supplementation: commentary. *J Clin Psychopharmacol.* 2018;38:7-10.

134. Reinares M, Rosa AR, Franco C, et al. A systematic review on the role of anticonvulsants in the treatment of acute bipolar depression. *Int J Neuropsychopharmacol.* 2013;16:485-496.

135. Yatham LN, Kennedy SH, Parikh SV, et al. Canadian Network for Mood and Anxiety Treatments (CANMAT) and International Society for Bipolar Disorders (ISBD) collaborative update of CANMAT guidelines for the management of patients with bipolar disorder: update 2013. *Bipolar Disord.* 2013;15:1-44.

136. El-Mallakh RS, Vöhringer PA, Ostacher MM, et al. Antidepressants worsen rapid-cycling course in bipolar depression: A STEP-BD randomized clinical trial. *J Affect Disord.* 2015;184:318-321.

137. El-Mallakh RS, Ghaemi SN, Sagduyu K, et al. Antidepressant-associated chronic irritable dysphoria (ACID) in STEP-BD patients. *J Affect Disord*. 2008;111:372-377.

138. Amsterdam JD, Brunswick DJ. Antidepressant monotherapy for bipolar type II major depression. *Bipolar Disord*. 2003;5:388-395.

139. Kupfer DJ, Chengappa KNR, Gelenberg AJ, et al. Citalopram as adjunctive therapy in bipolar depression. *J Clin Psychiatry*. 2001;62:985-990.

140. Altshuler LL, Sugar CA, McElroy SL, et al. Switch rates during acute treatment for bipolar II depression with lithium, sertraline, or the two combined: a randomized double-blind comparison. *Am J Psychiatry*. 2017;174(3):266-276.

141. Amsterdam JD, Shults J. Efficacy and safety of long-term fluoxetine versus lithium monotherapy of bipolar II disorder: a randomized, double-blind, placebo-substitution study. *Am J Psychiatry*. 2010;167:792-800.

142. Suppes T. Is there a role for antidepressants in the treatment of bipolar II depression? *Am J Psychiatry*. 2010;167:738-740.

143. Sachs GS, Nierenberg AA, Calabrese JR, et al. Effectiveness of adjunctive antidepressant treatment for bipolar depression. *N Engl J Med*. 2007;356:1711-1722.

144. American Psychiatric Association. Diagnostic and statistical manual of mental disorders (5th edn). Washington, DC: American Psychiatric Press; 2013.

145. Suppes T, Vieta E, Gustafsson U, Ekholm B. Maintenance treatment with quetiapine when combined with either lithium or divalproex in bipolar I disorder: analysis of two large randomized, placebo-controlled trials. *Depress Anxiety*. 2013;30:1089-1098.

146. Geddes JR, Gardiner A, Rendell J, et al. Comparative evaluation of quetiapine plus lamotrigine combination versus quetiapine monotherapy (and folic acid versus placebo) in bipolar depression (CEQUEL): a 2 x 2 factorial randomised trial. *Lancet Psychiatry*. 2016;3:31-39.

147. Vieta E, Suppes T, Eggens I, Persson I, Paulsson B, Brecher M. Efficacy and safety of quetiapine in combination with lithium or divalproex for maintenance of patients with bipolar I disorder (international trial 126). *J Affect Disord*. 2008;109:251-263.

148. Suppes T, Vieta E, Liu S, Brecher M, Paulsson B. Maintenance treatment for patients with bipolar I disorder: results from a north american study of quetiapine in combination with lithium or divalproex (trial 127). *Am J Psychiatry*. 2009;166:476-488.

149. van der Loos MLM, Mulder PGH, Hartong EGTM, et al. Efficacy and safety of lamotrigine as add-on treatment to lithium in bipolar depression: a multicenter, double-blind, placebo-controlled trial. *J Clin Psychiatry*. 2009;70:223-231.

150. Lorenzo-Luaces L, Amsterdam JD, Soeller I, DeRubeis RJ. Rapid versus non-rapid cycling bipolar II depression: response to venlafaxine and lithium and hypomanic risk. *Acta Psychiatr Scand*. 2016;133:459-469.

151. Leverich GS, Altshuler LL, Frye MA, et al. Risk of switch in mood polarity to hypomania or mania in patients with bipolar depression during acute and continuation trials of venlafaxine, sertraline, and bupropion as adjuncts to mood stabilizers. *Am J Psychiatry*. 2006;163:232-239.

152. Hammett S, Youssef NA. Systematic review of recent guidelines for pharmacological treatments of bipolar disorders in adults. *Ann Clin Psychiatry*. 2017;29:266-282.

153. Ciapparelli A, Dell'Osso L, Tundo A, et al. Electroconvulsive therapy in medication-nonresponsive patients with mixed mania and bipolar depression. *J Clin Psychiatry*. 2001;62:552-555.

154. Grunhaus L, Schreiber S, Dolberg OT, Hirshman S, Dannon PN. Response to ECT in major depression: are there differences between unipolar and bipolar depression? *Bipolar Disord*. 2002;4(Suppl 1):91-93.

155. Sampaio-Junior B, Tortella G, Borrione L, et al. Efficacy and safety of transcranial direct current stimulation as an add-on treatment for bipolar depression: a randomized clinical trial. *JAMA Psychiatry*. 2018;75:158-166.

156. Sit DK, McGowan J, Wiltrout C, et al. Adjunctive bright light therapy for bipolar depression: a randomized double-blind placebo- controlled trial. *Am J Psychiatry.* 2018;175:131-139.

157. McElroy SL, Martens BE, Mori N, et al. Adjunctive lisdexamfetamine in bipolar depression: a preliminary randomized, placebo- controlled trial. *Int Clin Psychopharmacol.* 2015;30:6-13.

158. Frye MA, Grunze H, Suppes T, et al. A placebo-controlled evaluation of adjunctive modafinil in the treatment of bipolar depression. *Am J Psychiatry.* 2007;164:1242-1249.

159. Ketter TA, Wang PW, Miller S. Bipolar therapeutics update 2014: a tale of 3 treatments. *J Clin Psychiatry.* 2015;76:69-70.

160. Goldberg JF, Burdick KE, Endick CJ. Preliminary randomized, double-blind, placebo-controlled trial of pramipexole added to mood stabilizers for treatment-resistant bipolar depression. *Am J Psychiatry.* 2004;161:564-566.

161. Zarate CA, Payne JL, Singh J, et al. Pramipexole for bipolar II depression: a placebo-controlled proof of concept study. *Biol Psychiatry.* 2004;56:54-60.

162. El-Mallakh RS, Penagaluri P, Kantamneni A, Gao Y, Roberts RJ. Long-term use of pramipexole in bipolar depression: a naturalistic retrospective chart review. *Psychiatr Q.*2010;81:207-213.

163. Dell'Osso B, Ketter TA, Cremaschi L, Spagnolin G, Altamura AC. Assessing the roles of stimulants/stimulant-like drugs and dopamine-agonists in the treatment of bipolar depression. *Curr Psychiatry Rep.* 2013;15:378.

164. Suppes T, Webb A, Paul B, Carmody T, Kraemer H, Rush AJ. Clinical outcome in a randomized 1-year trial of clozapine versus treatment as usual for patients with treatment-resistant illness and a history of mania. *Am J Psychiatry.* 1999;156:1164-1169.

165. Fehr BS, Ozcan ME, Suppes T. Low doses of clozapine may stabilize treatment-resistant bipolar patients. *Eur Arch Psychiatry Clin Neurosci.* 2005;255:10-14.

166. Ciapparelli A, Dell'Osso L, di Poggio AB, et al. Clozapine in treatment-resistant patients with schizophrenia, schizoaffective disorder, or psychotic bipolar disorder: a naturalistic 48-month follow-up study. *J Clin Psychiatry.* 2003;64:451-458.

167. Chang JS, Ha KS, Young Lee K, Sik Kim Y, Min AY. The effects of long-term clozapine add-on therapy on the rehospitalization rate and the mood polarity patterns in bipolar disorders. *J Clin Psychiatry.* 2006;67:461-467.

168. Saunders EF, Ramsden CE, Sherazy MS, Gelenberg AJ, Davis JM, Rapoport SI. Omega-3 and Omega-6 polyunsaturated fatty acids in bipolar disorder: a review of biomarker and treatment studies. *J Clin Psychiatry.* 2016;77:e1301-e1308.

169. Frangou S, Lewis M, McCrone P. Efficacy of ethyl-eicosapentaenoic acid in bipolar depression: randomised double-blind placebo- controlled study. *Br J Psychiatry.* 2006;188:46-50.

170. Sarris J, Mischoulon D, Schweitzer I. Omega-3 for bipolar disorder: meta-analyses of use in mania and bipolar depression. *J Clin Psychiatry.* 2012;73:81-86.

171. Ketter TA, Wang PW, Chandler RA, Culver JL, Alarcon AM. Adjunctive aripiprazole in treatment-resistant bipolar depression. *Ann Clin Psychiatry.* 2006;18:169-172.

172. McElroy SL, Suppes T, Frye MA, et al. Open-label aripiprazole in the treatment of acute bipolar depression: a prospective pilot trial. *J Affect Disord.* 2007;101:275-281.

173. Kelly T, Lieberman DZ. The utility of low-dose aripiprazole for the treatment of bipolar II and bipolar NOS depression. *J Clin Psychopharmacol.* 2017;37:99-101.

174. Dunn RT, Stan VA, Chriki LS, Filkowski MM, Ghaemi SN. A prospective, open-label study of Aripiprazole mono- and adjunctive treatment in acute bipolar depression. *J Affect Disord.* 2008;110:70-74.

175. Mazza M, Squillacioti MR, Pecora RD, Janiri L, Bria P. Beneficial acute antidepressant effects of aripiprazole as an adjunctive treatment or monotherapy in bipolar patients unresponsive to mood stabilizers: results from a 16-week open-label trial. *Expert Opin Pharmacother.* 2008;9:3145-3149.

176. Kemp DE, Dago PL, Straus JL, Fleck J, Karaffa M, Gilmer WS. Aripiprazole augmentation for treatment-resistant bipolar depression: sustained remission after 36 months. *J Clin Psychopharmacol.* 2007;27:304-305.

177. Sokolski KN. Adjunctive aripiprazole in bipolar I depression. *Ann Pharmacother*. 2007;41:35-40.

178. Thase ME, Bowden CL, Nashat M, et al. Aripiprazole in bipolar depression: a pooled, post-hoc analysis by severity of core depressive symptoms. *Int J Psychiatry Clin Pract*. 2012;16:121-131.

179. Benedetti F, Riccaboni R, Locatelli C, Poletti S, Dallaspezia S, Colombo C. Rapid treatment response of suicidal symptoms to lithium, sleep deprivation, and light therapy (chronotherapeutics) in drug-resistant bipolar depression. *J Clin Psychiatry*. 2014;75:133-140.

180. Wu JC, Kelsoe JR, Schachat C, et al. Rapid and sustained antidepressant response with sleep deprivation and chronotherapy in bipolar disorder. *Biol Psychiatry*. 2009;66:298-301.

181. Kelly T, Lieberman DZ. The use of triiodothyronine as an augmentation agent in treatment-resistant bipolar II and bipolar disorder NOS. *J Affect Disord*. 2009;116:222-226.

182. Goodman LA, Salyers MP, Mueser KT, et al. Recent victimization in women and men with severe mental illness: prevalence and correlates. *J Trauma Stress*. 2001;14:615-632.

183. Quarantini LC, Miranda-Scippa Â, Nery-Fernandes F, et al. The impact of comorbid posttraumatic stress disorder on bipolar disorder patients. *J Affect Disord*. 2010;123:71-76.

184. Wallace J. Treatment of trauma with lithium to forestall the development of posttraumatic stress disorder by pharmacological induction of a mild transient amnesia. *Med Hypotheses*. 2013;80:711-715.

185. Bajor LA, Ticlea AN, Osser DN. The psychopharmacology algorithm project at the Harvard South Shore Program: an update on post- traumatic stress disorder. *Harv Rev Psychiatry*. 2011;19: 240-258.

186. Hertzberg MA, Butterfield MI, Feldman ME, et al. A preliminary study of lamotrigine for the treatment of posttraumatic stress disorder. *Biol Psychiatry*. 1999;45:1226-1229.

187. Viktorin A, Rydén E, Thase ME, et al. The risk of treatmentemergent mania with methylphenidate in bipolar disorder. *Am J Psychiatry*. 2017;174:341-348.

188. Peruzzolo TL, Tramontina S, Rohde LA, Zeni CP. Pharmacotherapy of bipolar disorder in children and adolescents: an update. *Rev Bras Psiquiatr*. 2013;35:393-405.

189. Niemegeers P, Maudens KE, Morrens M, et al. Pharmacokinetic evaluation of armodafinil for the treatment of bipolar depression. *Expert Opin Drug Metab Toxicol*. 2012;8:1189-1197.

190. Gao K, Wu R, Kemp DE, et al. Efficacy and safety of quetiapine-XR as monotherapy or adjunctive therapy to a mood stabilizer in acute bipolar depression with generalized anxiety disorder and other co-morbidities: a randomized, placebo-controlled trial. *J Clin Psychiatry*. 2014;75:1062-1068.

191. Jentink J, Loane MA, Dolk H, et al. Valproic acid monotherapy in pregnancy and major congenital malformations. *N Engl J Med*. 2010;362:2185-2193.

192. Cummings C, Stewart M, Stevenson M, Morrow J, Nelson J. Neurodevelopment of children exposed in utero to lamotrigine, sodium valproate and carbamazepine. *Arch Dis Child*. 2011;96:643-647.

193. Cunnington M, Tennis P. International lamotrigine pregnancy registry scientific advisory C. Lamotrigine and the risk of malformations in pregnancy. *Neurology*. 2005;64:955-960.

194. Berwaerts K, Sienaert P, De Fruyt J. Teratogenic effects of lamotrigine in women with bipolar disorder. *Tijdschr Psychiatr*. 2009;51:741-750.

195. Clark CT, Klein AM, Perel JM, Helsel J, Wisner KL. Lamotrigine dosing for pregnant patients with bipolar disorder. *Am J Psychiatry*. 2013;170:1240-1247.

196. Dolk H, Wang H, Loane M, et al. Lamotrigine use in pregnancy and risk of orofacial cleft and other congenital anomalies. *Neurology*. 2016;86:1716-1725.

197. Vajda FJ, Dodd S, Horgan D. Lamotrigine in epilepsy, pregnancy and psychiatry–a drug for all seasons? *J Clin Neurosci*.2013;20:13-16.

198. Patorno E, Huybrechts KF, Bateman BT, et al. Lithium use in pregnancy and the risk of cardiac malformations. *N Engl J Med*. 2017;376:2245-2254.

199. Leiknes KA, Cooke MJ, Jarosch-von Schweder L, Harboe I, Hoie B. Electroconvulsive therapy during pregnancy: a systematic review of case studies. *Arch Womens Ment Health*. 2015;18(1):1-39.

200. McCauley-Elsom K, Gurvich C, Elsom SJ, Kulkarni J. Antipsychotics in pregnancy. *J Psychiatr Ment Health Nurs*. 2010;17:97-104.

201. Taylor DPC, Kapur S. South London and Maudsley NHS Trust. The Maudsley prescribing guidelines in psychiatry (11th edn). Chichester, West Sussex: John Wiley & Sons; 2012.

202. Maina G, Rosso G, Aguglia A, Bogetto F. Recurrence rates of bipolar disorder during the postpartum period: a study on 276 medication-free Italian women. *Arch Womens Ment Health.* 2014;17(5):367–372.

203. Bergink V, Kushner SA. Lithium during pregnancy. *Am J Psychiatry.* 2014;171:712-715.

204. Trixler M, Gati A, Fekete S,Tenyi T. Use of antipsychotics in the management of schizophrenia during pregnancy. *Drugs.* 2005;65:1193-1206.

205. Salloum IM, Cornelius JR, Daley DC, Kirisci L, Himmelhoch JM, Thase ME. Efficacy of valproate maintenance in patients with bipolar disorder and alcoholism: a double-blind placebo-controlled study. *Arch Gen Psychiatry.* 2005;62:37-45.

206. Brown ES, Gorman AR, Hynan LS. A randomized, placebo-controlled trial of citicoline add-on therapy in outpatients with bipolar disorder and cocaine dependence. *J Clin Psychopharmacol.* 2007;27:498-502.

207. Tolliver BK, Desantis SM, Brown DG, Prisciandaro JJ, Brady KT. A randomized, double-blind, placebo-controlled clinical trial of acamprosate in alcohol-dependent individuals with bipolar disorder: a preliminary report. *Bipolar Disord.* 2012;14:54-63.

208. Brown ES, Carmody TJ, Schmitz JM, et al. A randomized, double- blind, placebo-controlled pilot study of naltrexone in outpatients with bipolar disorder and alcohol dependence. *Alcohol Clin Exp Res.* 2009;33:1863-1869.

209. Chung AK, Chua SE. Effects on prolongation of Bazett's corrected QT interval of seven second-generation antipsychotics in the treatment of schizophrenia: a meta-analysis. *J Psychopharmacol.* 2011;25:646-666.

210. NICE, National Institute for Health and Care Excellence: Clinical Guideline No. 38. Bipolar disorders: the management of bipolar disorder in adults, children and adolescents, in primary and secondary care. In: British Psychological Society. ISBN: 978-1-4731-0721-2; 2014. https://www.nice.org.uk/

211. Malhi GS, Bassett D, Boyce P, et al. Royal Australian and New Zealand college of psychiatrists clinical practice guidelines for mood disorders. *Aust N Z J Psychiatry.* 2015;49:1087-1206.

212. Goodwin GM, Haddad PM, Ferrier IN, et al. Evidence-based guidelines for treating bipolar disorder: revised third edition recommendations from the British Association for Psychopharmacology. *J Psychopharmacol.* 2016;30(6):495–553.

213. Fountoulakis KN, Yatham L, Grunze H, et al. The International College of Neuro-Psychopharmacology (CINP) treatment guidelines for Bipolar disorder in adults (CINP-BD-2017), part 2: Review, grading of the evidence and a precise algorithm. *Int J Neuropsychopharmacol.* 2017;20:121-179.

How to cite this article: Wang D, Osser DN. The Psychopharmacology Algorithm Project at the Harvard South Shore Program: An update on bipolar depression. *Bipolar Disord.* 2019;00:1–18. https://doi.org/10.1111/bdi.12860

UPDATE

BIPOLAR DEPRESSION ALGORITHM

In the several months since the publication of the last version of this algorithm, the recommendations and flowchart remain the same. There have been no new studies that seem to change the overall sequences of the nodes. However, there are some additional and new studies deserving mention.

Node 2: The Patient with Bipolar Depression Is Not Currently on a Mood Stabilizer

In this long section of the algorithm paper, we discuss the merits of the various options for treatment of an acute bipolar depression if the patient is currently not on a mood stabilizer. One of the options is lamotrigine. It is noted that it may be helpful to obtain a plasma level of lamotrigine to optimize the oral dose, based on a small observational study suggesting that the best results were at about 4 mcg/mL. However, we found another small retrospective study that found that lamotrigine may have a therapeutic window of 5–11 mcg/mL.[1] Given the two studies, we are now suggesting that clinicians try to dose lamotrigine so the level will be between 4 and 11 mcg/mL.

Table 1: Options to Consider for Treatment-Resistant Bipolar Depression

There is misleading information in the brief discussion of the pramipexole studies - the 4th item in the table. It is stated that pramipexole "was poorly tolerated" in these two small studies. In the first study, done primarily in bipolar I depressed patients, 58% reported nausea vs 20% on placebo. However, this did not affect dropout rates in this 6 week study. In the second study which was exclusively in bipolar II patients, 60% of the pramipexole patients reported nausea vs 64% on placebo. Again, it didn't affect dropout rate: 90% of both groups completed the 6 week study. One patient on pramipexole developed a psychotic mania in the first study vs none on placebo, and in the bipolar IIs, one became hypomanic on active medication and two on placebo. The authors noted that studies are needed with longer-term treatment with pramipexole to see if there is more switching over time including switching to psychosis in vulnerable people.

The last item presented in this table is "Add triiodothyronine (T3)." A retrospective chart-review study from Canada presented positive data. Since that publication, a review of the literature on T3 augmentation in bipolar depression located several more studies including three open-label prospective investigations.[2] The percentages of patients improved were 56%, 75%, and 79%. The studies were all considered "flawed but promising" and there were suggestions that rapid cycling patients could benefit. Finally, there was a small double-blind comparison of adjunctive T3 compared with levothyroxine (T4) or placebo.[3] Thirty-two rapid-cycling treatment-resistant patients who had failed a trial of lithium were randomized to have one of these three treatments added to the lithium. They were followed for at least four months. The study was powered for 60 patients but given the difficulty of recruiting these refractory patients they were only able to study 32 and hence the statistical analyses had to be limited. The findings were that the T4 group fared better than the T3 group and the placebo. There was only a trend-level improvement for the T3 group versus the placebo, but it could have become significant if the N had been larger. T4 patients had a 33% increase in the time in euthymia compared to pretreatment, whereas the placebo group's time in euthymia declined by 6.5% ($p = 0.033$).

In conclusion, the evidence base for trying T3 instead of T4 is arguably more persuasive, but more research is needed before thyroid augmentation with either T3 or T4 should be located earlier in the algorithm for bipolar depression.

Table 2: Comorbidity and Other Features in Bipolar Depression: How They Affect the Algorithm

In this table, there is a discussion of considerations for women of childbearing potential. There is mention of a recent large National Institute of Mental Health-sponsored study of the risk of cardiac malformations including Ebstein's abnormality. Data has emerged that provided a more precise measure of what can be expected. The researchers found that the adjusted risk ratio for any cardiac abnormality was 1.65 compared to unexposed babies.[4] For Ebstein's, the risk ratio was 2.66, and in absolute numbers it was 0.6% for lithium-exposed infants versus 0.18% for those not exposed. The impact was dose-related, with higher ratios if the dose was over 900 mg daily. These results were included in a new meta-analysis of 13 high-quality studies published in January 2020.[5] This analysis found the odds ratio for any cardiac abnormality to be slightly higher—1.86. The risk was limited to fetuses exposed in the first trimester. The absolute risk was 1.2% for any cardiac abnormality. Note that these are comparisons between women with bipolar disorder who did or did not receive lithium, not between bipolar women on lithium and the general population of pregnant women. The fetuses of nonbipolar women have fewer cardiac abnormalities. The studies were generally unclear about whether they excluded women who were on other teratogenic medications or were misusing any substances like alcohol. The authors concluded that the risks of lithium exposure during pregnancy are low, though they are higher in the first trimester and doses should be kept in the lowest part of the therapeutic range, especially during that time. The risks and harms associated with mood episode relapse from stopping lithium or lowering the level below the therapeutic range appear, for most women, to exceed the harms of fetal abnormalities or other pregnancy complications associated with continuing lithium.

There is also a brief discussion of substance use disorders as a comorbidity in bipolar depression, and the recommendation is that remission from those use disorders should be a high treatment priority. We did not mention cannabis as one of the substances that could be a concern. The evidence available points clearly to an association between usage and worsening course of bipolar disorder over time. In a study of 4,915 subjects, there was (after control for many possible covariates) a strong increased risk of manic symptoms associated with the use of cannabis over a three-year follow-up period.[6] There was also an earlier age of onset of bipolar disorder, greater overall illness severity, more rapid cycling, poorer life functioning, and poorer adherence with prescribed treatments. In another study, the course of bipolar patients who stopped cannabis use after an illness episode was compared with a group who never had used cannabis and a group that continued to use.[7] The total sample was 1,922 patients. In a two-year period, the continued users had significantly lower rates of recovery, greater work impairment, and lower rates of living with a partner. The data were based on patient reports, so given likely underreporting, there was probably an underestimate of the strength of the association between cannabis use and lives worsened. A systematic review of the effects of cannabis on mood and anxiety disorders confirmed a negative association between cannabis use and long-term outcomes.[8] Thus, it seems that bipolar patients should stay away from cannabis in all its forms. Quitting cannabis should be on the short list of interventions to pursue if patients are not doing well. This is a tough sell in today's political environment regarding cannabis legalization. Many newspaper editorials and politicians are pushing it. Clinicians should not back off and accept patients' insistence on using this product but rather should continue efforts to educate and to consider the problem to be a serious one that potentially interferes with otherwise appropriate and effective bipolar treatments that may be offered.

REFERENCES

1. Katayama Y, Terao T, Kamei K, et al. Therapeutic window of lamotrigine for mood disorders: a naturalistic retrospective study. Pharmacopsychiatry 2014;47:111–4.
2. Parmentier T, Sienaert P. The use of triiodothyronine (T3) in the treatment of bipolar depression: a review of the literature. J Affect Disord 2018;229:410–4.
3. Walshaw PD, Gyulai L, Bauer M, et al. Adjunctive thyroid hormone treatment in rapid cycling bipolar disorder: a double-blind placebo-controlled trial of levothyroxine (L-T4) and triiodothyronine (T3). Bipolar Disord 2018;20:594–603.
4. Patorno E, Huybrechts KF, Bateman BT, et al. Lithium use in pregnancy and the risk of cardiac malformations. N Engl J Med 2017;376:2245–54.
5. Fornaro M, Maritan E, Ferranti R, et al. Lithium exposure during pregnancy and the postpartum period: a systematic review and meta-analysis of safety and efficacy outcomes. Am J Psychiatry 2020;177:76–92.
6. Henquet C, Krabbendam L, de Graaf R, ten Have M, van Os J. Cannabis use and expression of mania in the general population. J Affect Disord 2006;95:103–10.
7. Zorrilla I, Aguado J, Haro JM, et al. Cannabis and bipolar disorder: does quitting cannabis use during manic/mixed episode improve clinical/functional outcomes? Acta Psychiatr Scand 2015;131:100–10.
8. Mammen G, Rueda S, Roerecke M, Bonato S, Lev-Ran S, Rehm J. Association of cannabis with long-term clinical symptoms in anxiety and mood disorders: a systematic review of prospective studies. J Clin Psychiatry 2018;79.

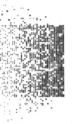

The Psychopharmacology Algorithm Project at the Harvard South Shore Program: An Algorithm for Acute Mania

Othman Mohammad, MD and David N. Osser, MD

Abstract: *This new algorithm for the pharmacotherapy of acute mania was developed by the Psychopharmacology Algorithm Project at the Harvard South Shore Program. The authors conducted a literature search in PubMed and reviewed key studies, other algorithms and guidelines, and their references. Treatments were prioritized considering three main considerations: (1) effectiveness in treating the current episode, (2) preventing potential relapses to depression, and (3) minimizing side effects over the short and long term. The algorithm presupposes that clinicians have made an accurate diagnosis, decided how to manage contributing medical causes (including substance misuse), discontinued antidepressants, and considered the patient's childbearing potential. We propose different algorithms for mixed and nonmixed mania. Patients with mixed mania may be treated first with a second-generation antipsychotic, of which the first choice is quetiapine because of its greater efficacy for depressive symptoms and episodes in bipolar disorder. Valproate and then either lithium or carbamazepine may be added. For nonmixed mania, lithium is the first-line recommendation. A second-generation antipsychotic can be added. Again, quetiapine is favored, but if quetiapine is unacceptable, risperidone is the next choice. Olanzapine is not considered a first-line treatment due to its long-term side effects, but it could be second-line. If the patient, whether mixed or nonmixed, is still refractory to the above medications, then depending on what has already been tried, consider carbamazepine, haloperidol, olanzapine, risperidone, and valproate first tier; aripiprazole, asenapine, and ziprasidone second tier; and clozapine third tier (because of its weaker evidence base and greater side effects). Electroconvulsive therapy may be considered at any point in the algorithm if the patient has a history of positive response or is intolerant of medications.*

Keywords: algorithm, bipolar disorder, management, mania, psychopharmacology

INTRODUCTION

Bipolar mania is a mood state characterized by distinctively and abnormally elevated mood or irritability. It has a recurrent course and, if not treated successfully, can be associated with significant cognitive and functional impairment, especially if associated with psychosis.[1] The successful treatment of a bipolar manic episode should

From Harvard Medical School; Boston Children's Hospital, Boston, MA (Dr. Mohammad); VA Boston Healthcare System, Brockton Division, Brockton, MA (Dr. Osser).

Original manuscript received 5March 2013; revised manuscript received 22 July 2013; accepted for publication 4 November 2013.

Correspondence: David N. Osser, MD, VA Boston Healthcare System, Brockton Division, 940 Belmont St., Brockton, MA 02301. Email: David.Osser@va.gov

DOI: 10.1097/HRP.0000000000000018

include three main goals: (1) treating the current episode, (2) choosing treatment that can prevent relapses to depression, and (3) whenever possible, choosing treatments that minimize side effects associated with psychopharmacology. Achieving these goals poses a significant challenge for the clinician because of the sometimes contradictory evidence about the efficacy of the different treatment options for bipolar disorder, coupled with a shifting understanding of the safety risks involved with different options. Also, in some treatment settings (e.g., inpatient in the managed care environment), the priority in selecting psychopharmacology may be to achieve effectiveness, or at least the appearance thereof, as quickly as possible, thereby facilitating the earliest possible discharge. For that purpose, two or three medications might be administered nearly at once, and without establishing the necessity or desirability of each for the long or even intermediate term. Decision making is also affected by clinical experience, which may be all that the clinician can rely on with very complex patients or in situations where evidence is lacking. But clinical experience can be overvalued, and it obviously needs to be reconsidered when evidence points in a different direction. In this article we present an evidence-based approach to the pharmacotherapy of acute mania—specifically in relation to the three goals stated above. This algorithm is part of the Psychopharmacology Algorithm Project at the Harvard South Shore Program (PAPHSS) and is meant to be considered in conjunction with this group's already published algorithm for the treatment of bipolar depression.[2]

METHODS

The current methods used in developing new and revised PAPHSS algorithms have been described previously.[2-6] In brief, the authors reviewed other algorithms and guidelines on bipolar mania and conducted literature searches using PubMed with keywords such as mania, algorithm, management, and psychopharmacology, focusing on new randomized, controlled trials (RCTs) not considered in previous reviews, in an attempt to survey the entire body of evidence. In constructing the decision tree, the authors gave preference in the early nodes to treatments that are effective for the current mania episode but that also may prevent subsequent depressive episodes. For the first episode, small advantages in efficacy for the acute mania were considered outweighed if a medication with slightly lesser efficacy had significant advantages in efficacy in bipolar depression. The second major consideration was medication safety. Since bipolar disorder is a recurrent and often chronic illness, early treatment with medications with relatively fewer long-term side effects was preferred. Applying these two preferences narrowed the number of choices in the early nodes of the algorithm and encouraged the use of monotherapy if possible. It also offered the potential to minimize the need for later medication switches (e.g., because of metabolic side effects) that can have a destabilizing effect. In later nodes, if the patient did not respond well to the earlier treatments, greater emphasis was placed on antimanic efficacy (while still including a heightened awareness of these agents' potential toxicities). This framework for risk-benefit assessment involves somewhat greater risk that recovery will be delayed or that a hospital admission may be longer than otherwise during the first or early episodes of mania, but taking the longer-term perspective seemed to be a responsible approach that respects the complexity of managing this illness. The British National Institute for Health and Clinical Excellence guidelines (2006) recommended maintenance treatment for bipolar disorder after a single severe manic episode with substantial risk of adverse outcome, or after two acute episodes with less severe mania.[7] In the case of bipolar II hypomania, maintenance was recommended in case of significant impairment in function, frequent episodes, or risk of self-harm.

All hierarchical and other clinical recommendations are the result of agreement by the two authors. Their conclusions were opinion-based distillations of a large body of evidence consisting of reviews, meta-analyses, and individual studies, large and small—which vary in quality and are subject to conflicting interpretation by experts. Hence, the peer review process that followed submission of this article is an essential part of the validation of this algorithm (and other PAPHSS algorithms). If the reasoning, based on the authors' interpretation of the pertinent evidence, was plausible to reviewers, then it was retained. When differences of opinion were present on any particular issue, adjustments were made or the relevant evidence further explored until consensus was achieved or the authors could present a stronger argument in support of their initial position.

DIAGNOSIS OF MANIA

This algorithm focuses on the treatment of acute mania in the context of bipolar disorder. Secondary mania may arise through various processes, including those related to substance abuse (e.g., the use of cocaine), physiologic conditions (e.g. hyperthyroidism), or the use of particular medications (e.g., adrenocorticosteroids). Hence, patients who present with manic symptoms should be carefully evaluated for any concomitant medical illness; their medication lists should be reviewed; and any possible abuse-prone substances or medications known to cause mania should be discontinued. The presence of these precipitants, however, does not exclude the possibility of an underlying predisposition to bipolar disorder that was triggered or kindled by those same precipitants.[8] If the patient is on an antidepressant, it should be tapered and discontinued since the antidepressant may be contributing to the maintenance of the manic state.[9]

Psychosis (more commonly delusions than hallucinations)[10] is present in at least 50% of patients with acute mania, and it contributes significantly to overall impairment.[11] Mania with psychotic features was considered an indicator of severity in the fourth edition of the *Diagnostic and Statistical Manual of Mental Disorders* [DSM-IV] and is a specifier in DSM-5. It is still one of the criteria for distinguishing mania and bipolar I disorder from hypomania and bipolar II. Classic studies of the course of untreated mania have demonstrated that psychotic features typically make their appearance only as the manic episode approaches peak severity,[12] although in DSM-5 they can occur at any time in the episode. However, patients with initial onset of psychosis or persisting psychosis after resolution of other manic symptoms will usually meet criteria for schizoaffective disorder or schizophrenia. Diagnostic ambiguity may be common with a first episode of mania and when the past history is unavailable.

Despite the apparent importance of psychosis in mania, one of the challenges in producing a psychopharmacology algorithm for bipolar mania is that the evidence base regarding optimal treatment of the psychosis is remarkably uninformative. Are antipsychotics more effective than other medications used for mood stabilization, such as lithium or anticonvulsants? Most empirical studies of medications for acute mania have either not provided data on differential outcomes in psychotic versus nonpsychotic mania or found no differences.[10,13] If one considers expert opinion, there does not appear to be a consensus.[8,14-16] In this algorithm, no difference is proposed for the treatment of psychotic versus nonpsychotic mania. However, if schizophrenia and schizoaffective disorder are not excluded as diagnostic possibilities, the prescribing clinician might want to commence treatment in accordance with evidence-supported practice for those disorders, which will usually mean starting with an antipsychotic.

FLOWCHART FOR THE ALGORITHM

A summary and overview of the algorithm appears in Figure 1. Each numbered "node" represents a decision point delineating patient populations ranging from unmedicated at the beginning to highly resistant at the bottom. The questions, evidence analysis, and reasoning that support the recommendations at each node will be presented below.

NODE 1: DOES THE PATIENT MEET DSM-5 CRITERIA FOR MANIA?

First, confirm a diagnosis based on DSM-5 criteria and note any co-occurring psychiatric or medical features and diagnoses that may be particularly important, including active substance abuse or dependence, anxiety or anxiety disorders, women with childbearing potential, and liver disease such as hepatitis C. Table 1 provides a brief summary of how these comorbidities and other considerations would affect the algorithm. A more thorough description of this important material is beyond the scope of this review, but the reader is encouraged to consult the references provided.

Next, the clinician should review past treatments. This may be easier said than done, as previous records may be unavailable or may not adequately document what was done or provide the rationale for what was done in a clear manner. However, if adequate trials of the treatments recommended in the early nodes of the algorithm have occurred with unsatisfactory results despite reasonable indication of adherence, or if the previous trials resulted in intolerance that was likely due to the recommended treatments, then consider selecting an option at the next node of the algorithm. If the patient is presently on a first-line recommendation, the response has been unsatisfactory, but the dose or level was not adequate, consider optimizing the dose and giving that medication more time before moving to the next option in the algorithm. If the patient is presently on a medication or medications not recommended at the beginning of the algorithm but seems to be having a partial benefit, consider adding the recommended treatment. If the results are favorable, try to discontinue the other medication(s).

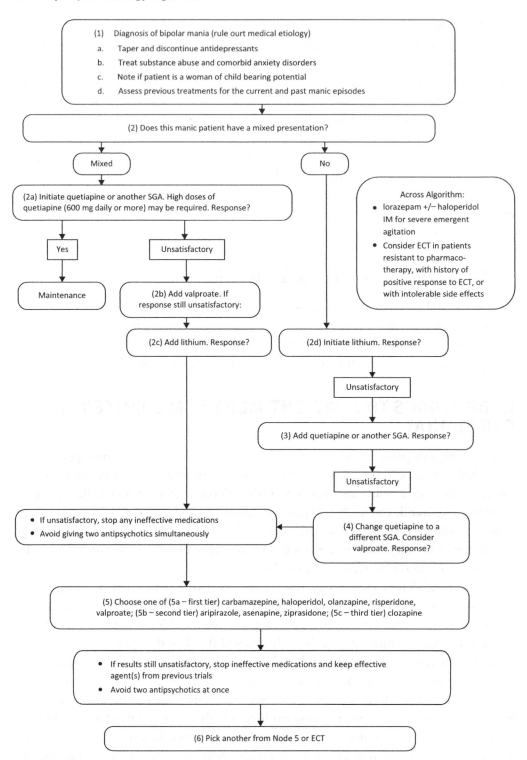

Figure 1. Flowchart for the algorithm for pharmacotherapy of acute mania. ECT, electroconvulsive therapy; SGA, second-generation antipsychotic.

Table 1 | Comorbidity and Other Features in Mania and How They Affect the Algorithm		
Comorbid Conditions	*Evidence considerations[a]*	*Recommendations*
Agitation requiring rapid management[17-22]	IM lorazepam, IM haloperidol, and IM atypicals are superior to placebo in controlling agitation Lorazepam + haloperidol was more beneficial than either haloperidol or lorazepam alone IM SGAs have a significantly lower risk of acute extrapyramidal symptoms compared to haloperidol when used without lorazepam or an antiparkinson agent; however, this risk difference becomes insignificant when adding an anticholinergic agent or lorazepam to haloperidol A Cochrane review evaluated chlorpromazine for psychosis-induced aggression and agitation.[23] Though the quantity and quality of evidence were limited, chlorpromazine was not more effective than haloperidol; the occurrence of serious hypotension suggested that "it may be best to avoid use of chlorpromazine" in view of the better-evaluated options available	In efficacy and safety, IM haloperidol + lorazepam is still the treatment of choice for rapid treatment of severe agitation (with imminent risk of harm to self or others) For less severe agitation, oral as-needed antipsychotics are often used but are usually unnecessary; benzodiazepines could be used instead Avoid the use of IM chlorpromazine
Delirious mania[24]	Bipolar mania can present as delirium in absence of evidence of any other medical condition Patients are mostly younger females; incontinence/inappropriate toileting and denudativeness are distinctive features of their presentation These cases are refractory to treatment with mood stabilizers or antipsychotics	ECT and benzodiazepines are the mainstays of treatment, rather than any particular antipsychotic or mood-stabilizing agent
Anxiety disorders[25]	Up to 75% of bipolar patients have at least one comorbid anxiety disorder at some point Comorbid anxiety disorders are associated with more frequent mood episodes and poorer treatment outcome	Antidepressants should probably be avoided SGAs with antianxiety properties (e.g., quetiapine), antianxiety agents (e.g., buspirone and benzodiazepines), and valproate may have a role in treatment Emphasize nonmedication approaches

(continued)

Table 1 | Comorbidity and Other Features in Mania and How They Affect the Algorithm (*continued*)

Comorbid Conditions	Evidence considerations[a]	Recommendations
Treatment of women of childbearing potential and women who become pregnant during treatment.[26-31]	Valproate is by far the most teratogenic medication used in bipolar disorder;[32] high dose folate (4-5 mg daily) has been recommended[30] but may not necessarily lower this risk; valproate (but not lamotrigine) lowers intelligence scores in young children exposed to it in utero[33] Carbamazepine is associated with increased spina bifida and (late in pregnancy) vitamin K deficiencies Lithium has fewer malformation risks than valproate or carbamazepine, but Ebstein's abnormality occurs in up to 1 in 1000 pregnancies: a low absolute risk but up to x20 the base rate[34] Although the safety of antipsychotics in pregnancy has not been firmly established (due to many limitations in the studies), they seem relatively safe[29] The SGAs that cause weight gain appear to increase risk of gestational metabolic complications (e.g., diabetes and babies large for gestational age); olanzapine may be associated with low and high birth weight, and a small risk of malformation (e.g., hip dysplasia, meningocele, ankyloblepharon, and neural tube defects)	Avoid valproate in any woman with the potential to become pregnant: should the patient become pregnant, cessation of valproate may occur too late to prevent harm Avoid carbamazepine Lithium is preferred over valproate and carbamazepine Antipsychotics are first choice[26] ECT is a relatively safe and effective treatment during pregnancy if steps are taken to decrease potential risks[35,36] Prescribe as few drugs as possible—ideally, just one When pregnancy occurs during treatment, it is usually best to continue the current therapy to avoid exposure to multiple agents—except for valproate or carbamazepine, in which case switching is probably best Adjust doses as pregnancy progresses (blood volume expands 30% in third trimester); plasma-level monitoring is helpful Consider the risk of relapse or withdrawal when switching medications or changing doses Anticholinergic drugs should not be prescribed to pregnant women except for acute, short-term need Depot antipsychotics should not be routinely used in pregnancy (infants may show extrapyramidal symptoms for several months)

Table 1 | Comorbidity and Other Features in Mania and How They Affect the Algorithm (*continued*)

Comorbid Conditions	Evidence considerations[a]	Recommendations
Active substance use disorders	Substance use disorders occur in as many as 65% of bipolar patients[37] Active substance misuse is associated with poorer outcome with medication treatments, but data are very limited[38] One prospective study of patients with active alcoholism on valproate maintenance for bipolar disorder found efficacy for the alcohol use disorder but not for the mood disorder[39] Citicoline added to standard treatment for comorbid cocaine dependence in manic patients led to reduced substance misuse[40]	Abstinence from substance misuse is a high treatment priority (if possible) Valproate and citicoline may have value as add-on treatments for some patients to help with the substance use component; however, other options (e.g., naltrexone or acamprosate for alcohol use disorders) might be preferred
Cardiac disease or presence of QTc-prolonging drugs[41]	In a meta-analysis of 15 studies comparing 6 SGAs for their effect on QTc prolongation, only aripiprazole had significantly less effect than the others[41] A seventh SGA, quetiapine, had 5 relevant studies, but the manufacturer refused to provide authors with QTc data; in 2011, however, the quetiapine package insert was amended with new QTc-prolongation warnings and requirements for monitoring	Consider aripiprazole as the antipsychotic of choice if the risk of further QTc prolongation is a significant concern; haloperidol, quetiapine, and ziprasidone would be relatively undesirable in that situation Review the patient's medications for other QTc-prolonging agents, and monitor for risk factors for Torsade's (e.g., bradycardia and electrolyte abnormalities)
Other medical comorbidities	Whenever possible, offer bipolar medications that do not worsen the patients' medical problems Monitor the impact of whatever is prescribed	In the presence of hepatitis or liver cirrhosis: avoid when possible agents that are known to irritate the liver and to raise liver function tests, including quetiapine, olanzapine, valproate, and carbamazepine In the presence of renal filtration impairment: avoid lithium In the presence of obesity, hyperlipidemia, or metabolic syndrome: consider aripiprazole, asenapine, carbamazepine, and ziprasidone (plus, to manage depression, lamotrigine)

ECT, electroconvulsive therapy; IM, intramuscular; SGA, second-generation antipsychotic.

[a] The evidence for "agitation requiring rapid management" (first row) is mostly derived from studies on mixed populations of schizophrenic and manic patients.

NODE 2: DOES THIS MANIC PATIENT HAVE A MIXED PRESENTATION?

Increasing evidence suggests that the treatment of bipolar mania in a mixed or "dysphoric" episode has a different psychopharmacological treatment than "pure" mania.[42-44] The evidence is almost entirely derived from post hoc analyses of trials that included both manic and mixed patients; only two prospective, randomized trials have focused on the mixed/dysphoric population.[45,46] This evidence deficiency is unfortunate because up to 40% of acute bipolar mania patients are in a mixed episode.[47] Another problem is that the criteria for mixed mania have varied. In DSM-IV, the criteria required that patients meet full criteria for mania and for major depression. These criteria did not capture the complexity and extreme variability of the clinical picture and the rapid mood shifts that are seen.[48] In DSM-5, the diagnosis has expanded to include patients who meet full criteria for mania or *hypomania* and have three or more depressive symptoms, but even this expansion may still not include the full spectrum of the disorder. In the treatment analyses, the criteria shortcomings are often addressed by monitoring clinical change on different rating scales for depression and mania. The variability in measures used, however, makes it difficult to compare the study outcomes.[48]

Despite these limitations with the evidence base and its interpretation, several recent reviews have reached the conclusion that mixed episodes, though more difficult to treat, especially with monotherapies, respond best to atypical antipsychotics and valproate as first-line options.[42-44] Lithium and carbamazepine seem less effective but are reasonable second-line agents to be used in combination with other medications.

Node 2a: Mixed Episodes. First Recommendation: Quetiapine or Another Second-Generation Antipsychotic

Among the second-generation antipsychotics (SGAs), quetiapine is the preferred choice in this algorithm. In a meta-analysis by Cipriani and colleagues,[49] quetiapine, when compared to its peers in this class of medications, had average efficacy in treating acute mania (in six placebo-controlled trials at a usual effective dose of around 600 mg daily). However, it is unique among SGAs approved for treating mania in that it is also effective as monotherapy for treating[50] and preventing[51] future episodes of bipolar depression. Therefore, given the emphasis we place in this algorithm on choosing treatments that not only deal with the present symptoms but address future mood changes, quetiapine is the first-choice SGA. Mixed patients were included in a recent, large, placebo-controlled RCT with 308 patients at a mean dose of 600 mg daily employing quetiapine XR.[52] Improvement was significant ($p < .001$) after three weeks on the primary outcome measure, the Young Mania Rating Scale (YMRS), and on all secondary measures. Quetiapine was also recently studied in comparison to paliperidone and placebo in a 12-week trial in 493 manic or mixed patients.[53] It produced greater symptom improvement in depression than paliperidone and was comparable on manic symptoms. A recent, small, placebo-controlled, 8-week prospective trial of adjunctive quetiapine in 55 bipolar II mixed hypomania patients found significant improvement in the Clinical Global Impression and the Montgomery-Åsberg Depression Rating Scale (MADRS) but no difference from placebo in the YMRS.[46] Hypomania improved in both groups. Adding this set of new data, we think it reasonable to consider quetiapine to have advantages over other atypical antipsychotics for acute mixed mania. Some mixed patients, however, may need higher than average doses.[54]

Other antipsychotics could be considered if quetiapine is unsuitable because of metabolic side effects, QTc prolongation, or other risks associated with it. Two antipsychotics that should be mentioned right away are olanzapine and risperidone. They are often favored by clinicians, who perceive them as having strong efficacy in mania. Like most other SGAs, olanzapine and risperidone have FDA approval for both mixed and nonmixed mania. Overall, the two had somewhat larger effect sizes than quetiapine in Cipriani and colleagues' meta-analysis:[49] 0.43 standardized mean difference from placebo for olanzapine and 0.50 for risperidone, versus 0.37 for quetiapine. Close inspection of the data on response to olanzapine in mixed patients, however, reveals that the comparative efficacy is not that substantial. In one post hoc analysis of two large, pivotal RCTs, sleep and paranoia improved on olanzapine, but almost all symptoms related to depression did not.[55] Other, more positive reports in mixed populations had significant methodological limitations, making it impossible to be sure if olanzapine had clear antidepressant properties in these patients.[48,56]

Olanzapine did recently demonstrate statistically significant ($p < .04$) benefits as a monotherapy for bipolar depression in a large RCT (n = 514).[57] The two-point difference in MADRS scores at six weeks and the changes on individual core depressive items on the MADRS, however, seem clinically insignificant. The largest improvements, by far, were in the sleep and appetite items.

Another objection that can be raised regarding the initial use of olanzapine concerns its long-term side effects—an important positioning factor in this algorithm. Olanzapine has the highest risk among the atypical antipsychotics for weight gain and metabolic disorders, including (eventually) diabetes. Weight gain over one year in schizophrenia patients was almost twice as high as with quetiapine and risperidone, which are considered to have intermediate risk for weight gain.[58] Glucose dysregulation and insulin resistance occur early, even in the absence of weight gain, and place the patient at risk for later diabetes.[59] Many guidelines and algorithms for treating schizophrenia, including the PAPHSS algorithm, do not find olanzapine appropriate for first-line use in that disorder.[3] In mania, the Texas Medication Algorithm Project separated olanzapine from the first-line options for all mania patients (euphoric and mixed).[60] The World Federation of Societies of Biological Psychiatry guidelines declared in 2009 that olanzapine is "not to be used first" in mania, because of the risks.[61]

In mania studies, limited attention has focused on risperidone's efficacy for mixed patients. No adequate evaluation has been done,[43,48] and no studies have been published for bipolar depression. Hence, risperidone does not seem to be a good candidate for initial use in mixed mania despite its FDA approval.

In summary, on the issue of ability to deal with mixed mania and bipolar depression, quetiapine's evidence seems superior to that of olanzapine or risperidone.

A second choice for an SGA might be ziprasidone. In a post hoc analysis of 179 dysphoric manic patients pooled from two ziprasidone mania studies, the patients' manic and also depressive symptoms showed significant improvement.[62] Ziprasidone was not found effective for bipolar depression, however, in two recent placebo-controlled RCTs.[63] The authors proposed that methodological weaknesses may have limited the ability to detect a difference in the treatments.

Aripiprazole deserves some consideration, again according to post hoc analysis of data in mixed patients.[64] It also has had two failed trials, however, in bipolar depression.[65]

Further discussion of alternative antipsychotics for acute mania will be found at Node 3, when quetiapine is again preferred for nonmixed patients.

Clinicians are advised to have a detailed discussion with their manic patients about the risks and benefits of the medications under consideration, as discussed here, and also of any other medications relevant to the individual case. This discussion should include mention of which medications are FDA approved and which are off-label, and why medications that are not FDA approved might be recommended. This discussion should be documented in the record.

Node 2b: What If the Response to Quetiapine (or to Another SGA, If Used) Is Unsatisfactory? Recommendation: Add Valproate

As noted earlier, reviewers have concluded that mixed mania will often require combination therapy of an antipsychotic with a mood stabilizer. The mood stabilizer with the best evidence is valproate. In a retrospective analysis of 145 patients, Zarate and colleagues[66] noted that the combination of quetiapine and valproate seemed particularly effective in mixed states. In a subsequent placebo-controlled RCT, divalproex monotherapy was used to treat 364 patients, 44% of whom had a mixed syndrome.[67] The dose averaged 3350 mg daily. Results were positive, though not robustly, and outcomes seemed comparable in the mixed and nonmixed patients. Studies in which antipsychotics (including haloperidol, olanzapine, and risperidone) were added after initial unsatisfactory response to valproate have generally shown positive results from the combination compared to adding placebo.[43] Taken together, these studies appear to provide support for recommending valproate as an augmentation strategy to the antipsychotic in mixed mania.

Nevertheless, the preference in this algorithm is to use the fewest medications that are necessary. Valproate has many side effects, and it certainly should be avoided in women of childbearing potential (see Table 1). Almost all of the studies of combination treatment in mania that have found superior results with the combination versus placebo have started with patients who were on the first medication for two weeks or more and had not responded to it.[8] Patients who had started on a monotherapy and done well on it would not have entered those studies. Therefore, it is reasonable to give the first medication at least a few days in the inpatient setting (and longer for outpatients under good supervision) to see if a trend toward effectiveness begins on monotherapy.

It is important to keep in mind that most studies of medications for treating mania measure outcome at three weeks or more. Typical results with antipsychotics are that improvement (as indicated by, for example, a 50% drop in the YMRS) occurs in about 50% of patients by that time.[68,69] With placebo, a typical result is that 30% of patients improve in three weeks. Remissions require much more time. Thus, substantial improvement in the first few days of treatment on an inpatient unit is usually due to a combination of the antimanic medication starting to work and (more importantly) the effect of the supportive milieu, psychotherapy, and any nonspecific sedatives that are administered in the early days (see Table 1). The clinician should use these other resources liberally, rather than adding unnecessary antimanic medications (or rushing to high doses), since no evidence suggests that these extra measures speed improvement in the core disorder. In a recent RCT of intramuscular sedative treatments for 100 agitated patients in an emergency room setting (36 of whom were manic), haloperidol 2.5 mg plus the benzodiazepine midazolam 7.5 mg had the best outcome with the fewest side effects at all time points (30, 60, and 90 minutes).[22] The other options were haloperidol plus promethazine 25 mg (which produced less sedation and almost four times more extrapyramidal reactions), olanzapine 10 mg (which had 1.6 times more side effects than haloperidol plus midazolam), and ziprasidone 10 mg (which had low sedative effectiveness). It should be noted that intramuscular olanzapine should not be combined with benzodiazepines, due to the increased risk of respiratory depression.[70] Benzodiazepines also present some risk of complicating the mania with delirium. After stopping any anticholinergic agents, electroconvulsive therapy (ECT) may be helpful in that situation.[24] Clinicians should be cognizant of the risk of tardive dyskinesia with the long-term use of any typical neuroleptic, such as haloperidol, for mania. Mood-disordered patients have a higher risk of this side effect from neuroleptics.[71]

It is routine to add an oral benzodiazepine such as lorazepam or clonazepam to antipsychotics for additional short-term sedation as an alternative to increasing the dose of the primary antimanic agent(s).[8,15] The evidence supporting this practice with mania patients, however, is sparse.[21] Busch and colleagues[72] found in a retrospective study (n = 30) that adding a benzodiazepine (average dose = 1.6 mg/day of lorazepam equivalents) to a moderate dose of neuroleptic (300 mg of chlorpromazine equivalents) led to fewer seclusions and restraints in manic patients.

Carbamazepine also could be considered, instead of valproate, as a potential addition to the antipsychotic at this node. Although it did not perform as well in mixed as in nonmixed patients in the pivotal studies leading for FDA approval for acute mania, it seemed to be of some benefit, especially by the third week of treatment.[43]

Node 2c: What If the Response to Antipsychotic Plus Anticonvulsant Is Unsatisfactory? Recommendation: Add Lithium

Though, as noted earlier, the results with lithium in mixed states are generally regarded as disappointing, the data are sparse.[43] Lithium is a well-established antimanic treatment (see more detailed review of lithium in Node 2d), and it has been suggested that it not be eliminated from consideration in the population with mixed symptoms.[44] Another factor is that mixed-episode patients have increased suicidality and are more likely to have future mixed states than other patients,[42] and data have shown that lithium can be effective for preventing suicidal behavior even when it is not effective for preventing affective episodes.[73] Therefore, the recommendation is to add lithium at this point if the patient is still manic.

Node 2d: For Most Other Manic Patients Who Are Not Mixed: Recommendation Is to Initiate Lithium

In a 2004 review of 101 studies of medications for bipolar disorder,[74] only lithium was found to be effective in treating acute mania, in preventing recurrences of mania, and also in treating and preventing recurrences of bipolar depression.[74] Other recent studies and analyses confirm and extend these conclusions, and add that none of the atypical antipsychotics, despite some having FDA approval for use in maintenance, has convincing evidence of efficacy for that purpose.[75,76] Ghaemi[75] and Goodwin and colleagues[76] argue that the flaw in the methodology of all the maintenance studies of SGAs is that they start with preselected acute responders to the SGA being tested for maintenance. This "enriched" population of responders is then randomly assigned to either stay on the SGA or switch (often abruptly) to placebo or an active comparator (e.g., lithium). It is argued that this research design is not a test of maintenance but, instead, a demonstration of withdrawal effects.

Lithium may also be the only medication for bipolar disorder with evidence of ability to reduce the risk of suicide and suicide attempts.[77-79] As noted, its antisuicidal effect appears distinct from its mood-stabilizing properties.[80] However, the STEP-BD study did not confirm that lithium had an antisuicidal effect, but the lack of confirmation may reflect the patient sample, which had a low risk of suicide.[81] Lithium's neuroprotective effects also seem unique. Excellent lithium responders (about one-third of lithium-treated patients) appear to have preserved, in contrast to other lithium-treated patients (who had results comparable to non-bipolar controls), spatial working memory, sustained attention on long-term maintenance, and higher plasma levels of brain-derived neurotrophic factor.[82] Growing neuroimaging evidence suggests that lithium, but not valproate, increases cortical gray matter and maintains hippocampal volume compared to patients not treated[83,84] (who seem to suffer from hippocampal volume loss related to the illness). Lithium also normalizes concentrations of N-acetyl aspartate in prefrontal cerebral cortex, which is a proposed marker of neuronal activity in bipolar patients.[85-87] Antipsychotics, by contrast, reduce cortical gray matter and glial cell volume by as much as 20% more than in controls, in studies performed in Macaque monkeys.[88,89] Observations in humans also strongly suggest similar harms, at least in patients diagnosed with schizophrenia.[90]

Unfortunately, cognitive impairment associated with bipolar disorder can persist despite lithium in some patients.[91]

Further support for choosing lithium first comes from a multivariate modeling study of a community sample of bipolar patients. Baldessarini and colleagues[92] found that patients receiving lithium as monotherapy were less likely to need any alterations of their drug regimens during the following year when compared to patients receiving anticonvulsants (e.g., valproate), antipsychotics, or antidepressants. Also, in a large (n = 4268) observational cohort study from Denmark, the rate of patients needing switches or additions of psychotropic medication was much greater when on valproate than on lithium (hazard ratio = 1.86).[93] Admissions were also greater when on valproate, both for mania and depression.

Good evidence supports the short-term efficacy of lithium in cases of acute mania with moderate psychotic symptoms.[71] One study compared response to lithium versus valproate in four subtypes of mania (anxious-depressive, psychotic, classic, and irritable-dysphoric subtypes). In the psychotic type, lithium was significantly more likely to lower mania ratings by 50%.[94,95]

Based on the results of one early, heavily promoted comparison with valproate,[96] some have argued that lithium is not first-line for mania when the patient has a history of rapid cycling. A subsequent meta-analysis of studies involving 905 rapid-cycling patients found no disadvantage for lithium.[97] One observational study of 360 bipolar patients found no difference in lithium response in the rapid versus the non-rapid cyclers.[98] Controlled maintenance studies also showed no advantage of valproate over lithium for rapid cyclers.[99] Two other studies compared lithium to valproate and found no significant difference between them except for more adverse events with valproate.[100,101]

Lithium use may result, however, both in marked increases in rates of suicidal behavior and in early recurrences of bipolar episodes following abrupt or rapid (less than two weeks) discontinuation.[102,103] Clinicians need to initiate an ongoing discussion with patients on the importance of adherence and on the risks associated with sudden interruptions of all long-term psychotropic drug treatments (but especially lithium), and be available to offer treatment alternatives should patients find lithium to be intolerable.[104]

In summary, lithium appears to have strong support for being the first-line treatment for acute nonmixed mania with or without mild to moderate psychosis. Patient and physician biases against it need to be addressed.[75]

Because of its narrow therapeutic index, trough serum concentrations of lithium should be closely monitored. The British National Institute for Health and Clinical Excellence guidelines (2006) recommend that levels be taken seven days after initiation and then seven days after every dose or formulation change and the introduction or discontinuation of interacting medications.[7] Levels should be taken 12 hours after the last dose. Treatment of acute mania may require lithium levels of 0.8 mEq/L or more, but the suggested optimal target maintenance level for preventing recurrences of manic or depressive episodes is 0.60-0.75 mEq/L.[2,105]

Other possible first-line pharmacotherapeutic agents for treating a first episode of mania with or without moderate psychosis include valproate, SGAs, and carbamazepine. We will comment further on each of these.

Valproate Valproate in its various forms (e.g., divalproex) is chosen by many clinicians as an initial treatment for acute mania. Examination of a forest plot of valproate efficacy, however, indicates that in the four subsequent placebo-controlled RCTs since the first large trial in 1994 that led to FDA approval, the effect size has been progressively diminishing.[106] In the last two RCTs, one in adolescents[107] and one in adults,[108] VPA produced no better results than placebo. In Cipriani and colleagues' meta-analysis of antimanic agents,[49] the effect size of valproate was only –0.16, which barely met statistical significance. Moreover, valproate has not been found efficacious for maintenance treatment of either mania or depression[109] and does not have FDA approval for maintenance of bipolar disorders. Consequently, valproate does not seem to be an appropriate first-line option in this evidence-focused algorithm for nonmixed mania, even though clinical experience and results in trials not involving placebo seem to support its value. It was proposed as a reasonable choice for mixed mania in Node 2b and will be proposed as an option in subsequent nodes.

Second-Generation Antipsychotics   As noted earlier, most SGAs have been found effective for acute mania, and most are FDA approved for this indication (and for mixed mania).[49] We have noted that of these, only quetiapine has been found effective and is FDA approved as a monotherapy for acute depression in bipolar disorder. Some evidence suggests, moreover, that quetiapine monotherapy can prevent future episodes of depression.[51] For these reasons, and because of the importance we place on prevention, quetiapine may be seen as competing with lithium as a first-line treatment for acute mania. That said, the quality of the Nolen and Weisler maintenance study,[110] like others done with SGAs, is suspect. In that study, which compared quetiapine with lithium and placebo for maintenance, all patients were initial quetiapine responders. They were randomized to either stay on quetiapine or switch to lithium or placebo. Given that the patients were not known to be responders to lithium, the fact that lithium did as well as quetiapine (with both better than placebo) for maintenance seems to be a more impressive result for lithium than for quetiapine. Indeed, in a recent post hoc analysis of data from that study, patients did even better on lithium maintenance, compared to the lithium group as a whole, if levels were a more adequate 0.6 mEq/L or greater. The FDA has not approved quetiapine as a monotherapy maintenance treatment for bipolar disorder. It has approved quetiapine as an adjunctive maintenance therapy when added to another mood stabilizer, because of other data.[111]

Adverse effects are significant with both lithium and quetiapine, but since the publication of our previous, 2010 analysis of their comparative risks,[2] QTc prolongation has been identified as a potential new risk with quetiapine. A manufacturer's package-insert warning in July 2011 cautioned against combining quetiapine with 12 other cardiac depressants and emphasized the need for clinical monitoring for cardiac safety. Furthermore, a recent meta-analysis of 77 studies concluded that the side effects of lithium are generally moderate and appear acceptable when compared to the risks of antipsychotics.[112,113] Short-term weight gain, for example, was three times greater with quetiapine compared to lithium in one head-to-head trial in mania.[114] Lithium also causes less weight gain than valproate.[96] In the CAFE study of early psychosis, quetiapine was second only to olanzapine for weight gain and metabolic morbidity,[115] as discussed further in Node 4. Renal disease, however, is a major concern with lithium. The number needed to harm for severe renal damage associated with lithium was approximately 300, with an estimated absolute placebo-adjusted risk of about 3.3/1000 treated cases.[116]

Carbamazepine Carbamazepine is effective in mania,[49,117] with recent FDA approval for acute mania and mixed states of a new slow-release formulation. It has many drug interactions, however; due to the induction of several oxidative and glucuronidation enzymes, it increases the clearance of many other agents. It also induces its own metabolism, which produces falling serum concentrations and creates difficulties in adjusting dose. Other adverse effects include hyponatremia, liver toxicity, teratogenesis (e.g., neural tube defects), and blood dyscrasias. The evidence supporting its effectiveness for treating or preventing bipolar depression comes only from uncontrolled studies.

NODE 3: WHAT IF THE RESPONSE TO LITHIUM IN ACUTE NONMIXED MANIA IS UNSATISFACTORY? RECOMMENDATION: ADD QUETIAPINE OR ANOTHER SGA

If the results are unsatisfactory with lithium, the next option would be to introduce an SGA. This might be done quickly in some cases, as discussed in Node 2b (regarding the addition of a mood-stabilizing anticonvulsant to the initial SGA for mixed patients). Moreover, as discussed in Node 2d, quetiapine comes closest to lithium in possessing a broad mood-stabilizing capacity, though it was argued that the evidence regarding quetiapine is less convincing than that for lithium. In Node 2a, we also discussed the reasons for preferring quetiapine, instead of other SGAs, such as olanzapine and risperidone, that have somewhat greater potency in managing acute mania. In summary, it was noted there that quetiapine is reasonably effective in acute mania if used at adequate doses of 600 mg daily, and that the slightly superior efficacy of the others may not be visible to clinicians in the acute inpatient setting because of the confounding effect of the other concomitant treatments, including therapeutic containment, psychotherapy, IM "chemical restraints," and sedating oral adjunctive medications such as benzodiazepines. In the case of olanzapine, important acute (e.g., insulin resistance) and long-term (metabolic syndrome) side effects render it undesirable for first-line use in mania. According to several meta-analyses, however, risperidone has the numerically largest effect size of the SGAs in acute mania and has a more acceptable side-effect profile than olanzapine.[49,106,118] Hence, risperidone is a reasonable option at this node instead of quetiapine if the prescriber prefers to focus on initial efficacy without worrying about long-term maintenance—which in some manic patients may be less critical. First-generation neuroleptics such as haloperidol (though not FDA approved) are also highly effective for acute mania and may even work faster than any SGAs.[49,119] They are generally unacceptable, however, because of a high risk of inducing neuroleptic dysphoria or depression and because of the greater risk of tardive dyskinesia in bipolar patients.[120,121]

Quetiapine has evidence of efficacy versus placebo when added to lithium for acute treatment of mania (after at least two weeks of unsatisfactory response to lithium), and it helps to prevent future episodes.[111,122]

Some clinicians might consider adding valproate rather than an antipsychotic to lithium. We reviewed in Node 2d the evidence that valproate seems less effective than previously assumed. The recent "game changing" 2010 BALANCE study should also be noted. In comparing the results over two years of combining valproate and lithium versus using either treatment alone, the combination showed very little additional benefit compared to lithium alone.[109] Hence, valproate is not recommended as the first-line addition after unsatisfactory results with lithium.

NODE 4: HAS THE RESPONSE TO LITHIUM AND QUETIAPINE BEEN UNSATISFACTORY? RECOMMENDATION: CHANGE QUETIAPINE TO A DIFFERENT SGA. CONSIDER AN ANTICONVULSANT MOOD STABILIZER

Having utilized without success lithium and quetiapine, the two agents with the broadest spectrum of efficacy in bipolar disorder, we would now give greater consideration to the options that seem to have efficacy limited to acute mania. These options include the anticonvulsants valproate and carbamazepine as well as other SGAs. Other anticonvulsants, including gabapentin, lamotrigine, levetiracetam, and topiramate, have little or no apparent efficacy in the manic phase of bipolar disorder, and oxcarbazepine remains inadequately evaluated.[49] First-generation antipsychotics are still not desirable because they increase risk of tardive dyskinesia, to which bipolar patients are highly susceptible, and they may increase the risk of bipolar depression.[30] ECT is a consideration addressed below.

When introducing a Node 4 medication, eliminate any current medication that has been considered ineffective, although such medication might be retained if it has demonstrated efficacy for preventing future episodes of mania or bipolar depression.

A switch to one of the SGAs that is more effective in mania is the first recommended option. Since this manic episode can now be characterized as treatment resistant, the priority becomes the termination of the episode. Risperidone, if not already tried, and olanzapine are SGAs with larger effect sizes in the meta-analyses and are the best options here. It is unfortunate that no randomized trials have evaluated whether, after failure on an adequate trial of one SGA for acute mania (e.g., quetiapine), switching to another SGA would produce a different outcome. The best evidence we have are the comparative trials in non-treatment-resistant cases, which suggest a hierarchy of acute efficacy in which risperidone and olanzapine are the leaders among the SGAs.[49]

Risperidone was approved for treatment of acute mania in the United States in 2003. The dose range that has proved effective in reducing YMRS scores more than placebo is 1-6 mg daily.[123] In one study, remission rates (defined as a sustained YMRS score <8 for three weeks) at 10 months were 42% for risperidone and 13% for placebo.[123] A 2006 Cochrane review found equal efficacy in psychotic and non- psychotic mania.[124] In that analysis, risperidone was equally sedating as olanzapine, produced more extrapyramidal and sexual side effects, but resulted in less weight gain.

Olanzapine was approved in the United States in 2000. The usually effective doses ranged between 5 and 20 mg, with three-week improvement rates in pooled analysis averaging 55% versus 30% with placebo. Three-week remission rates were 18% versus 7%, respectively.[68] These findings illustrate the point made earlier that one cannot expect re-mission in three-week trials in acute mania, even from the most effective antimanic med-ications. It takes many weeks or sometimes months. If patients improve sooner than that, the credit probably should be shared with the other treatments offered in the therapeutic environment of the hospital. For further perspective on olanzapine, it is worth noting a new three-week, placebo-controlled RCT comparing olanzapine and lithium for acute ma-nia in 40 women from Iran. Mania scores on the Manic State Rating Scale were reduced 20.3 points on lithium at a mean blood level of 0.8 meq/L versus 7.6 points on olanzapine at a mean dose of 20.5 mg daily (p = .0002 favoring lithium).[125] In the two other com-parisons of these agents, olanzapine was superior in one, and no efficacy difference was found in the other.[49]

Other options that could be considered at this node include the anticonvulsant mood stabilizers. Valproate was reviewed as an option in Node 2d, and we noted the marginal or negative results in recent RCTs in adolescents and adults with acute mania.[107,108] In their recent study of valproate in adults, Hirschfeld and colleagues[108] proposed that the problem could have been use of a "moderate" dose of 2200 mg daily. In their previous, modestly positive study, they had used a mean dose of 3350 mg daily.[67] In the earlier study, how-ever, the side effects of somnolence, nausea, vomiting, and dizziness were much more common. Also, the authors noted that the protocol of the later study encouraged earlier hospital discharge, which may have affected outcomes. The later study also allowed longer use of adjunctive lorazepam, which may have decreased the drug/placebo differences. Pres-sure for shorter hospital stays are a reality today, however, and, as noted, experts encourage liberal use of adjunctive benzodiazepines. Thus, some of the conditions that may poten-tially explain valproate's lack of efficacy in the study by Hirschfeld and colleagues are likely to be present in typical hospital practice.

Other reasons for postponing valproate include the results of the BALANCE study.[109] The large (n = 330), open-label, two-year maintenance RCT found that valproate was far less effective than lithium and that it added little to lithium in combination therapy. In conjunction with the unimpressive data on acute efficacy (see discussion under Node 2d), this important study reduces the preference for valproate in this algorithm, in which main-tenance is a central priority. Similar results favoring lithium over valproate were reported in an observational cohort study, cited earlier, from a Danish registry of bipolar patients.[93] Another matter of concern is that valproate use has been associated with neurotoxicity when used in patients with dementia, in whom it accelerated brain volume loss over one year of treatment and did not, when compared to placebo, reduce behavioral dysregula-tion, agitation, or psychosis.[126,127] This risk of neurotoxicity contrasts with lithium, which, as mentioned earlier, demonstrates a neuro- protective effect in a variety of neurological conditions, though lithium carries its own risk of neurotoxicity, including delirium in the elderly. Finally as noted in Table 1, valproate is a medication of last choice in women of childbearing potential because of severe teratogenicity and impairment of subsequent cog-nitive ability in exposed fetuses.

Despite these negative considerations, the initial trials of valproate in mania were strongly positive, leading to FDA approval.[96,128,129] There is evidence that valproate may be

effective in a different set of bipolar patients than lithium: one analysis concluded that valproate was sometimes more effective than lithium in treating acute mania with dysphoria,
irritability, impulsivity, and hostility.[94] Many clinicians who use it regularly today have experiences convincing them that it is effective in a variety of patients and has an acceptable
margin of safety. Valproate also might be effective in acute bipolar depression. Three small
published RCTs were positive (total n = 142), but publication bias may have affected the
results; larger studies are needed before conclusions can be drawn.[130] Nevertheless, these
positive considerations suggest that valproate is a possible choice at Node 4, following the
failure of lithium and quetiapine or the unacceptability of the better SGA options because
of the patient's side-effect vulnerabilities.

Additional safety concerns with valproate not mentioned previously include liver
toxicity, drug interactions (e.g., with lamotrigine), and masculinizing effects in young
women.[131] In one report, triglycerides were severely elevated when valproate was added to
quetiapine.[132] Potential explanations include cytochrome P450 isoenzyme 3A4 inhibition
by valproate, protein binding displacement, or a pharmacodynamic effect. Systematic
research is needed to elucidate the frequency and causes of this interaction between two
medications that are commonly combined.

Nutritional deficits induced by valproate might have a role in the outcome of mania
treatment. In one study, folic acid given with valproate resulted in significantly greater reductions of mania symptom ratings than valproate alone, specifically in areas of language
disorder, thought content, and disruptive-aggressive behavior.[133]

According to the British National Institute for Health and Clinical Excellence guidelines, serum concentrations of valproate should be monitored only if toxicity, lack of
response, or poor adherence is suspected.[7] No clear-cut therapeutic range has been established, and expert opinion indicates that the therapeutic index for valproate, compared to
lithium, is fairly wide. It has been suggested that plasma levels for acute mania fall in the
range of 50 to 125 ng/mL.[15]

Carbamazepine is an option again here, as it was in node 3. It is more frequently prescribed than valproate in Japan (where Okuma carried out important early clinical trials of
this agent for bipolar disorder) and in regions of Europe. In the United States, clinicians
use it much less often than valproate because of the safety and dosing issues noted earlier
and also, one suspects, because of the aggressive marketing of valproate in the decade after
FDA approval. The relatively low risk of weight gain with carbamazepine compared to
other options[134] can be an advantage.

If the patient is medically unstable or needs rapid relief of mania-related psychosis or
delirium, ECT can be considered here or earlier in the algorithm. Also consider ECT for
women in their first month of pregnancy, when organogenesis is taking place and the risk
of teratogenicity is highest. The evidence for ECT's effectiveness in treating mania is not
secure, however, due to difficulties in conducting trials with appropriate randomization and
blinding, and in obtaining informed consent from some patients, including those with possibly compromised legal competence. A recent review of the evidence for ECT in treating
mania concluded that no study is consistently adequate methodologically.[135] Nevertheless,
one prospective study found ECT to be more effective than lithium in the first eight weeks
of treatment of acute mania.[136] Other studies are mostly retrospective analyses, finding

that ECT treatment for mania was as effective as lithium or chlorpromazine (the only first-generation antipsychotic that is FDA approved for treating mania, though we do not recommend it, because of safety issues related to alpha blockade and hypotension).[137,138]

NODE 5: WHAT IF THREE RECOMMENDED TREATMENTS FOR EITHER BIPOLAR MIXED OR NONMIXED MANIC PATIENTS HAVE BEEN INEFFECTIVE OR ONLY PARTIALLY EFFECTIVE? RECOMMENDATION: MANY OPTIONS

Three tiers of options are proposed, based on the quantity of supporting evidence for their efficacy in less treatment-resistant patients. The first tier of options includes the high-efficacy SGAs (e.g., olanzapine or risperidone if not already tried) and the anticonvulsants valproate and carbamazepine. The merits and drawbacks of all these options have already been reviewed. Haloperidol could also be considered because of its very strong efficacy.[49] Second-tier agents for consideration at Node 5 include aripiprazole, asenapine, and ziprasidone. Clozapine could be a third-tier choice, though it has multiple, and potentially severe, adverse effects.

As indicated in Figure 1, the flowchart of this algorithm, it is suggested at this point that any medications that appear to be ineffective be stopped before adding new ones. The idea here is to avoid unnecessary accumulated side effects, which is one of the key goals and priorities for algorithm sequencing. While discontinuing such medications would appear to be a reasonable principle of conservative practice, no good evidence actually shows that one can remove an apparently ineffective medication during treatment of acute mania without any impact on the effectiveness of what will be added. Indeed, as noted earlier, in the design of just about all the studies of adding new medications, the previous ineffective medication is continued, and either the new one or a control medication (or none) is added.[139] Hence, here at Node 5, if you have discontinued a medication before adding another medication that does not then produce satisfactory results or that causes further decompensation, you could consider resuming the discontinued medication to see if that could be helpful.

It is recommended to avoid combining two antipsychotics (other than during crossover from one to another), due to both the lack of any evidence of added efficacy and the increased risk of side effects, including metabolic syndrome, extrapyramidal symptoms, hyperprolactinemia, sexual dysfunction, sedation/somnolence, cognitive impairment, diabetes, and tardive dyskinesia.[140] We provide below additional discussion of some of these agents as monotherapies and in combination with lithium and anticonvulsants—if they were not reviewed in sufficient detail before.

Carbamazepine

In 2004, the FDA approved the extended-release form of carbamazepine for treating acute mania. As discussed under Node 4, the efficacy of carbamazepine as an antimanic agent is established, with doses of the recently introduced long- acting formulation ranging from

600 to 1600 mg daily. In a review of RCTs comparing carbamazepine and lithium, and combining results in meta-analyses when possible, the two were similar in efficacy for acute mania as well as in safety and the ability to prevent relapses.[141] Notably, carbamazepine is not FDA approved for long-term use, and the review found that in maintenance studies, carbamazepine patients were more likely than patients on lithium to withdraw from the studies due to adverse effects.[141] Patients with rapid cycling might benefit from adding carbamazepine to lithium: in one study, the long-term response was better with the combination than with either of the medications alone (28% response with lithium, 19% with carbamazepine, and 56% with the combination).[142] A similar study found better results with the combination but more side effects and increased need for additional adjunctive medications.[143] For acute mania with prominent agitation, the combination might also be more helpful than monotherapy with an antipsychotic;[144] in one study, adding carbamazepine to lithium produced benefits comparable to those from adding haloperidol to lithium.[145]

Aripiprazole

The use of aripiprazole for treating acute mania was approved by the FDA in 2004. Compared to other SGAs, aripiprazole has a more benign side-effect profile regarding weight gain, cardiac and metabolic effects, and some extrapyramidal symptoms, although it frequently causes akathisia and, because of its partial dopamine-agonist effect, may worsen Parkinson's disease. The evidence regarding its efficacy in acute mania is less strong than for other SGAs, and in several published studies it failed to outperform placebo.[106,146,147] Aripiprazole can be added to lithium or valproate, and such combinations have yielded superior response and remission rates among outpatients than with either agent alone.[148] Although approved in the United States for maintenance treatment of bipolar disorder, most of the support for that indication is based on a single, relatively brief (six-month) study that showed benefits only for preventing mania and not for the more common depressive episodes of the illness.[149] Only 12% of the patients continued to take aripiprazole for the full six months, suggesting a lack of patient acceptability.[149]

Ziprasidone

The use of ziprasidone for treating acute mania was approved by the FDA in 2004. Two RCTs compared ziprasidone to placebo for acute mania and found significantly better response with this SGA than with placebo.[150,151] One RCT for acute mania compared ziprasidone to haloperidol; the latter produced higher rates of response and remission (54.7% vs. 36.9%, and 31.9% vs. 22.7%, respectively).[152] Inferior results with ziprasidone in comparison to other antipsychotics (its effect size was only –0.20 in Cipriani and colleagues' meta-analysis),[49] which also can be seen in studies of patients with schizophrenia, may in part be due to suboptimal dosing, the requirement for taking it with 500 kcal meals, and (for outpatients) problems complying with twice-daily administration. A recent study failed to find any effectiveness for ziprasidone as an add-on to lithium or valproate in acute mania, but methodological problems were offered to explain this finding.[153,154] On the positive side for ziprasidone, it may not only cause less weight gain in obese patients but produce better mania outcomes when added to the existing regimens of such patients.[155] Also, a recent six-week RCT in acute bipolar mixed depression at a dose of 130 mg daily found significant benefit (p = .004) in depression scores.[156] These patients were not manic, but the study suggests a role for ziprasidone in preventing depressive episodes.

Asenapine

The use of asenapine as a treatment for acute mania was approved by the FDA in 2009 and as an adjunctive treatment to augment lithium or valproate in 2012. As an adjunctive treatment for acute mania, asenapine performed no better than placebo on all primary outcome measures at week 3 but did separate at week 12.[157] Two placebo-controlled RCTs of asenapine monotherapy are also available. In one study, it was significantly superior to placebo, but not to olanzapine, in reducing YMRS mania symptom ratings, and in the other, it was not more effective than placebo in either response or remission rates.[158-161] Asenapine is administered twice daily as sublingual tablets, which may not be as simple to use as ordinary oral preparations. It has a favorable side-effect profile, however, with respect to weight gain, metabolic problems, extrapyramidal symptoms, prolactin elevation, and cardiovascular toxicity.

Clozapine

Clozapine is not approved in the United States for bipolar disorder but is sometimes used off-label to manage treatment-resistant mania. No RCTs of clozapine in mania have been published, but uncontrolled clinical trials suggest that clozapine might be a reasonable option for patients at node 5 and beyond.[162-165]

NODE 6: WHAT IF ALL THE ABOVE AGENTS HAVE NOT BEEN EFFECTIVE?

It seems unlikely that a patient could reach this point and still remain in a manic state if the diagnosis is correct and if the algorithm has been followed rigorously with adequate trials. Certainly, a reconsideration of diagnosis is appropriate. Indeed, diagnostic reconsideration should actually occur after every step of this and any other algorithm when the response is unsatisfactory and no clear explanation is apparent. For example, there might be some unidentified organic cause, or strong psychosocial stresses could be preventing the mood disorder from stabilizing. Nevertheless, it is possible that unexpected positive results could occur with further adjustment of medications. It is suggested that the clinician review the options offered in Node 5 and consider picking another from those.

We would also note here some experimental approaches to mania treatment that have been reported. Selected examples are listed in Table 2, but we have no particular recommendations regarding when or whether any should be tried in preference to the more established treatments.

Table 2	New and Experimental Treatments Proposed for Acute Mania		
Medication	**Action**	**Comments**
Gabapentin	Antiepileptic	No evidence for efficacy as a primary or secondary treatment despite numerous trials and widespread use in the past[166]
Levetiracetam	Antiepileptic	No RCTs in mania May be helpful when added to haloperidol[167] No added benefit when combined with valproate[168]
Oxcarbazepine	Antiepileptic	One RCT as monotherapy with response rate 42% vs. placebo 26%; no data on remission rates[169] As adjunct to lithium in 52 patients, more effective and better tolerated than carbamazepine[170] A Cochrane review found that the trials were insufficient to make a recommendation[171]
Topiramate	Antiepileptic	Multiple RCTs failed to find any efficacy in acute mania as primary or secondary agent[49,172,173] May help patients on olanzapine (and perhaps other SGAs) lose some weight[174]
Amisulpride[a]	Antipsychotic	In an RCT, when added to valproate, had results comparable to haloperidol + valproate; haloperidol + valproate had more side effects[175]
Paliperidone	Antipsychotic	Metabolite of risperidone Has been tested and found effective for mania in two RCTs[13] Surprisingly, not effective when used as an adjunct to lithium[176] Has no significant advantages over generic risperidone
Allopurinol	Hypouricemic agent	Three placebo-controlled RCTs as adjunct to lithium; more improvement on allopurinol at doses of 600 mg daily; well-tolerated[177-179] May work better if patients abstain from caffeine[178]
Aspirin	Nonsteroidal anti-inflammatory agent	Netherlands database showed that low-dose aspirin (up to 80 mg daily) is associated with 17% reduction of risk of relapse on maintenance lithium[180]
Omega-3 fatty acids (e.g., in fish oils)	Lipid supplement	A Cochrane review of 5 RCTs found some positive results for bipolar depression but not for mania[181] A more recent study was negative[182] May possibly help prevent depression
Tamoxifen	Estrogen receptor modulator and protein kinase C inhibitor	Two RCTs with placebo controls and some pilot studies support effectiveness in mania at doses of 20 to 80 mg daily[117,183-186] Has been used as monotherapy and as adjunct to lithium No information about its role in depression or in maintenance treatment
Transcranial magnetic stimulation		Though it may be more promising for bipolar depression, some emerging data support its use for bipolar mania[187]

RCT, randomized, controlled trial; SGA, second-generation antipsychotic.
[a]Not available in the United States.

COMPARISON WITH OTHER GUIDELINE AND ALGORITHM RECOMMENDATIONS

This algorithm for selecting psychopharmacological treatment for acute mania is in accord with most features of other recently published guidelines and algorithms. There are also various points of disagreement, however, in part because the current algorithm incorporates the results of studies not available earlier. For example, we concluded that olanzapine is not a first-line treatment for acute mania—which is in agreement with some guidelines but not others. One unique difference in this algorithm is the de-emphasis on valproate as an option, due to the newer evidence suggesting inferior efficacy. Table 3 summarizes four guidelines and algorithms published by different groups in recent years. We have noted some points of contrast between their recommendations and ours.

Table 3 | Comparison of Present Algorithm to Other Recent Algorithms and Guidelines for Acute Mania			
Algorithm/guideline	*Year*	*Other algorithms/guidelines*	*Present algorithm*
Canadian Network for Mood and Anxiety Treatments guidelines for managing patients with bipolar disorders, as updated in collaboration with International Society for Bipolar Disorders[188]	2013	No distinction in early nodes between different subtypes of bipolar mania No preference is given among the first-line agents; SGAs, valproate, lithium, or their combinations can be first-line	Makes this distinction early in the algorithm and accordingly suggests narrower, subtype-specific treatment options Suggests starting with a monotherapy trial Gives priority to lithium in nonmixed mania and to quetiapine in mixed mania
British Association for Psychopharmacology evidence-based guidelines for treating bipolar disorder, revised second edition[189]	2009	Has different treatment suggestions depending on the level of severity Makes the assumption that in severe mania, lithium is not a first-line agent Suggests the use of SGAs Lists valproate as a first-line agent in severe mania Does not favor any SGA over another	Makes a distinction early in the algorithm between mixed and nonmixed states, and suggests narrower, subtype-specific treatment options Review found that lithium can be effective in severe mania and suggests adding an adjunct SGA for partial response, thus favoring lithium-based combinations Review of recent evidence resulted in valproate being dropped to lower nodes in the algorithm for nonmixed mania and being second-line for mixed mania Favors the use of quetiapine and recommends considering olanzapine later as an option due to safety/side-effect profile

(continued)

Table 3	Comparison of Present Algorithm to Other Recent Algorithms and Guidelines for Acute Mania (*continued*)			
Algorithm/guideline	*Year*	*Other algorithms/guidelines*	*Present algorithm*
World Federation of Societies of Biological Psychiatry guidelines for the biological treatment of bipolar disorders: update on treating acute mania[61]	2009	Detailed discussion and clear hierarchy based on level of evidence and side-effect profile of each medication No distinction in medication choice based on mania subtype, although clinicians are encouraged to make diagnostic distinction Aripiprazole, risperidone, and valproate (except for women of childbearing potential) are first-line agents in terms of efficacy and risk/benefit ratio	Makes subtype-specific recommendations such as preferring lithium first-line for nonmixed mania due to its broad efficacy, antisuicidal properties, neuroprotective benefits, and other advantages
The Texas implementation of medication algorithms: update to the algorithms for treating bipolar *1* disorder[190]	2005	After making a distinction between mixed and nonmixed mania, gives a wider variety of agents to use as first-line in both states Excludes quetiapine and favors other SGAs and valproate as first-line agents in mixed mania	Provides narrower choices based on appraised evidence in both mixed and nonmixed states Recommends use of quetiapine as first-line in mixed states and makes valproate second-line

SGA, second-generation antipsychotic.

CONCLUSIONS AND FINAL COMMENT

The psychopharmacological treatment of mania in bipolar disorder is replete with challenges. Though many medications are effective or partly effective for acute episodes, relatively few are of benefit in all phases of the disorder and have the effect of truly stabilizing mood and behavior. Even fewer treatments offer satisfactory safety, especially in the long term. Clinicians, typically under pressure of limited time, often resort to targeting symptoms with different medicines in complex and largely untested combinations, often without satisfactory clinical results. Many experts believe that patients may do better with a more systematic approach that emphasizes the most evidence-supported, safest treatments and fewer medications per patient. The recommendations provided here offer a reasonable, but tentative, path to improved outcomes of pharmacotherapy, with fewer complications, for patients with mania. Nevertheless, the proposals are subject to ongoing revision as additional research findings become available.

Declaration of interest: The authors report no conflicts of interest. The authors alone are responsible for the content and writing of the article.

The authors thank Drs. Ross J. Baldessarini and Mark S. Bauer for their comments and suggestions on an early draft of this article.

REFERENCES

1. Levy B, Weiss RD. Neurocognitive impairment and psychosis in bipolar I disorder during early remission from an acute episode of mood disturbance. J Clin Psychiatry 2010;71:201-6.
2. Ansari A, Osser DN. The psychopharmacology algorithm project at the Harvard South Shore Program: an update on bipolar depression. Harv Rev Psychiatry 2010;18:36-55.
3. Osser DN, Jalali-Roudsari M, Manschreck T. The Psychopharmacology Algorithm Project at the Harvard South Shore Program: an update on schizophrenia. Harv Rev Psychiatry 2013;21:18-40.
4. Bajor LA, Ticlea AN, Osser DN. The Psychopharmacology Algorithm Project at the Harvard South Shore Program: an update on posttraumatic stress disorder. Harv Rev Psychiatry 2011;19:240-58.
5. Hamoda HM, Osser DN. The Psychopharmacology Algorithm Project at the Harvard South Shore Program: an update on psychotic depression. Harv Rev Psychiatry 2008;16:235-47.
6. Osser DN, Dunlop LR. The Psychopharmacology Algorithm Project at the Harvard South Shore Program: an update on generalized social anxiety disorder. Psychopharm Rev 2010;45:91-8.
7. National Collaborating Centre for Mental Health; National Institute for Health and Clinical Excellence. Bipolar disorder: the management of bipolar disorder in adults, children, and adolescents in primary and secondary care. London: NICE, 2006.
8. Goodwin FK, Jamison KR. Manic-depressive illness: bipolar disorders and recurrent depression. 2nd ed. New York: Oxford University Press, 2007.
9. Rosa AR, Cruz N, Franco C, et al. Why do clinicians maintain antidepressants in some patients with acute mania? Hints from the European Mania in Bipolar Longitudinal Evaluation of Medication (EMBLEM), a large naturalistic study. J Clin Psychiatry 2010;71:1000-6.
10. McElroy SL, Keck PE Jr, Strakowski SM. Mania, psychosis, and antipsychotics. J Clin Psychiatry 1996;57 suppl 3: 14-26; discussion 47-9.
11. Swann AC, Daniel DG, Kochan LD, Wozniak PJ, Calabrese JR. Psychosis in mania: specificity of its role in severity and treatment response. J Clin Psychiatry 2004;65:825-9.
12. Carlson GA, Goodwin FK. The stages of mania. A longitudinal analysis of the manic episode. Arch Gen Psychiatry 1973; 28:221-8.
13. Yildiz A, Vieta E, Tohen M, Baldessarini RJ. Factors modifying drug and placebo responses in randomized trials for bipolar mania. Int J Neuropsychopharmacol 2011;14:863-75.
14. Schatzberg AF, Cole JO, DeBattista C. Manual of clinical psychopharmacology. 7th ed. Washington, DC: American Psychiatric Press, 2010.
15. Janicak PG, Marder SR, Pavuluri MN. Principles and practice of psychopharmacotherapy. 5th ed. Philadelphia: Lippincott Williams & Wilkins, 2011.
16. American Psychiatric Association. American Psychiatric Association practice guidelines for the treatment of psychiatric disorders. Arlington, VA: American Psychiatric Publishing, 2006.
17. Battaglia J, Moss S, Rush J, et al. Haloperidol, lorazepam, or both for psychotic agitation? A multicenter, prospective, double-blind, emergency department study. Am J Emerg Med 1997;15:335-40.
18. Garza-Trevino ES, Hollister LE, Overall JE, Alexander WF. Efficacy of combinations of intramuscular antipsychotics and sedative-hypnotics for control of psychotic agitation. Am J Psychiatry 1989;146:1598-601.
19. Andrezina R, Josiassen RC, Marcus RN, et al. Intramuscular aripiprazole for the treatment of acute agitation in patients with schizophrenia or schizoaffective disorder: a double-blind, placebo-controlled comparison with intramuscular haloperidol. Psychopharmacology (Berl) 2006;188:281-92.
20. Satterthwaite TD, Wolf DH, Rosenheck RA, Gur RE, Caroff SN. A meta-analysis of the risk of acute extrapyramidal symptoms with intramuscular antipsychotics for the treatment of agitation. J Clin Psychiatry 2008;69:1869-79.
21. Zeller SL, Rhoades RW. Systematic reviews of assessment measures and pharmacologic treatments for agitation. Clin Ther 2010;32:403-25.
22. Mantovani C, Labate CM, Sponholz A Jr, et al. Are low doses of antipsychotics effective in the management of psychomotor agitation? A randomized, rated-blind trial of 4 intramuscular interventions. J Clin Psychopharmacol 2013;33:306-12.

23. Ahmed U, Jones H, Adams CE. Chlorpromazine for psychosis induced aggression or agitation. Cochrane Database Syst Rev 2010;(4):CD007445.

24. Karmacharya R, England ML, Ongur D. Delirious mania: clinical features and treatment response. J Affect Disord 2008; 109:312-6.

25. Provencher MD, Guimond AJ, Hawke LD. Comorbid anxiety in bipolar spectrum disorders: a neglected research and treatment issue? J Affect Disord 2012;137:161-4.

26. Trixler M, Gati A, Fekete S, Tenyi T. Use of antipsychotics in the management of schizophrenia during pregnancy. Drugs 2005;65:1193-206.

27. Gentile S. Clinical utilization of atypical antipsychotics in pregnancy and lactation. Ann Pharmacother 2004;38:1265-71.

28. Collins KO, Comer JB. Maternal haloperidol therapy associated with dyskinesia in a newborn. Am J Health Syst Pharm 2003;60:2253-5.

29. Reis M, Kallen B. Maternal use of antipsychotics in early pregnancy and delivery outcome. J Clin Psychopharmacol 2008; 28:279-88.

30. Taylor D, Paton C, Kapur S. The Maudsley prescribing guidelines in psychiatry. 11th ed. Chichester, UK: Wiley-Blackwell, 2012.

31. McKean M. Psychiatric care during pregnancy and postpartum. Part 1: diagnosis and management of mood disorders. Psychopharm Rev 2013;48:17-24.

32. Jentink J, Loane MA, Dolk H, et al. Valproic acid monotherapy in pregnancy and major congenital malformations. N Engl J Med 2010;362:2185-93.

33. Cummings C, Stewart M, Stevenson M, Morrow J, Nelson J. Neurodevelopment of children exposed in utero to lamotrigine, sodium valproate and carbamazepine. Arch Dis Child 2011; 96:643-7.

34. Cohen LS, Friedman JM, Jefferson JW, Johnson EM, Weiner ML. A reevaluation of risk of in utero exposure to lithium. JAMA 1994;271:146-50.

35. Miller LJ. Use of electroconvulsive therapy during pregnancy. Hosp Community Psychiatry 1994;45:444-50.

36. Yonkers KA, Wisner KL, Stowe Z, et al. Management of bipolar disorder during pregnancy and the postpartum period. Am J Psychiatry 2004;161:608-20.

37. McElroy SL, Altshuler LL, Suppes T, et al. Axis I psychiatric comorbidity and its relationship to historical illness variables in 288 patients with bipolar disorder. Am J Psychiatry 2001; 158:420-6.

38. Pettinati HM, O'Brien CP, Dundon WD. Current status of cooccurring mood and substance use disorders: a new therapeutic target. Am J Psychiatry 2013;170:23-30.

39. Salloum IM, Cornelius JR, Daley DC, Kirisci L, Himmelhoch JM, Thase ME. Efficacy of valproate maintenance in patients with bipolar disorder and alcoholism: a double-blind placebo- controlled study. Arch Gen Psychiatry 2005;62:37-45.

40. Brown ES, Gorman AR, Hynan LS. A randomized, placebo- controlled trial of citicoline add-on therapy in outpatients with bipolar disorder and cocaine dependence. J Clin Psychopharmacol 2007;27:498-502.

41. Chung AK, Chua SE. Effects on prolongation of Bazett's corrected QT interval of seven second-generation antipsychotics in the treatment of schizophrenia: a meta-analysis. J Psychopharmacol 2011;25:646-66.

42. Swann AC, Lafer B, Perugi G, et al. Bipolar mixed states: an international society for bipolar disorders task force report of symptom structure, course of illness, and diagnosis. Am J Psychiatry 2013;170:31-42.

43. Fountoulakis KN, Kontis D, Gonda X, Siamouli M, Yatham LN. Treatment of mixed bipolar states. Int J Neuropsychopharmacol 2012;15:1015-26.

44. McIntyre RS, Yoon J. Efficacy of antimanic treatments in mixed states. Bipolar Disord 2012;14 suppl 2:22-36.

45. Houston JP, Tohen M, Degenhardt EK, Jamal HH, Liu LL, Ketter TA. Olanzapine-divalproex combination versus divalproex monotherapy in the treatment of bipolar mixed episodes: a double-blind, placebo-controlled study. J Clin Psychiatry 2009;70:1540-7.

46. Suppes T, Ketter TA, Gwizdowski IS, et al. First controlled treatment trial of bipolar II hypomania with mixed symptoms: quetiapine versus placebo. J Affect Disord 2013;150:37-43.
47. Dunner DL. Atypical antipsychotics: efficacy across bipolar disorder subpopulations. J Clin Psychiatry 2005;66 suppl 3:20-7.
48. Kruger S, Trevor Young L, Braunig P. Pharmacotherapy of bipolar mixed states. Bipolar Disord 2005;7:205-15.
49. Cipriani A, Barbui C, Salanti G, et al. Comparative efficacy and acceptability of antimanic drugs in acute mania: a multipletreatments meta-analysis. Lancet 2011;378:1306-15.
50. Janicak PG, Rado JT. Quetiapine for the treatment of acute bipolar mania, mixed episodes and maintenance therapy. Expert Opin Pharmacother 2012;13:1645-52.
51. Weisler RH, Nolen WA, Neijber A, Hellqvist A, Paulsson B. Continuation of quetiapine versus switching to placebo or lithium for maintenance treatment of bipolar I disorder (Trial 144: a randomized controlled study). J Clin Psychiatry 2011; 72:1452-64.
52. Cutler AJ, Datto C, Nordenhem A, Minkwitz M, Acevedo L, Darko D. Extended-release quetiapine as monotherapy for the treatment of adults with acute mania: a randomized, double-blind, 3-week trial. Clin Ther 2011;33:1643-58.
53. Vieta E, Nuamah IF, Lim P, et al. A randomized, placebo- and active-controlled study of paliperidone extended release for the treatment of acute manic and mixed episodes of bipolar I disorder. Bipolar Disord 2010;12:230-43.
54. Khazaal Y, Tapparel S, Chatton A, Rothen S, Preisig M, Zullino D. Quetiapine dosage in bipolar disorder episodes and mixed states. Prog Neuropsychopharmacol Biol Psychiatry 2007;31:727-30.
55. Baker RW, Tohen M, Fawcett J, et al. Acute dysphoric mania: treatment response to olanzapine versus placebo. J Clin Psychopharmacol 2003;23:132-7.
56. Gonzalez-Pinto A, Lalaguna B, Mosquera F, et al. Use of olanzapine in dysphoric mania. J Affect Disord 2001;66:247-53.
57. Tohen M, McDonnell DP, Case M, et al. Randomised, double-blind, placebo-controlled study of olanzapine in patients with bipolar I depression. Br J Psychiatry 2012;201:376-82.
58. McEvoy JP, Lieberman JA, Perkins DO, et al. Efficacy and tolerability of olanzapine, quetiapine, and risperidone in the treatment of early psychosis: a randomized, double-blind 52week comparison. Am J Psychiatry 2007;164:1050-60.
59. Hahn MK, Wolever TM, Arenovich T, et al. Acute effects of single-dose olanzapine on metabolic, endocrine, and inflammatory markers in healthy controls. J Clin Psychopharmacol 2013;33:740-6.
60. Suppes T, Dennehy EB, Hirschfeld RM,et al. The Texas implementation of medication algorithms: update to the algorithms for treatment of bipolar I disorder. J Clin Psychiatry 2005;66: 870-86.
61. Grunze H,Vieta E, Goodwin GM, et al. The World Federation of Societies of Biological Psychiatry (WFSBP) guidelines for the biological treatment of bipolar disorders: update 2009 on the treatment of acute mania. World J Biol Psychiatry 2009; 10:85-116.
62. Stahl S, Lombardo I, Loebel A, Mandel FS. Efficacy of ziprasidone in dysphoric mania: pooled analysis of two double-blind studies. J Affect Disord 2010;122:39-45.
63. Lombardo I, Sachs G, Kolluri S, Kremer C, Yang R. Two 6-week, randomized, double-blind, placebo-controlled studies of ziprasidone in outpatients with bipolar I depression: did baseline characteristics impact trial outcome? J Clin Psychopharmacol 2012;32:470-8.
64. Suppes T, Eudicone J, McQuade R, Pikalov A 3rd, Carlson B. Efficacy and safety of aripiprazole in subpopulations with acute manic or mixed episodes of bipolar I disorder. J Affect Disord 2008;107:145-54.
65. Thase ME, Jonas A,Khan A, et al. Aripiprazole monotherapy in nonpsychotic bipolar I depression: results of 2 randomized, placebo- controlled studies. J Clin Psychopharmacol 2008;28:13-20.
66. Zarate CA Jr, Rothschild A, Fletcher KE, Madrid A, Zapatel J. Clinical predictors of acute response with quetiapine in psychotic mood disorders. J Clin Psychiatry 2000;61:185-9.
67. Bowden CL, Swann AC, Calabrese JR, et al. A randomized, placebo-controlled, multicenter study of divalproex sodium extended release in the treatment of acute mania. J Clin Psychiatry 2006;67:1501-10.

68. Chengappa KN, Baker RW, Shao L, et al. Rates of response, euthymia and remission in two placebo-controlled olanzapine trials for bipolar mania. Bipolar Disord 2003;5:1-5.

69. Keck PE Jr, Marcus R, Tourkodimitris S, et al. A placebo- controlled, double-blind study of the efficacy and safety of aripiprazole in patients with acute bipolar mania. Am J Psychiatry 2003;160:1651-8.

70. Marder SR, Sorsaburu S, Dunayevich E, et al. Case reports of post-marketing adverse event experiences with olanzapine intramuscular treatment in patients with agitation. J Clin Psychiatry 2010;71:433-41.

71. Keck PE Jr, Mendlwicz J, Calabrese JR, et al. A review of randomized, controlled clinical trials in acute mania. J Affect Disord 2000;59 suppl 1:S31-S7.

72. Busch FN, Miller FT, Weiden PJ. A comparison of two adjunctive treatment strategies in acute mania. J Clin Psychiatry 1989;50:453-5.

73. Muller-Oerlinghausen B. Arguments for the specificity of the antisuicidal effect of lithium. Eur Arch Psychiatry Clin Neurosci 2001;251 suppl 2:II72-5.

74. Bauer MS, Mitchner L. What is a "mood stabilizer"? An evidence-based response. Am J Psychiatry 2004;161:3-18.

75. Ghaemi SN. From BALANCE to DSM-5: taking lithium seriously. Bipolar Disord 2010;12:673-7.

76. Goodwin FK, Whitham EA, Ghaemi SN. Maintenance treatment study designs in bipolar disorder: do they demonstrate that atypical neuroleptics (antipsychotics) are mood stabilizers? CNS Drugs 2011;25:819-27.

77. Goodwin FK, Fireman B, Simon GE, Hunkeler EM, Lee J, Revicki D. Suicide risk in bipolar disorder during treatment with lithium and divalproex. JAMA 2003;290:1467-73.

78. Baldessarini RJ, Tondo L, Davis P, Pompili M, Goodwin FK, Hennen J. Decreased risk of suicides and attempts during long-term lithium treatment: a meta-analytic review. Bipolar Disord 2006;8:625-39.

79. Cipriani A, Pretty H, Hawton K, Geddes JR. Lithium in the prevention of suicidal behavior and all-cause mortality in patients with mood disorders: a systematic review of randomized trials. Am J Psychiatry 2005;162:1805-19.

80. Ahrens B, Muller-Oerlinghausen B. Does lithium exert an independent antisuicidal effect? Pharmacopsychiatry 2001;34:132-6.

81. Marangell LB, Dennehy EB, Wisniewski SR, et al. Case-control analyses of the impact of pharmacotherapy on prospectively observed suicide attempts and completed suicides in bipolar disorder: findings from STEP-BD. J Clin Psychiatry 2008; 69:916-22.

82. Rybakowski JK, Suwalska A. Excellent lithium responders have normal cognitive functions and plasma BDNF levels. Int J Neuropsychopharmacol 2010;13:617-22.

83. Lyoo IK, Dager SR, Kim JE, et al. Lithium-induced gray matter volume increase as a neural correlate of treatment response in bipolar disorder: a longitudinal brain imaging study. Neuropsychopharmacology 2010;35:1743-50.

84. Moore GJ, Cortese BM, Glitz DA, et al. A longitudinal study of the effects of lithium treatment on prefrontal and subgenual prefrontal gray matter volume in treatment-responsive bipolar disorder patients. J Clin Psychiatry 2009;70:699-705.

85. Hajek T, Bauer M, Pfennig A, et al. Large positive effect of lithium on prefrontal cortexN-acetylaspartate in patients with bipolar disorder: 2-centre study. J Psychiatry Neurosci 2012; 37:185-92.

86. Hajek T, Cullis J, Novak T, et al. Hippocampal volumes in bipolar disorders: opposing effects of illness burden and lithium treatment. Bipolar Disord 2012;14:261-70.

87. Hajek T, Kopecek M, Hoschl C, Alda M. Smaller hippocampal volumes in patients with bipolar disorder are masked by exposure to lithium: a meta-analysis. J Psychiatry Neurosci 2012;37:333-43.

88. Konopaske GT, Dorph-Petersen KA, Pierri JN, Wu Q, Sampson AR, Lewis DA. Effect of chronic exposure to antipsychotic medication on cell numbers in the parietal cortex of macaque monkeys. Neuropsychopharmacology 2007;32:1216-23.

89. Konopaske GT, Dorph-Petersen KA, Sweet RA, et al. Effect of chronic antipsychotic exposure on astrocyte and oligodendrocyte numbers in macaque monkeys. Biol Psychiatry 2008; 63:759-65.

90. Ho BC, Andreasen NC, Ziebell S, Pierson R, Magnotta V. Long-term antipsychotic treatment and brain volumes: a longitudinal study of first-episode schizophrenia. Arch Gen Psychiatry 2011;68:128-37.

91. Mora E, Portella MJ, Forcada I, Vieta E, Mur M. Persistence of cognitive impairment and its negative impact on psychosocial functioning in lithium-treated, euthymic bipolar patients: a 6-year follow-up study. Psychol Med 2013;43:1187-96.

92. Baldessarini RJ, Leahy L, Arcona S, Gause D, Zhang W, Hennen J. Patterns of psychotropic drug prescription for U.S. patients with diagnoses of bipolar disorders. Psychiatr Serv 2007;58:85-91.

93. Kessing LV, Hellmund G, Geddes JR, Goodwin GM, Andersen PK. Valproate v. lithium in the treatment of bipolar disorder in clinical practice: observational nationwide register-based cohort study. Br J Psychiatry 2011;199:57-63.

94. Swann AC, Bowden CL, Calabrese JR, Dilsaver SC, Morris DD. Pattern of response to divalproex, lithium, or placebo in four naturalistic subtypes of mania. Neuropsychopharmacology 2002;26:530-6.

95. Lenox RH, Gould TD, Manji HK. Endophenotypes in bipolar disorder. Am J Med Genet 2002;114:391-406.

96. Bowden CL, Brugger AM, Swann AC, et al. Efficacy of divalproex vs lithium and placebo in the treatment of mania. The Depakote Mania Study Group. JAMA 1994;271:918-24.

97. Tondo L, Hennen J, Baldessarini RJ. Rapid-cycling bipolar disorder: effects of long-term treatments. Acta Psychiatr Scand 2003;108:4-14.

98. Baldessarini RJ, Tondo L, Floris G, Hennen J. Effects of rapid cycling on response to lithium maintenance treatment in 360 bipolar I and II disorder patients. J Affect Disord 2000;61:13-22.

99. Calabrese JR, Rapport DJ, Youngstrom EA, Jackson K, Bilali S, Findling RL. New data on the use of lithium, divalproate, and lamotrigine in rapid cycling bipolar disorder. Eur Psychiatry 2005;20:92-5.

100. Hirschfeld RM, Allen MH, McEvoy JP, Keck PE Jr, Russell JM. Safety and tolerability of oral loading divalproex sodium in acutely manic bipolar patients. J Clin Psychiatry 1999; 60:815-8.

101. Kowatch RA, Suppes T, Carmody TJ, et al. Effect size of lithium, divalproex sodium, and carbamazepine in children and adolescents with bipolar disorder. J Am Acad Child Adolesc Psychiatry 2000;39:713-20.

102. Suppes T, Baldessarini RJ, Faedda GL, Tondo L, Tohen M. Discontinuation of maintenance treatment in bipolar disorder: risks and implications. Harv Rev Psychiatry 1993;1:131-44.

103. Goodwin GM. Recurrence of mania after lithium withdrawal. Implications for the use of lithium in the treatment of bipolar affective disorder. Br J Psychiatry 1994;164:149-52.

104. Cavanagh J, Smyth R, Goodwin GM. Relapse into mania or depression following lithium discontinuation: a 7-year follow-up. Acta Psychiatr Scand 2004;109:91-5.

105. Severus WE, Kleindienst N, Seemuller F, Frangou S, Moller HJ, Greil W. What is the optimal serum lithium level in the long-term treatment of bipolar disorder—a review? Bipolar Disord 2008;10:231-7.

106. Tamayo JM, Zarate CA Jr, Vieta E, Vazquez G, Tohen M. Level of response and safety of pharmacological monotherapy in the treatment of acute bipolar I disorder phases: a systematic review and meta-analysis. Int J Neuropsychopharmacol 2010;13:813-32.

107. Wagner KD, Ridden L, Kowatch RA, et al. A double-blind randomized, placebo-controlled trial of divalproex extended- release in the treatment of bipolar disorder in children and adolescents. J Am Acad Child Adolesc Psychiatry 2009;48: 519-32.

108. Hirschfeld RM, Bowden CL, Vigna NV, Wozniak P, Collins M. A randomized, placebo-controlled, multicenter study of divalproex sodium extended-release in the acute treatment of mania. J Clin Psychiatry 2010;71:426-32.

109. Geddes JR, Goodwin GM, Rendell J, et al. Lithium plus valproate combination therapy versus monotherapy for relapse prevention in bipolar I disorder (BALANCE): a randomised open-label trial. Lancet 2010;375:385-95.

110. Nolen WA, Weisler RH. The association of the effect of lithium in the maintenance treatment of bipolar disorder with lithium plasma levels: a post hoc analysis of a double-blind study comparing switching to lithium or placebo in patients who responded to quetiapine (Trial 144). Bipolar Disord 2013; 15:100-9.

111. Yatham LN, Paulsson B, Mullen J, Vagero AM. Quetiapine versus placebo in combination with lithium or divalproex for the treatment of bipolar mania. J Clin Psychopharmacol 2004; 24:599-606.

112. McKnight RF, Adida M, Budge K, Stockton S, Goodwin GM, Geddes JR. Lithium toxicity profile: a systematic review and meta-analysis. Lancet 2012;379:721-8.

113. Malhi GS, Berk M. Is the safety of lithium no longer in the balance? Lancet 2012;379:690-2.

114. Bowden CL, Grunze H, Mullen J, et al. A randomized, double-blind, placebo-controlled efficacy and safety study of quetiapine or lithium as monotherapy for mania in bipolar disorder. J Clin Psychiatry 2005;66:111-21.

115. Patel JK, Buckley PF, Woolson S, et al. Metabolic profiles of second-generation antipsychotics in early psychosis: findings from the CAFE study. Schizophr Res 2009;111:9-16.

116. Bendz H, Schon F, Attman PO, Aurell M. Renal failure occurs in chronic lithium treatment but is uncommon. Kidney Int 2010;77:219-24.

117. Yildiz A, Vieta E, Leucht S, Baldessarini RJ. Efficacy of antimanic treatments: meta-analysis of randomized, controlled trials. Neuropsychopharmacology 2011;36:375-89.

118. Correll CU, Sheridan EM, DelBello MP. Antipsychotic and mood stabilizer efficacy and tolerability in pediatric and adult patients with bipolar I mania: a comparative analysis of acute, randomized, placebo-controlled trials. Bipolar Disord 2010; 12:116-41.

119. Goikolea JM, Colom F, Capapey J, et al. Faster onset of antimanic action with haloperidol compared to second-generation antipsychotics. A meta-analysis of randomized clinical trials in acute mania. Eur Neuropsychopharmacol 2013;23:305-16.

120. Tohen M, Zarate CA Jr. Antipsychotic agents and bipolar disorder. J Clin Psychiatry 1998;59 suppl 1:38-48; discussion 9.

121. Zarate CA Jr, Tohen M. Double-blind comparison of the continued use of antipsychotic treatment versus its discontinuation in remitted manic patients. Am J Psychiatry 2004; 161:169-71.

122. Yatham LN, Maj M. Bipolar disorder: clinical and neurobiological foundations. Chichester, UK: Wiley, 2010.

123. Gopal S, Steffens DC, Kramer ML, Olsen MK. Symptomatic remission in patients with bipolar mania: results from a doubleblind, placebo-controlled trial of risperidone monotherapy. J Clin Psychiatry 2005;66:1016-20.

124. Rendell JM, Gijsman HJ, Bauer MS, Goodwin GM, Geddes GR. Risperidone alone or in combination for acute mania. Cochrane Database Syst Rev 2006;(1):CD004043.

125. Shafti SS. Olanzapine vs. lithium in management of acute mania. J Affect Disord 2010;122:273-6.

126. Tariot PN, Schneider LS, Cummings J, et al. Chronic divalproex sodium failed to attenuate agitation and clinical progression of Alzheimer disease. Arch Gen Psychiatry 2011;68:853-61.

127. Fleisher AS, Truran D, Mai JT, et al. Chronic divalproex sodium use and brain atrophy in Alzheimer disease. Neurology 2011;77:1263-71.

128. Pope HG Jr, McElroy SL, Keck PE Jr, Hudson JI. Valproate in the treatment of acute mania. A placebo-controlled study. Arch Gen Psychiatry 1991;48:62-8.

129. Muller J, Luderer HJ. [DEWIPA—a standardized questionnaire for assessing knowledge about symptoms, etiology and psychopharmacologic treatment in patients with depressive episodes]. Psychiatr Prax 1999;26:167-70.

130. Reinares M, Rosa AR, Franco C, et al. A systematic review on the role of anticonvulsants in the treatment of acute bipolar depression. Int J Neuropsychopharmacol 2013;16:485-96.

131. Akdeniz F, Taneli F, Noyan A, Yuncu Z, Vahip S. Valproate- associated reproductive and metabolic abnormalities: are epileptic women at greater risk than bipolar women? Prog Neuropsychopharmacol Biol Psychiatry 2003;27:115-21.

132. Liang CS, Yang FW, Lo SM. Rapid development of severe hypertriglyceridemia and hypercholesterolemia during augmentation of quetiapine with valproic acid. J Clin Psychopharmacol 2011;31:242-3.

133. Behzadi AH, Omrani Z, Chalian M, Asadi S, Ghadiri M. Folic acid efficacy as an alternative drug added to sodium valproate in the treatment of acute phase of mania in bipolar disorder: a double-blind randomized controlled trial. Acta Psychiatr Scand 2009;120:441-5.

134. Ketter TA, Kalali AH, Weisler RH. A 6-month, multicenter, open-label evaluation of beaded, extended-release carbamazepine capsule monotherapy in bipolar disorder patients with manic or mixed episodes. J Clin Psychiatry 2004;65:668-73.

135. Versiani M, Cheniaux E, Landeira-Fernandez J. Efficacy and safety of electroconvulsive therapy in the treatment of bipolar disorder: a systematic review. J ECT 2011;27:153-64.

136. Small JG, Klapper MH, Kellams JJ, et al. Electroconvulsive treatment compared with lithium in the management of manic states. Arch Gen Psychiatry 1988;45:727-32.

137. Thomas J, Reddy B. The treatment of mania. A retrospective evaluation of the effects of ECT, chlorpromazine, and lithium. J Affect Disord 1982;4:85-92.

138. McCabe MS, Norris B. ECT versus chlorpromazine in mania. Biol Psychiatry 1977;12:245-54.

139. Geoffroy PA, Etain B, Henry C, Bellivier F. Combination therapy for manic phases: a critical review of a common practice. CNS Neurosci Ther 2012;18:957-64.

140. Gallego JA, Nielsen J, De Hert M, Kane JM, Correll CU. Safety and tolerability of antipsychotic polypharmacy. Expert Opin Drug Saf 2012;11:527-42.

141. Ceron-Litvoc D, Soares BG, Geddes J, Litvoc J, de Lima MS. Comparison of carbamazepine and lithium in treatment of bipolar disorder: a systematic review of randomized controlled trials. Hum Psychopharmacol 2009;24:19-28.

142. Denicoff KD, Smith-Jackson EE, Disney ER, Ali SO, Leverich GS, Post RM. Comparative prophylactic efficacy of lithium, carbamazepine, and the combination in bipolar disorder. J Clin Psychiatry 1997;58:470-8.

143. Baethge C, Baldessarini RJ, Mathiske-Schmidt K, et al. Longterm combination therapy versus monotherapy with lithium and carbamazepine in 46 bipolar I patients. J Clin Psychiatry 2005; 66:174-82.

144. Klein E, Bental E, Lerer B, Belmaker RH. Carbamazepine and haloperidol v placebo and haloperidol in excited psychoses. A controlled study. Arch Gen Psychiatry 1984;41:165-70.

145. Small JG, Klapper MH, Marhenke JD, Milstein V, Woodham GC, Kellams JJ. Lithium combined with carbamazepine or haloperidol in the treatment of mania. Psychopharmacol Bull 1995;31:265-72.

146. Perlis RH, Welge JA, Vornik LA, Hirschfeld RM, Keck PE Jr. Atypical antipsychotics in the treatment of mania: a metaanalysis of randomized, placebo-controlled trials. J Clin Psychiatry 2006;67:509-16.

147. Fountoulakis KN, Vieta E. Efficacy and safety of aripiprazole in the treatment of bipolar disorder: a systematic review. Ann Gen Psychiatry 2009;8:16.

148. Vieta E, T'joen C, McQuade RD, et al. Efficacy of adjunctive aripiprazole to either valproate or lithium in bipolar mania patients partially nonresponsive to valproate/lithium monotherapy: a placebo-controlled study. Am J Psychiatry 2008; 165:1316-25.

149. Tsai AC, Rosenlicht NZ, Jureidini JN, Parry PI, Spielmans GI, Healy D. Aripiprazole in the maintenance treatment of bipolar disorder: a critical review of the evidence and its dissemination into the scientific literature. PLoS Med 2011;8:e1000434.

150. Keck PE Jr, Versiani M, Potkin S, West SA, Giller E, Ice K. Ziprasidone in the treatment of acute bipolar mania: a three-week, placebo-controlled, double-blind, randomized trial. Am J Psychiatry 2003;160:741-8.

151. Potkin SG, Keck PE Jr, Segal S, Ice K, English P. Ziprasidone in acute bipolar mania: a 21-day randomized, double-blind, placebo-controlled replication trial. J Clin Psychopharmacol 2005;25:301-10.

152. Vieta E, Ramey T, Keller D, English PA, Loebel AD, Miceli J. Ziprasidone in the treatment of acute mania: a 12-week, placebo-controlled, haloperidol-referenced study. J Psychopharmacol 2010;24:547-58.

153. Sachs GS, Vanderburg DG, Edman S, et al. Adjunctive oral ziprasidone in patients with acute mania treated with lithium or divalproex, part 2: influence of protocol-specific eligibility criteria on signal detection. J Clin Psychiatry 2012;73:1420-5.

154. Sachs GS, Vanderburg DG, Edman S, et al. Adjunctive oral ziprasidone in patients with acute mania treated with lithium or divalproex, part 1: results of a randomized, double-blind, placebo-controlled trial. J Clin Psychiatry 2012;73:1412-9.

155. Miller S, Ittasakul P, Wang PW, et al. Enhanced ziprasidone combination therapy effectiveness in obese compared to nonobese patients with bipolar disorder. J Clin Psychopharmacol 2012; 32:814-9.

156. Patkar A, Gilmer W, Pae CU, et al. A 6 week randomized double-blind placebo-controlled trial of ziprasidone for the acute depressive mixed state. PLoS One 2012;7:e34757.

157. Szegedi A, Calabrese JR, Stet L, Mackle M, Zhao J, Panagides J. Asenapine as adjunctive treatment for acute mania associated with bipolar disorder: results of a 12-week core study and 40-week extension. J Clin Psychopharmacol 2012;32:46-55.

158. McIntyre RS. Asenapine: a review of acute and extension phase data in bipolar disorder. CNS Neurosci Ther 2011;17:645-8.

159. McIntyre RS, Cohen M, Zhao J, Alphs L, Macek TA, Panagides J. Asenapine for long-term treatment of bipolar disorder: a double-blind 40-week extension study. J Affect Disord 2010; 126:358-65.

160. McIntyre RS, Cohen M, Zhao J, Alphs L, Macek TA, Panagides J. Asenapine in the treatment of acute mania in bipolar I disorder: a randomized, double-blind, placebo-controlled trial. J Affect Disord 2010;122:27-38.

161. McIntyre RS, Cohen M, Zhao J, Alphs L, Macek TA, Panagides J. A 3-week, randomized, placebo-controlled trial of asenapine in the treatment of acute mania in bipolar mania and mixed states. Bipolar Disord 2009;11:673-86.

162. McElroy SL, Dessain EC, Pope HG Jr, et al. Clozapine in the treatment of psychotic mood disorders, schizoaffective disorder, and schizophrenia. J Clin Psychiatry 1991;52:411-4.

163. Calabrese JR, Kimmel SE, Woyshville MJ, et al. Clozapine for treatment-refractory mania. Am J Psychiatry 1996;153:759-64.

164. Barbini B, Scherillo P, Benedetti F, Crespi G, Colombo C, Smeraldi E. Response to clozapine in acute mania is more rapid than that of chlorpromazine. Int Clin Psychopharmacol 1997;12:109-12.

165. Suppes T, Webb A, Paul B, Carmody T, Kraemer H, Rush AJ. Clinical outcome in a randomized 1-year trial of clozapine versus treatment as usual for patients with treatment-resistant illness and a history of mania. Am J Psychiatry 1999;156:1164-9.

166. Melvin CL, Carey TS, Goodman F, Oldham JM, Williams JW Jr, Ranney LM. Effectiveness of antiepileptic drugs for the treatment of bipolar disorder: findings from a systematic review. J Psychiatr Pract 2008;14 suppl 1:9-14.

167. Grunze H, Langosch J, Born C, Schaub G, Walden J. Levetiracetam in the treatment of acute mania: an open add-on study with an on-off-on design. J Clin Psychiatry 2003;64:781-4.

168. Kruger S, Sarkar R, Pietsch R, Hasenclever D, Braunig P. Levetiracetam as monotherapy or add-on to valproate in the treatment of acute mania—a randomized open-label study. Psychopharmacology (Berl) 2008;198:297-9.

169. Wagner KD, Kowatch RA, Emslie GJ, et al. A double-blind, randomized, placebo-controlled trial of oxcarbazepine in the treatment of bipolar disorder in children and adolescents. Am J Psychiatry 2006;163:1179-86.

170. Vieta E, Cruz N, Garcia-Campayo J, et al. A double-blind, randomized, placebo-controlled prophylaxis trial of oxcarbazepine as adjunctive treatment to lithium in the long-term treatment of bipolar I and II disorder. Int J Neuropsychopharmacol 2008;11:445-52.

171. Vasudev A, Macritchie K, Vasudev K, Watson S, Geddes J, Young AH. Oxcarbazepine for acute affective episodes in bipolar disorder. Cochrane Database Syst Rev 2011;(12): CD004857.

172. Kushner SF, Khan A, Lane R, Olson WH. Topiramate monotherapy in the management of acute mania: results of four double-blind placebo-controlled trials. Bipolar Disord 2006; 8:15-27.

173. Vigo DV, Baldessarini RJ. Anticonvulsants in the treatment of major depressive disorder: an overview. Harv Rev Psychiatry 2009;17:231-41.

174. Arnone D. Review of the use of topiramate for treatment of psychiatric disorders. Ann Gen Psychiatry 2005;4:5.

175. Thomas P, Vieta E. Amisulpride plus valproate vs haloperidol plus valproate in the treatment of acute mania of bipolar I patients: a multicenter, open-label, randomized, comparative trial. Neuropsychiatr Dis Treat 2008;4:675-86.

176. Berwaerts J, Lane R, Nuamah F, et al. Paliperidone XR as adjunctive therapy to lithium or valproate in the treatment of acute mania: a randomized, placebo-controlled study. J Affect Disord 2011;129:252-60.

177. Machado-Vieira R, Soares JC, Lara DR, et al. A doubleblind, randomized, placebo-controlled 4-week study on the efficacy and safety of the purinergic agents allopurinol and dipyridamole adjunctive to lithium in acute bipolar mania. J Clin Psychiatry 2008;69:1237-45.

178. Fan A, Berg A, Bresee C, Glassman LH, Rapaport MH. Allopurinol augmentation in the outpatient treatment of bipolar mania: a pilot study. Bipolar Disord 2012;14:206-10.

179. Akhondzadeh S, Milajerdi MR, Amini H, Tehrani-Doost M. Allopurinol as an adjunct to lithium and haloperidol for treatment of patients with acute mania: a double-blind, randomized, placebo-controlled trial. Bipolar Disord 2006; 8:485-9.

180. Stolk P, Souverein PC, Wilting I, et al. Is aspirin useful in patients on lithium? A pharmacoepidemiological study related to bipolar disorder. Prostaglandins Leukot Essent Fatty Acids 2010;82:9-14.

181. Montgomery P, Richardson AJ. Omega-3 fatty acids for bipolar disorder. Cochrane Database Syst Rev 2008;(2):CD005169.

182. Murphy BL, Stoll AL, Harris PQ, et al. Omega-3 fatty acid treatment, with or without cytidine, fails to show therapeutic properties in bipolar disorder: a double-blind, randomized add-on clinical trial. J Clin Psychopharmacol 2012;32:699-703.

183. Yildiz A, Guleryuz S, Ankerst DP, Ongur D, Renshaw PF. Protein kinase C inhibition in the treatment of mania: a double-blind, placebo-controlled trial of tamoxifen. Arch Gen Psychiatry 2008;65:255-63.

184. Kulkarni J, Garland KA, Scaffidi A, et al. A pilot study of hormone modulation as a new treatment for mania in women with bipolar affective disorder. Psychoneuroendocrinology 2006;31:543-7.

185. Zarate CA Jr, Singh JB, Carlson PJ, et al. Efficacy of a protein kinase C inhibitor (tamoxifen) in the treatment of acute mania: a pilot study. Bipolar Disord 2007;9:561-70.

186. Amrollahi Z, Rezaei F, Salehi B, et al. Double-blind, randomized, placebo-controlled 6-week study on the efficacy and safety of the tamoxifen adjunctive to lithium in acute bipolar mania. J Affect Disord 2011;129:327-31.

187. Gilmer WS, Zarnicki JN. Review of transcranial magnetic stimulation for bipolar disorder. Psychopharm Rev 2012; 47:25-30.

188. Yatham LN1, Kennedy SH, Parikh SV, et al. Canadian Network for Mood and Anxiety Treatments (CANMAT) and International Society for Bipolar Disorders (ISBD) collaborative update of CANMAT guidelines for the management of patients with bipolar disorder: update 2013. Bipolar Disord 2013;15:1-44.

189. Goodwin GM; Consensus Group of the British Association for Psychopharmacology. Evidence-based guidelines for treating bipolar disorder: revised second edition—recommendations from the British Association for Psychopharmacology. J Psychopharmacol 2009;23:346-88.

190. Suppes T, Dennehy EB, Hirschfeld RM, et al.; Texas Consensus Conference Panel on Medication Treatment of Bipolar Disorder. The Texas implementation of medication algorithms: update to the algorithms for treatment of bipolar I disorder. J Clin Psychiatry 2005;66:870-86.

UPDATE

ACUTE BIPOLAR MANIA ALGORITHM

I n the last five years since the publication of this algorithm, the recommendations and flowchart remain mostly the same. There have been no new studies that seem to change the overall sequences of the nodes. However, there have been a variety of studies usually adding support to what was proposed in the 2014 algorithm, but sometimes making adjustments to the risk to benefit analysis for certain recommendations. There is one new medication approved for acute mania—cariprazine in 2015 (a second-generation antipsychotic, previously approved for schizophrenia). Also, there have been some new developments that if confirmed and expanded by more studies might result in changes to the algorithm.

New data have emphasized the prognostic significance of a first attack of mania and the importance of evidence-supported treatment. In a review of eight studies, the rate of recurrence of mania after a first episode over the next four years was 60%.[1] Younger age of onset was associated with higher recurrence rates. Other evidence (mentioned in the original algorithm) suggests early and adequate treatment can improve outcome. The new data highlight the prognostic importance of a single manic episode and that it should be taken seriously. There was also an editorial worth noting that cautioned against contributing to the development of "the malignant transformation of bipolar disorder" into a disabling and rapid cycling condition through application of less than an expert level of care following the onset of the disorder.[2] The author (Robert Post, who contributed to formulating the "kindling" model of how bipolar disorder can progress) argued that the comparison with cancer was appropriate because of the high suicide rate in bipolar disorder.

Node 1: Diagnosis and Other Features in Mania That Might Affect the Algorithm

In Table 1, there is a discussion of considerations for women of child-bearing potential. In a recent large National Institute of Mental Health-sponsored study of the risk of cardiac malformations including Ebstein's abnormality, data emerged that provided a more precise measure of what can be expected. The researchers found that the adjusted risk ratio for any cardiac abnormality was 1.65 compared to unexposed babies.[3] For Ebstein's, the risk ratio was 2.66, and in absolute numbers it was 0.6% for lithium-exposed infants versus 0.18% for those not exposed. The impact was dose-related, with higher ratios if the dose was over 900 mg daily. These results were included in a meta-analysis of 13 high-quality studies published in

January 2020.[4] This analysis found the odds ratio for any cardiac abnormality to be slightly higher—1.86. The risk was limited to fetuses exposed in the first trimester. The absolute risk was 1.2% for any cardiac abnormality. Note that these comparisons are with women with bipolar disorder who did not receive lithium, not with the general population of pregnant women. The fetuses of nonbipolar women have fewer cardiac abnormalities. The studies were generally unclear about whether they excluded women who were on other teratogenic medications or were misusing any substances like alcohol. The authors concluded that the risks of lithium exposure during pregnancy are low, though they are higher in the first trimester and doses should be kept in the lowest part of the therapeutic range especially during that time. The risks and harms associated with mood episode relapse from stopping lithium or lowering the level below the therapeutic range appear, for most women, to far exceed the harms of fetal abnormalities or other pregnancy complications associated with continuing lithium.

In the same row, we discussed the severe teratogenicity of valproate for women of childbearing potential and suggested it should be nearly a last choice for treating mania in such women. An editorial in 2017 strongly confirmed that recommendation.[5]

Finally, in this row, there were old citations suggesting a relatively favorable impression of using electroconvulsive therapy (ECT) for pregnant women with bipolar disorder. However, a study compiling all known case reports of use of ECT as of 2015 found that there was a surprising and concerning 7% mortality rate in the fetuses.[6] ECT should now be considered a last resort and certainly riskier than previously thought.

Node 2d: The First-Line Treatment for Nonmixed, Classic Mania Is Still Lithium

In addition to all the reasons given in the algorithm paper, there are some new citations confirming the remarkable and unique neuroprotective effects of lithium that should be added.[7,8]

Node 3: What to Add to Lithium If the Response Is Unsatisfactory in Classic Mania

Nothing is changed here, but there is a new citation of work by Goikolea and colleagues adding support to the contention that use of haloperidol is ill-advised because of the very high rate of haloperidol-treated patients slipping into depression after resolution of the mania.[9]

Node 5: First-Tier Next Options After Three Trials and Unsatisfactory Response in Acute Mania

Cariprazine was approved in 2015 for acute mania and mixed mania at doses of 3 to 6 mg once daily.[10] It is a partial dopamine agonist, like aripiprazole and brexpiprazole. There has been little attention paid to it and many pharmacy benefit managers have not been including it in their formularies because new products have high costs. However, it does add to the relatively few options for mania that are mild in weight gain and metabolic side effects. It seemed reasonable to add it as one of the options at Node 5. However, the latest development is that it was also approved by the FDA for acute bipolar depression, in June

2019 based on four studies, three published so far, and three that were positive for the product.[11] The approved doses were 1.5 and 3 mg, with the 1.5 mg dose appearing to be best in benefit to harm ratio.[11] It now joins quetiapine as one of only two medications specifically approved for both acute bipolar depression and acute mania. However, the best dose for depression is significantly lower than the best doses for mania, so it is unclear how much mania protection is going to be afforded by the antidepressant dose, and it is unclear if the initial treatment with a high dose for mania is going to have a preventive effect on subsequent depressions and be tolerable over the long term. More research and experience are needed before a firmer and higher spot on the algorithm can be considered for cariprazine. However, the advantage in weight gain could influence patients and their clinicians to want to consider it earlier if it is available.

Table 1: Comorbidity and Other Features in Mania and How They Affect the Algorithm

There is a brief discussion of substance use disorders as a comorbidity in mania and the recommendation is that remission from those use disorders should be a high treatment priority. We did not mention cannabis as one of the substances that could be a concern. The evidence available points clearly to an association between usage and worsening course of bipolar disorder over time. In a study of 4915 subjects, Henquet and colleagues (after control for many possible covariates) found a strong increased risk of manic symptoms associated with the use of cannabis over a three-year follow-up period.[12] They also found an earlier age of onset of bipolar disorder, greater overall illness severity, more rapid cycling, poorer life functioning, and poorer adherence with prescribed treatments. Zorrilla and colleagues evaluated the subsequent course of bipolar patients who stopped cannabis use after an illness episode, and compared their outcome with bipolar patients who never had used cannabis and a group that continued to use.[13] The total sample was 1922 patients. In a two-year period, the continued users had significantly lower rates of recovery, greater work impairment, and lower rates of living with a partner. The data were based on patient reports, so given likely underreporting, there was probably an underestimate of the strength of the association between cannabis use and lives worsened. A systematic review of the effects of cannabis on mood and anxiety disorders confirmed a negative association between cannabis use and long-term outcomes.[14] Thus, it seems that bipolar patients should stay away from cannabis in all its forms. Quitting cannabis should be on the short list of interventions to pursue if patients are not doing well. This is a tough sell in today's political environment regarding cannabis legalization. Many newspaper editorials and politicians are pushing it. Clinicians should not back off and accept patients' insistence on using this product but rather should continue efforts to educate and to consider the problem to be a serious one that potentially interferes with otherwise appropriate and effective bipolar treatments that may be offered.

Table 2: New and Experimental Treatments Proposed for Acute Mania

One intriguing proposed addition to this list is the use of probiotic microorganisms that might modulate inflammatory mechanisms contributing to the pathophysiology of bipolar disorder. A pilot randomized, placebo-controlled trial in 66 recently hospitalized manic patients found fewer rehospitalization days for the probiotic treatment group compared to placebo over 24 weeks (2.8 vs. 8.3 days, p = .017).[15] This clearly needs replication and extension, and the specific probiotics used may or may not be the only ones that could be effective.

Another interesting direction for research stems from the fact that light therapy can help depression. Could dark therapy help mania? A study of 23 patients hospitalized for mania were randomized to wear orange-tinted blue-light-blocking glasses or clear glasses from 6 PM to 8 AM for seven nights.[16] Retinal ganglion cells contain melanopsin, which is blue light sensitive, and these cells convey daylight information to the brain. It was proposed that the blue-light-blocking glasses could be equivalent to the effect of total darkness but still enable the person to see enough to participate in activities. The blue-blocking glasses caused a dramatic 14-point drop in YMRS compared to 2 points with the control glasses. All patients were also on standard pharmacotherapy.

REFERENCES

1. Gignac A, McGirr A, Lam RW, Yatham LN. Recovery and recurrence following a first episode of mania: a systematic review and meta-analysis of prospectively characterized cohorts. J Clin Psychiatry 2015;76:1241-8.
2. Post RM. Preventing the malignant transformation of bipolar disorder. JAMA 2018;319:1197-8.
3. Patorno E, Huybrechts KF, Bateman BT, et al. Lithium use in pregnancy and the risk of cardiac malformations. N Engl J Med 2017;376:2245-54.
4. Fornaro M, Maritan E, Ferranti R, et al. Lithium exposure during pregnancy and the postpartum period: a systematic review and meta-analysis of safety and efficacy outcomes. Am J Psychiatry 2020;177:76-92.
5. Balon R, Riba M. Should women of childbearing potential be prescribed valproate? A call to action. J Clin Psychiatry 2016;77:525-6.
6. Leiknes KA, Cooke MJ, Jarosch-von Schweder L, Harboe I, Hoie B. Electroconvulsive therapy during pregnancy: a systematic review of case studies. Arch Womens Ment Health 2015;18:1-39.
7. Giakoumatos CI, Nanda P, Mathew IT, et al. Effects of lithium on cortical thickness and hippocampal subfield volumes in psychotic bipolar disorder. J Psychiatr Res 2015;61:180-7.
8. Gildengers AG, Butters MA, Aizenstein HJ, et al. Longer lithium exposure is associated with better white matter integrity in older adults with bipolar disorder. Bipolar Disord 2015;17:248-56.
9. Goikolea JM, Colom F, Torres I, et al. Lower rate of depressive switch following antimanic treatment with second-generation antipsychotics versus haloperidol. J Affect Disord 2013;144:191-8.
10. Calabrese JR, Keck PE Jr, Starace A, et al. Efficacy and safety of low- and high-dose cariprazine in acute and mixed mania associated with bipolar I disorder: a double-blind, placebo-controlled study. J Clin Psychiatry 2015;76:284-92.
11. Citrome L. Cariprazine for bipolar depression: what is the number needed to treat, number needed to harm and likelihood to be helped or harmed? Int J Clin Pract 2019;73:e13397.
12. Henquet C, Krabbendam L, de Graaf R, ten Have M, van Os J. Cannabis use and expression of mania in the general population. J Affect Disord 2006;95:103-10.
13. Zorrilla I, Aguado J, Haro JM, et al. Cannabis and bipolar disorder: does quitting cannabis use during manic/mixed episode improve clinical/functional outcomes? Acta Psychiatr Scand 2015;131:100-10.
14. Mammen G, Rueda S, Roerecke M, Bonato S, Lev-Ran S, Rehm J. Association of cannabis with long-term clinical symptoms in anxiety and mood disorders: a systematic review of prospective studies. J Clin Psychiatry 2018;79.
15. Dickerson F, Adamos M, Katsafanas E, et al. Adjunctive probiotic microorganisms to prevent rehospitalization in patients with acute mania: a randomized controlled trial. Bipolar Disord 2018;20:614-21.
16. Henriksen TE, Skrede S, Fasmer OB, et al. Blue-blocking glasses as additive treatment for mania: a randomized placebo-controlled trial. Bipolar Disord 2016;18:221-32.

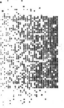

The Psychopharmacology Algorithm Project at the Harvard South Shore Program: An Update on Unipolar Nonpsychotic Depression

Christoforos Iraklis Giakoumatos, MD and David Osser, MD

Background: *The Psychopharmacology Algorithm Project at the Harvard South Shore Program presents evidence-based recommendations considering efficacy, tolerability, safety, and cost. Two previous algorithms for unipolar nonpsychotic depression were published in 1993 and 1998. New studies over the last 20 years suggest that another update is needed.*

Methods: *The references reviewed for the previous algorithms were reevaluated, and a new literature search was conducted to identify studies that would either support or alter the previous recommendations. Other guidelines and algorithms were consulted. We considered exceptions to the main algorithm, as for pregnant women and patients with anxious distress, mixed features, or common medical and psychiatric comorbidities.*

Summary: *For inpatients with severe melancholic depression and acute safety concerns, electroconvulsive therapy (or ketamine if ECT refused or ineffective) may be the first-line treatment. In the absence of an urgent indication, we recommend trialing venlafaxine, mirtazapine, or a tricyclic antidepressant. These may be augmented if necessary with lithium or T3 (triiodothyronine). For inpatients with non-melancholic depression and most depressed outpatients, sertraline, escitalopram, and bupropion are reasonable first choices. If no response, the prescriber (in collaboration with the patient) has many choices for the second trial in this algorithm because there is no clear preference based on evidence, and there are many individual patient considerations to take into account. If no response to the second medication trial, the patient is considered to have a medication treatment-resistant depression. If the patient meets criteria for the atypical features specifier, a monoamine oxidase inhibitor could be considered. If not, reconsider (for the third trial) some of the same options suggested for the second trial. Some other choices can also considered at this stage. If the patient has comorbidities such as chronic pain, obsessive-compulsive disorder, attention-deficit/hyperactivity disorder, or posttraumatic stress disorder, the depression could be secondary; evidence-based treatments for those disorders would then be recommended.*

Keywords: algorithm, depression, psychopharmacology, treatment, unipolar depression

From Harvard Medical School and VA Boston Healthcare System, Brockton Division, Brockton, MA.
Original manuscript received 4 December 2017, accepted for publication subject to revision 4 February 2017; revised manuscript received 4 March 2017.
Correspondence: Christoforos Iraklis Giakoumatos, MD, VA Boston Healthcare System, 940 Belmont St., Brockton, MA 02301. Email: cigiakoumatos@gmail.com

DOI: 10.1097/HRP.0000000000000197

As reported by the World Health Organization in its 2004 update on the global burden of disease, unipolar nonpsychotic depression was the third largest cause of disease burden worldwide.[1] It was the eighth largest cause of disease burden in low-income countries and the largest cause in middle- and high-income countries. Around the same time, a United States national household survey showed that 6.7% of adults had experienced a major depressive episode in the previous 12 months.[2] In 2016, Olfson and colleagues[3] showed that 8.4% of adults in the United States screened positively for depression but that only 28.7% received any treatment even if they had visited their primary care provider within the previous year. When treated, the modality was an antidepressant 87% of the time. The primary care system may have the best opportunity to diagnose and treat depression.

Kessler and colleagues[2] reported that the lifetime prevalence of depression was 16.2%. Their group showed that just 51.6% of the depressed patients received treatment and that, among them, only 41.9% were adequately treated. Furthermore, approximately 50% of depressed patients failed to achieve response to the first adequate trial of an antidepressant agent.

The efficacy of antidepressants has been a subject of debate. Unpublished negative studies, when included in metaanalyses, have markedly lowered effect sizes.[4] Kirsch and colleagues[5,6] reviewed the data and reported that the overall efficacy of the new-generation antidepressants is below the National Institute for Health and Care Excellence criteria for clinical relevance. Investigators challenged this study and considered the Kirsch analysis to be flawed; many methodological weaknesses of antidepressant trials have been identified.[7,8] Most experts think that antidepressants do work moderately well in properly selected patients entered into well-conducted trials.[9] Among the poorer responders are the following: patients with subthreshold depression (i.e., not fully meeting *Diagnostic and Statistical Manual of Mental Orders* [DSM] criteria);[10] patients whose depression is secondary to intense dyadic discord (stress or conflict within an important or intimate relationship);[11] patients with bipolar spectrum depressions (including those with mixed features),[12,13] anxious distress,[14] or onset in the context of some debilitating medical illnesses.[15] Also, the Sequenced Alternatives to Relieve Depression (STAR*D) study found that response to antidepressants and their augmentations diminishes with successive trials having unsatisfactory response.[16] Therefore, to get the best results with medication, clinicians should start with an accurate diagnosis and consider important predictors of response. Clinical experience will likely be an insufficient basis for decision making, given the high placebo response in many depressed patient populations. An analysis of four long-term, placebo-controlled antidepressant trials suggested that the great majority of relapses in patients who continued to take their antidepressants were in the patients whose initial response was a placebo effect.[17] The clinician may remember the positive initial effect and fail to notice or not be around when the treatment fails, with the clinician therefore prescribing the same ineffective treatment over and over. Michael O'Donnell, former editor of the *British Medical Journal,* offered a definition of clinical experience: "making the same mistakes over and over with increasing confidence over an impressive number of years."[18]

Evidence-supported psychopharmacology algorithms could simplify the process of choosing medications, especially for clinicians, such as primary care physicians, not strongly familiar with the evidence base.[19] Algorithms are more prescriptive than guidelines and easier to incorporate into practice. The need for such algorithms can be better appreciated when taking into account the study done by Observational Health Data Sciences and Informatics, which is an international collaboration of more than 120 researchers from 12 countries.[20] They looked at the medical records of 250 million patients treated for depression and found hundreds of different sequences of first, second, and third antidepressants used by various prescribers. Eleven percent of patients with depression had a treatment pathway that was unique. Algorithm-guided treatment could help minimize this gross level of practice variation in clinical care and improve clinical outcomes by achieving remission in shorter amounts of time and with fewer medication changes than with treatment as usual.[21,22] Also, algorithms have the potential to produce more cost-effective results if generic options are recommended over more expensive, brand-name products when there is no apparent disadvantage in outcome or safety.

Since 1995, the Psychopharmacology Algorithm Project at the Harvard South Shore Program (PAPHSS) has been creating evidence-derived treatment algorithms. Seven peer-reviewed PAPHSS algorithms have been published and can be accessed through a publicly available website (www.psychopharm. mobi). This article updates previous versions of algorithms for unipolar nonpsychotic depression, as published by one of the authors (DO).

This and all the other PAPHSS algorithms focus on psychopharmacological treatment, but this focus should not be taken to suggest that the authors do not consider psychotherapeutic or other nonpharmacological treatments for depression unimportant. Indeed, in many cases, psychotherapy could be first-line or combined at any point with pharmacotherapy.[23] The intention is only to suggest, if psychopharmacology is chosen as a treatment approach, what would be the best-supported and safest options for the first, second, and further trials, and what considerations would alter these preferences.

METHODS

Prior publications have described the PAPHSS methods of algorithm development.[24–29] The algorithms are created in a way to simulate a curbside psychopharmacological consultation. They present a series of questions describing the clinical situation (diagnoses and history of previous treatment) that the consultant might ask. Then, recommendations are made that are derived from an analysis of the literature pertinent to that clinical scenario. The authors reviewed their previously published unipolar nonpsychotic depression algorithms,[19,30] consulted other recent algorithms and guidelines,[31–34] and focused on key randomized, controlled trials (RCTs), especially recent ones not considered in previous reviews. In constructing the decision tree, the authors considered efficacy, tolerability, safety, and cost as the main bases for prioritizing treatments. All recommendations were the result of agreement by the two authors. Their conclusions were opinion-based distillations of the body of evidence reviewed—which could be subject to conflicting interpretations by other experts. However, the peer review process that follows initial submission of the article adds some validation to the reasoning in this algorithm and other PAPHSS algorithms. If the reasoning, based on the authors' interpretation of the pertinent evidence, is plausible to reviewers, then it is retained. When differences of opinion occur, the authors make adjustments to achieve consensus with the reviewers or probe the relevant evidence further in order to present a stronger argument in support of their position. At each decision point, different but approximately equivalent options are offered for consideration, enabling prescribers to select what seems best and most acceptable to the patient in each particular clinical situation.

FLOWCHART FOR THE ALGORITHM

A summary and overview of the algorithm appears in Figure 1. Each "node" represents a clinical scenario where a treatment choice must be made. The algorithm delineates patient populations ranging from those beginning treatment to those, at the end, who are highly treatment resistant. The questions, evidence review, and reasoning that support the recommendations at each node will be presented below.

NODE 1: DIAGNOSIS OF UNIPOLAR NONPSYCHOTIC DEPRESSION

The treatment recommendations of this algorithm apply only to patients who have been diagnosed with unipolar nonpsychotic depression based on the DSM-5 criteria.[35] Though the validity of these criteria may be questioned, the psychopharmacology evidence base is almost entirely tied to these criteria. One can only speculate about the psychopharmacological responsiveness of depressions diagnosed in other ways. Notably, treatment recommendations may differ depending on the specifier of the depressive disorder (with anxious distress, atypical features, mixed features, melancholic features, or seasonal pattern).[36] We will discuss these recommendation differences at appropriate points in the algorithm. The default recommendations apply to patients with no specifiers or significant comorbidities.

Table 1 presents considerations and recommendations when some frequently encountered medical and psychiatric comorbidities or other circumstances are present that could change the basic algorithm recommendations. In cases with significant medical conditions, it is advised that care be coordinated among the different specialists involved in the patient's care.

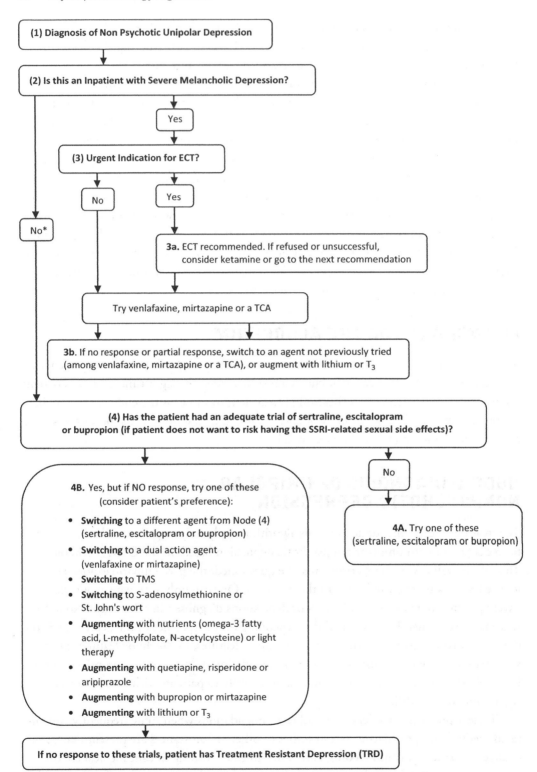

Figure 1. Flowchart of the algorithm for nonpsychotic unipolar depression.
ECT, electroconvulsive therapy; MAOI, monoamine oxidase inhibitor; SSRI, selective serotonin reuptake inhibitors; T_3, triiodothyronine; TCA, tricyclic antidepressant; TMS, transcranial magnetic stimulation.
*Inpatients without melancholia and outpatients with or without melancholia.

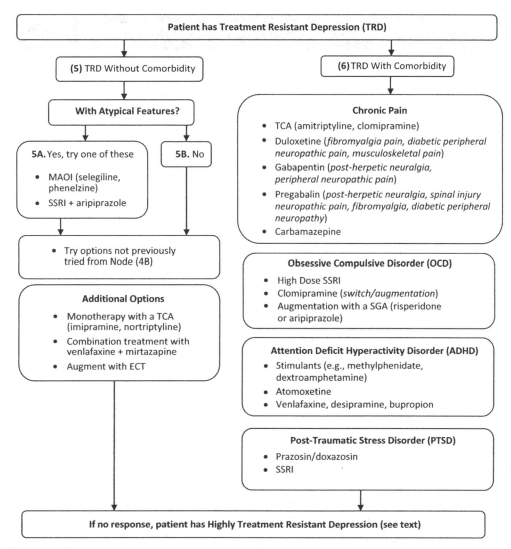

Figure 1. (*Continued*)

Table 1	Comorbidity and Other Features in Major Depression and How They Affect the Algorithm		
Comorbidity and other circumstances	*Considerations*	*Recommendations*
Coronary artery disease	Untreated depression worsens prognosis in cardiovascular disease[37]	SSRIs may protect against myocardial infarction[15]
		Data with sertraline indicated that effectiveness is limited to patients with a history of major depressions that predated the onset of the CAD[38]
		Escitalopram was shown to be safe and effective for depression in patients with CAD, but the relationship with time of onset of the depression was not evaluated[39]

(*continued*)

Table 1 | Comorbidity and Other Features in Major Depression and How They Affect the Algorithm (continued)

Comorbidity and other circumstances	Considerations	Recommendations
Chronic kidney disease	Sertraline might not be effective in patients with CKD not requiring dialysis[40]	Skip Node 4 and go directly to Node 4B
Cardiac arrhythmias	TCAs and MAOIs may cause cardiac arrhythmias due to their effects on cardiac sodium and potassium channels[41]	Avoid TCAs and MAOIs EKG monitoring of TCA-treated patients is a more accurate way to detect toxicity than plasma-level monitoring Sertraline appears to be safe in patients at risk of arrhythmia following myocardial infarction[38] We do not recommend citalopram, because of concerns about QTc prolongation[42]
Gastrointestinal bleeding	SSRIs increase hemorrhage risk Gastrointestinal bleeding can be increased 9-fold by SSRIs combined with NSAIDs[43] Other antidepressants such as mirtazapine and bupropion are not well studied but may not be safer[44]	Adding proton-pump inhibitors such as omeprazole decreases the risk to only slightly above controls not on SSRIs[43]
Older adults (greater than 65 years of age)	SSRIs may increase risk of bleeding; however, in a Cochrane meta-analysis of poststroke patients, bleeding risk was nonsignificant[45] SSRIs and venlafaxine are associated with higher rates of hyponatremia secondary to SIADH in older adults;[46] in a meta-analysis of 15 RCTs, venlafaxine and duloxetine were associated with increased risk of dizziness in the elderly compared to SSRIs;[47] SSRIs, TCAs, and other antidepressant classes have been associated with increased risk of falls, particularly in frail older women[48] Right, unilateral, ultra-brief ECT has been shown to have good efficacy and favorable tolerability in older adults with severe depression[49] Evidence to support the effectiveness of methylphenidate as an adjuvant to SSRIs in treatment-resistant depression is limited;[50] additionally, methylphenidate carries an FDA black-box warning for increased cardiovascular mortality[51]	Consider side-effect profiles of antidepressant medications prior to initiation or titration in elderly adults In patients with intolerable hyponatremia secondary to SSRI use, consider mirtazapine[46] Consider ECT, particularly right unilateral ultra-brief ECT, in older adults with severe depression Risks and benefits of adding methylphenidate to an SSRI in treatment-resistant depression in the elderly should be carefully considered, in light of limited evidence of efficacy and FDA black-box warning.

Table 1 | Comorbidity and Other Features in Major Depression and How They Affect the Algorithm (continued)		
Comorbidity and other circumstances	**Considerations**	**Recommendations**
Women of childbearing potential and pregnant women	About 10% of pregnant women will experience depression[52] Untreated or suboptimally treated depression during pregnancy leads to poor adherence with prenatal care Relapse of major depressive disorder during pregnancy is common (43%) and can occur significantly more often in women who discontinued their medication just prior to conception or during early stages of the pregnancy[53]	Patients on antidepressants at high risk of relapse are best maintained on an antidepressant during and after pregnancy Risk of exposure to medications must be weighed against the risks of untreated depression, which can affect both mother and child Late exposure (after 20th week of pregnancy) is associated with increased risk of prematurity, postpartum hemorrhage,[54] and persistent pulmonary hypertension of the newborn;[55] these could be due to confounding by indication SSRI use during pregnancy may increase risk for speech, language, and motor disorders;[56] again, there could be confounding by indication Avoid paroxetine because of risk of atrial septal defects (odds ratio = 1.8 [95% CI, 1.1–3.0]);[57] if already on it, consider risks involved with switching
Depression with mixed features	This new specifier in DSM-5 is for patients with three comorbid manic symptoms on most days of the depression; most commonly, these include racing thoughts, pressured speech, decreased need for sleep, and increased energy Bipolar depression must be ruled out (by past history of hypomania or mania, though this history is easy to miss); bipolar depression would involve a different treatment algorithm[26] Unipolar depression with mixed features may be an intermediate condition on a spectrum from unipolar to bipolar disorder or may be indicative of a patient who is going to become bipolar at some point Antidepressants seem much less effective for mixed states and are potentially harmful especially if the patient has an underlying bipolar disorder.[12,58]	Only one randomized, controlled study of a medication for this new diagnostic category exists: lurasidone was more effective than placebo (number needed to treat = 3), especially if there were only two manic features (effect size = 1.0) rather than three, as required in DSM-5 (effect size = 0.5)[59] In the absence of evidence of effectiveness of other (usually less expensive) medications for major depression with mixed features, and given the robust benefit shown in this study, the recommendation at this time is lurasidone, despite the cost
Depression with anxious distress or high levels of anxiety	STAR*D and other studies find this situation to be common and associated with poorer response to antidepressants and most augmenters[14]	Sedating atypical antipsychotics such as quetiapine can be effective as monotherapy or as augmenters of antidepressants, though with considerable side-effect burden;[60,61] aripiprazole is effective as an augmenter[36]

NODE 2: IS THIS AN INPATIENT WITH SEVERE MELANCHOLIC DEPRESSION?

Having diagnosed the patient with a DSM-5 major depression and having considered the comorbidities and conditions in Table 1 that might change the basic algorithm, the next step to further differentiate treatment is to determine if the patient is hospitalized with severe depression and the melancholia specifier. The specifier requires that the patient have both prominent loss of pleasure and reactivity to usually pleasurable stimuli and additional somatic manifestations, including psychomotor agitation or retardation, weight loss, diurnal variation (worse in morning), and excessive guilt.

Some evidence indicates that such inpatients require different somatic and pharmacological therapy than other inpatients with non-melancholic depression and outpatients with either melancholic or non-melancholic depression. Evidence suggests, for example, that inpatients with melancholia respond less well to selective serotonin reuptake inhibitors (SSRIs) than tricyclic antidepressants (TCAs).[62] Evidence of good efficacy in these inpatients is also available for venlafaxine and mirtazapine—agents with dual actions that include norepinephrine reuptake inhibition, like TCAs.[63] In outpatients with the melancholia specifier, however, meta-analyses have found no difference between the efficacy of SSRIs and TCAs. Hence, a different algorithm is proposed for these inpatients, though it does not always start with medication.

NODE 3: IN TREATING A PATIENT WITH SEVERE MELANCHOLIC DEPRESSION, IS THERE AN URGENT INDICATION FOR ECT?

Node 3A: If Yes, ECT or Ketamine

Electroconvulsive therapy (ECT) is urgently indicated in patients with severe suicidality, catatonia, insufficient oral intake, or medical conditions (e.g., pregnancy) that may limit the use of psychotropics. Therefore, before considering any medication, severely ill melancholic patients at acute risk of suicide should be considered for ECT. The Consortium for Research in ECT reported a 75% remission rate among 217 patients who completed a short course of ECT during an acute episode of depression, with 65% of patients having remission by the fourth week of therapy.[64] Despite this strong evidence of effectiveness, cognitive side effects such as amnesia, which are commonly reported as adverse effects of ECT, may influence patients' decisions to accept it.[65] Several studies have failed to show a difference in effectiveness between high-dose right unilateral ECT and bilateral ECT, and have indicated that unilateral electrode placement on the right side is associated with a lower incidence of cognitive side effects.[66,67] Patients with the longest episodes of depression may be the most likely to respond to ECT.[68]

As previously mentioned, ECT is the treatment of choice for inpatients with severe melancholic depression at imminent risk of suicide. If the patient refuses a trial of ECT or if such is unsuccessful, however, ketamine can be considered.[69] Some evidence suggests that ketamine can produce desirable rapid results, even within an hour, but such results may be shortlived.[69–71] Maintenance studies have not been done. The use of ketamine for this indication is not yet approved by the U.S. Food and Drug Administration (FDA). In this clinical scenario, however—with an imminent risk of self-harm, with contraindications for ECT, with the patient refusing ECT, or with ECT's having been unsuccessful—ketamine can be considered and may be acceptable to the patient as a bridging therapy to lower the acute suicidal risk and help stabilize the patient until another form of treatment can be administered. It should be noted that the benefits of ketamine may not be limited to suicidal depressed patients with melancholia; there is at least one report of response in a nonsuicidal melancholic patient.[72]

Node 3B: If No, Try Venlafaxine, Mirtazapine, or a TCA

If an inpatient with severe melancholia does not have an urgent indication for ECT or ketamine, the first-line psychopharmacology recommendation options are (as noted above) venlafaxine, mirtazapine, or a TCA. The last of these may be preferred because of their evidence of superiority to placebo and SSRIs for treating inpatients with melancholic depression.[62] TCAs, however, come with potential cardiac-conduction side effects, and the risk of death from overdose is greater than with other agents.[73,74]

Venlafaxine also shows some evidence of effectiveness in this type of depression. Benkert and colleagues[75] reported a significantly faster response and a significant difference in the proportion of sustained responders when venlafaxine was compared to imipramine in inpatients with melancholia. Since venlafaxine has a risk of increase in blood pressure, blood pressure needs to be monitored in patients taking this agent, and the risk of death by overdose is higher than with SSRIs.[74] The effectiveness of venlafaxine in hospitalized patients with melancholic depression was further supported by Guelfi and colleagues,[76] who reported a significantly greater response rate of venlafaxine compared to placebo.

A multicenter, randomized, double-blind study in hospitalized, severely depressed patients with melancholic features compared the efficacy of mirtazapine and venlafaxine. Although the differences were not statistically significant, mirtazapine produced more responders and remitters than venlafaxine, and with fewer dropouts due to adverse events.[63] Notably, the mean daily doses used in this study were high (49.5 ± 8.3 mg/day for mirtazapine and 255.0 ± 59.8 mg/day for venlafaxine).

Thus, mirtazapine, venlafaxine, and TCAs can be effective for treating inpatients with severe melancholic depression. We consider mirtazapine and venlafaxine to be preferred, however, due to their better tolerability and safety profiles compared to TCAs.

Augmentation, the addition of an agent to an antidepressant regimen in order to improve efficacy,[77] is also a potential option. Two well-studied augmenters of TCAs are lithium and T3 (triiodothyronine). A meta-analysis of ten placebo-controlled studies found that lithium augmentation of TCAs was significantly more effective than placebo augmentation.[78] Two meta-analyses of T3 augmentation showed enhanced response of patients who did not fully respond to a trial of TCAs alone.[79,80]

The data for lithium or T3 augmentation of SSRIs is not as convincing as their evidence in TCA augmentation. In the STAR*D study, remission rates following lithium and T3 augmentation of citalopram were not very robust and did not differ significantly, though a trend favored T3 (25% remissions vs. 15% with lithium).[81] Rapid effects are sometimes observed in T3 and lithium augmentation of TCAs, but this effect does not seem to occur to the same degree with SSRIs.[82] The lower adverse effects and ease of administration of T3 augmentation give it a slight advantage over lithium augmentation as a choice at this point.

Since TCAs and the dual-action agents with noradrenergic properties are the recommended first-line treatments for severely ill inpatients with melancholia, the preference for augmenters is centered on agents that have a good evidence base for augmenting TCAs—namely, lithium and T3. Their effect as augmenters for the dual-action agents must be considered speculative, however, in that no controlled trials are available for these specific combinations.

NODE 4: IN TREATING OUTPATIENTS WITH DEPRESSION, HAS THE PATIENT HAD AN ADEQUATE TRIAL OF SERTRALINE, ESCITALOPRAM, OR, IF PATIENT DOES NOT WANT TO RISK HAVING SSRI-RELATED SEXUAL SIDE EFFECTS, BUPROPION?

Node 4A: If No, Proceed with Trial

If the patient is not an inpatient with severe melancholic depression, you arrive at Node 4 (see Figure 1). This is where the rest of the population of depressed patients can be found, including all outpatients (even if having the melancholic specifier) and other depressed inpatients without melancholia. If none of the comorbidity and other circumstances described in Table 1 apply, then the first-line recommendation for pharmacotherapy of these patients is an SSRI.[32,83–90] Cipriani and colleagues,[91,92] in their two meta-analyses of head-to-head comparative studies and placebo-controlled studies of antidepressants, found that sertraline and escitalopram had slight advantages over most other antidepressants for efficacy and tolerability. Further support for escitalopram as a possibly superior SSRI for first-line use comes from the Combination Medication to Enhance Depression Outcomes (CO-MED) study.[93] This large (n = 665), prospective, comparative study was designed to address the question of whether it would be better to start depressed patients on two antidepressants at once rather than using just one. Escitalopram was chosen as the monotherapy. It was compared to escitalopram plus bupropion and to mirtazapine plus venlafaxine. Placebo was added to the escitalopram. The study found no difference in outcomes (39% remissions) and more side effects with the combinations. No other monotherapy was compared to escitalopram, but escitalopram monotherapy held up well against what was expected to be tough competition; the results can be seen as supporting escitalopram as a first-line choice at Node 4. Many studies compared TCAs to newer antidepressants, especially SSRIs, but with the exception of inpatients with severe melancholia, the meta-analyses identified no difference in efficacy between them but more serious side effects with TCAs.[8,94]

Another option for first-line use is bupropion. Zimmerman and colleagues[95] reviewed the evidence and concluded that bupropion is as effective as SSRIs and TCAs, and wondered why bupropion is not the first choice antidepressant in usual practice, given its lack of sexual side effects. Trivedi and colleagues[96] showed that it produces equal improvement in comorbid anxiety symptoms and has the same amount of activation side effects, such as insomnia, as SSRIs. In STAR*D, which included a comparison of augmenting citalopram with bupropion versus buspirone, a trend favored bupropion when patients had high levels of anxiety (18% remissions of depression on bupropion vs. 9% on buspirone)[14]—again suggesting that bupropion is not unreasonable as an option, even in anxious depressions. So: why is bupropion not used more often? One explanation is concern about its association with the risk of lowering the seizure threshold. The risk of seizures with the sustained release (SA) formulation was 0.1%, however, which is comparable to, or better than, SSRIs and other antidepressants, at least at doses up to 300 mg daily.[97,98] Importantly, on the positive side regarding adverse effects, bupropion is associated with a lower risk of weight gain than other augmenters.[99] Bupropion is, indeed, the least likely agent to cause sexual side effects, and it may even improve sexual functioning in patients who had developed sexual side effects while taking SSRIs. Sexual dysfunction is one of the major causes of disability and treatment dropouts in the outpatient treatment of depression in primary care.[100] It occurs in 40%-80% of patients treated with SSRIs or serotonin norepinephrine reuptake inhibitors (SNRIs), compared to 14% on placebo.[101] Spontaneous remission of sexual dysfunction occurs in only about 10%, and partial remission in 11%, of patients.[102]

In conclusion, this discussion of the risks and benefits of SSRIs versus bupropion could form the basis of the discussion with the patient. If a male patient chooses to start an SSRI and he develops sexual side effects, he can either be switched to bupropion or may need sildenafil (or related agents) added to the regimen, which is the most effective medication to improve SSRI-induced erectile dysfunction in men.[103] The frequent need for an inconvenient and (currently) expensive medication to address this side effect involving the disabling of a central human physiological function is an important consideration in deciding whether to choose an SSRI or SNRI for major depression rather than bupropion.

Other possible first-line medications for major depression include mirtazapine, paroxetine, or trazodone. The weight gain associated with the first two, however, and the sedation with the last render them inferior Node 4 choices unless either of those side effects would actually be desirable. A once-daily formulation of trazodone is available that might cause less sedation, but a similar controlled-release formulation was not more tolerable than regular-release trazodone in a large study.[104] Other newer, expensive, brand-name antidepressant products are available, but none has shown evidence of superiority in efficacy or safety to justify the additional cost. Vortioxetine has generated some interest regarding its possible special efficacy for cognitive impairment in the context of depression.[105] These improvements in cognition were greater in patients currently working.[106] The FDA psychopharmacology advisory committee reportedly voted to approve an indication for this symptom in patients with major depression. The FDA leadership, however, has been reluctant to grant new drug indications targeting specific symptoms of a syndrome like depression, and did not agree. They want to see more and better comparative studies showing the effect to occur consistently. A final question is whether duloxetine is better for patients with pain as a symptom along with their depression. A meta-analysis of five studies addressing this question by Spielmans and colleagues[107] showed that the effect size for the pain-reduction effect was 0.115 by Cohen's d, which is a clinically insignificant effect—despite FDA approval having been granted for neuropathic pain and pain associated with fibromyalgia. The authors concluded that the claims being made in advertising and detailing regarding this effect on pain are not justified by the evidence, though successful marketing resulted in annual sales in the billions of dollars before duloxetine became available as a generic. More recently, in a meta-analysis of 14 placebo-controlled antidepressant trials with SSRIs and SNRIs, none of the medications demonstrated relative superiority for pain relief.[108] Each had a significant, but small, impact on pain, and for the SNRIs it strongly correlated with improved mood.

Some guidelines and clinicians think it reasonable to select other SNRIs such as venlafaxine for first-line use in outpatients. No advantages in efficacy have been demonstrated, however, and the evidence indicates the likelihood of greater harms from SNRIs in the cardiovascular realm, including hypertension, tachycardia, strokes, and (in some populations) even deaths.[109]

Node 4B. If the Response to the Option Selected at Node 4A Is Unsatisfactory, Try One of These (Consider Patient's Preference)

Very few data are available on what is best to do after the first medication fails despite an adequate trial.[110] In the literature, the consensus of what constitutes an adequate trial appears to be a 8-week period on an antidepressant at a therapeutic dose, though some would say it should be 12 weeks.[111] Many augmentation or switching options exceed placebo in randomized trials, but few head-to-head comparisons are available concerning efficacy or safety—and even fewer with placebo controls.[112] Note that the recent important VA [Veterans Affairs] Augmentation and Switching Treatments for Improving Depression Outcomes (VAST-D) clinical trial enrolled depressed patients who had an unsatisfactory response to an average of 2.3–2.5 trials. Because Node 4B patients would have failed only one trial, these VAST-D results are more pertinent to the next node of this algorithm and will be discussed there.[99]

Given the lack of a strong evidence basis for identifying a preferred medication for the second trial, it was decided that patient preference should be a particularly strong consideration. That was, to some extent, what was done in STAR*D: after failure with the initial antidepressant citalopram, subjects decided whether they wanted a switch or an augmentation—for example, if they thought they had a partial response and the side effects were acceptable, they might pick augmentation. Then, they were randomized to one of two options for the augmentation. In applying the present algorithm, prescribers are encouraged to present to patients some of the most studied available options for augmentation or for switching if the patient prefers a switch. Individual patients may, or may not, want to choose an option that has had a smaller number of efficacy studies if that means avoiding the risk of potential side effects associated with other options that have undergone more studies, have FDA approval, and therefore have been intensively marketed.

Many have wondered if it is better to augment or switch after one antidepressant trial with unsatisfactory results. Gaynes and colleagues[113] evaluated the patients in STAR*D who chose augmentation and matched them retrospectively with a control group of patients with similar demographics and severity who chose to be in the switch study in the Level 2 trial. They found an odds ratio of 1.14 favoring augmentation, which was not statistically or clinically significant.

This algorithm provides four choices for switching and four choices for augmenting the initial antidepressant. The prescriber may present some or all of them to the patient for consideration. The authors do not have a preference, and the order of presentation should not be taken as indicating such a preference.

Switch Options One could switch to one of the other two first-line recommendations not yet tried (among sertraline, escitalopram, or bupropion). Monotherapy switches (up to three) have been found to produce improvement rates as high as 60%-70%.[114] Some studies support switch within, and some between, classes of antidepressants.[115,116] The STAR*D study and various evidence reviews have found essentially no difference in outcome between switching within the same class or to a different class.[117,118]

Switching to a dual-action agent—that is, one that has effects on both serotonin and norepinephrine (e.g., SNRIs or mirtazapine) is a second switch option. At least some reports suggest that patients on or switched to venlafaxine were more likely to experience remission than patients on or switched to an SSRI.[119–121] Most of these studies were funded by the dual-action agent manufacturer. STAR*D found a numerical, but not statistically significant, advantage to switching to venlafaxine rather than to sertraline or bupropion (25% remissions vs. 18% and 21%, respectively). Disadvantages of venlafaxine include the risk of blood pressure elevation, the risk of discontinuation syndromes that are more frequent or more severe than with many other antidepressants, and the difficulty of some patients in tolerating the nausea and other gastrointestinal side effects, even on the extended-release formulation.[122] Mirtazapine has demonstrated efficacy in placebo-controlled studies and has shown superiority to SSRIs in treating moderately to severely depressed patients.[63] Again, these studies were funded by the manufacturer of mirtazapine. In a metaanalysis, mirtazapine showed a faster onset of action than SSRIs at 2 weeks; however, no significant differences were observed in remission at the end of 6 to 12 weeks of treatment except in comparison to paroxetine.[123] The patient should be actively informed of the risk of weight gain, and agranulocytosis is probably only a rare concern despite the package insert warning suggesting an alarming rate of 2:3000 in the registration studies.

The third switching option that might be considered is switching to repetitive transcranial magnetic stimulation (rTMS). It involves repeated subconvulsive magnetic stimulation to the brain, particularly the dorsolateral prefrontal cortex as the primary target, an area that neuroimaging studies suggest is hypoactive in depressed patients.[124,125] rTMS is less invasive than other neuromodulatory interventions, and it has been associated with a better cognitive side-effect profile than ECT. A randomized, controlled trial comparing rTMS and ECT to placebo sham treatment found it to be not as effective as ECT.[126] The FDA has approved rTMS for use after one failed trial of an antidepressant but not after two trials (based on the submitted trial data). Hence, it is proposed as an option at this point in the algorithm. A multicenter, randomized, controlled trial of patients who failed at least one but no more than four adequate antidepressant treatments showed remission rates for rTMS at 7%-14% after at least three weeks of treatment and less than 18% after six weeks of treatment.[127]

Finally, for patients who might prefer a neutraceutical or herbal option, S-adenosylmethionine (SAMe) and St. John's wort have reasonable evidence of efficacy as monotherapies for depression and have generally fewer side effects than antidepressants.[128,129]

Augmentation Options The first set of proposed augmenting options is to select a nutraceutical agent (omega-3 fatty acid, L-methylfolate, or n-acetylcysteine) or light therapy.[130–134] These options have the important advantage of minimal side effects, but efficacy is much less well established than some other options. Yet, insufficient evidence is available to conclude that these options are less effective than the others, and the side effect profiles could make them appealing to some patients.

The effect size of omega-3 fatty acid products in treating depression may be smaller than the others in this category. Doses have ranged widely in the studies, but a median seems to be about 1 gram twice daily. L-methylfolate is backed by a small quantity of more impressive data in non- or partial responders to SSRIs, at a dose of 15 mg (but not 7.5 mg) daily. Folate (which is much less expensive) might also work. It is unclear from the inconclusive studies what the best dose would be, but it might be on the order of 1 mg daily.[135] One placebo-controlled trial found improvement on secondary outcome measures only, at 1000 mg twice daily.[131] An association has been found between light therapy and reduced depressive symptoms when compared to placebo and control treatment, even in patients without a seasonal pattern.[136]

The second category of augmentation options is to use a second-generation antipsychotic. Three are FDA approved: aripiprazole, brexpiprazole (not included in our recommendations as it has similar efficacy to aripiprazole but a much higher cost), and quetiapine. The fixed combination of fluoxetine and olanzapine, which has FDA-approval, is not included in our recommendations because of the significant weight gain and metabolic side effects associated with olanzapine. Evidence also suggests that risperidone is an effective augmentation option.[137] Extensive industry- sponsored marketing to prescribers and patients has highlighted the second-generation psychotic augmentation option in the minds of many clinicians and patients. However, thought provoking meta-analyses of the data on efficacy, balanced by consideration of the side effects of these medications, indicate that they should not be the automatic choice among the augmentations.[61,138,139] The number needed to treat for efficacy is a modest 8 in exchange for considerable metabolic, akathisic, extrapyramidal, and other side effects. Long-term efficacy is unknown, and the side effects often become more significant with time.

A third augmentation option would be to use the antidepressants bupropion or mirtazapine. In STAR*D, bupropion produced 30% remissions as an augmentation, which was equal to buspirone on the primary outcome measure (Hamilton Rating Scale for

Depression). On some secondary measures (Quick Inventory of Depressive Symptomatology Self-Report [QIDS-SR], side-effect burden, patient satisfaction), however, bupropion seemed somewhat more effective.[140] Mirtazapine has been shown to be an effective augmentation for SSRIs in several small randomized trials but can cause significant weight gain.[141,142] Mirtazapine can also be an effective switching option for sexual dysfunction caused by SSRIs.[143]

The fourth option to consider is augmentation with lithium or T3. These are the oldest and among the best-evidenced augmentation strategies, though as noted in the Node 3 discussion, lithium's evidence is more robust as an augmenter of TCAs. Tricyclics are used much less often today, however, and are not recommended at Node 4 because of their side-effect burden. Lithium is itself associated with a significant side-effect burden, though the doses used for augmentation (usually 600–900 mg daily) are somewhat lower than for treating bipolar disorder. T3 has had a mild side-effect burden in the published studies, though clinicians still worry about the potential consequences of doses that for some patients can become supraphysiological. As mentioned above, the data for lithium or T3 augmentation of SSRIs are not as convincing as the data for TCA augmentation.[78,79,81]

TREATMENT-RESISTANT DEPRESSION

If the patient did not respond satisfactorily to the chosen Node 4B option (switch or augmentation), then for the purposes of this algorithm, the patient is considered to have a treatment-resistant depression (TRD). At least two adequate pharmacotherapy trials of reasonable mainstream options have taken into account safety and patient preferences. The STAR*D study found that the odds of the depression remitting with a third or fourth trial are much diminished, and even if remissions occur, the chances of relapse within the next year are 65% or greater.[16] Ivanova and colleagues[144] showed that patients with TRD (defined somewhat differently), when compared to patients with non-TRD, had at least four times more psychiatric hospitalizations and approximately three times more emergency room visits. It should be emphasized here that before proceeding with more medication trials, it would be important to make another thorough review of medical, psychological, and environmental/social factors (e.g., dyadic discord) that could account for the unsatisfactory results so far.[11] Also, it would be wise to review Table 1 again.

NODE 5: DOES THE PATIENT HAVE TRD WITHOUT COMORBIDITIES BUT WITH ATYPICAL FEATURES?

The Columbia criteria for atypical depression codified in DSM-5 include having significant mood reactivity combined with two of the following clinical characteristics: hyperphagia, hypersomnia, leaden paralysis, and pathological rejection sensitivity. Atypical depression is a pattern seen more often in bipolar depression than unipolar. Clinicians should reconsider the diagnosis, as the treatment would be different from what is proposed in this algorithm if the patient has bipolar disorder.[26,145]

Node 5A: Patient Has the Atypical Features Specifier for Major Depression

Up to now, the atypical features (ATF) has not been utilized to define a unique treatment pathway in this algorithm. This is because SSRIs or bupropion are generally effective in treating ATF,[146,147] and they are early recommendations in Nodes 4A and 4B. At this point they probably would have been tried. Monoamine oxidase inhibitors (MAOIs) are also effective in treating ATF, but they have many side effects and for this reason were not previously recommended in the default algorithm. But now, if the patient meets criteria for the ATF specifier, it might be time to consider MAOIs. A metaanalysis in patients with atypical depression found that MAOIs are more effective than TCAs.[148] Phenelzine has been the most studied MAOI in atypical depression. It seems also to have maintenance efficacy.[149] It requires, however, the use of a tyramine-restricted diet. Side effects include weight gain, postural hypotension, and sexual dysfunction.[150] It is necessary to wait two to five weeks after discontinuing an SSRI (five weeks for fluoxetine) before an MAOI may be started, because of the danger of the potentially fatal serotonin syndrome. The transdermal formulation of selegiline may provide similar efficacy without so many adverse events and without requiring dietary restrictions except in doses over 6 mg per 24 hours.[151–153] The risk of serotonin syndrome, albeit very rare, remains a concern.[154]

Another option, besides an MAOI, would be to add aripiprazole to an SSRI. In one of the studies evaluating aripiprazole as an augmentation for SSRIs, response in atypical depression was included as an outcome measure.[36] The response in those subjects was particularly robust: indeed, it was more significant than in the subjects with non-atypical depression (p <.001 vs. p <.05).

Node 5B: TRD Without Comorbidities and Without Atypical Features (Consider Patient's Preference)

As was the case for selection of the second treatment trial (Node 4B), little data are available to guide the choice of the third trial. STAR*D remains as a source of relevant information, having suggested possible effectiveness of switches to a TCA or mirtazapine, or augmentation with lithium or T3 for a third trial. Some informative signals have also come from the 2017 VAST-D study noted briefly at Node 4.[99] In that large study of 1500 depressed veterans (85% male, 47% with comorbid PTSD), who had an average of 2.4 previous medication trials without satisfactory outcome, three randomized treatment options were available: augmentation of their current antidepressants with aripiprazole (raised to 10 mg daily), augmentation with bupropion (raised to 400 mg daily), and switch to bupropion monotherapy up to 400 mg daily. Patients could not have been on bupropion before. They were treated for 12 weeks. Remission rates were 29% on aripiprazole augmentation, 27% on bupropion augmentation, and 22% on switch to bupropion. Number needed to treat for the superiority of aripiprazole augmentation over bupropion switch was 14—indicating that this difference, though statistically significant, is clinically small. These differences in effectiveness have to be balanced by consideration of the side effects of each treatment. Notably, 25% of the aripiprazole augmentation patients gained substantial (7%) body weight, versus 5% on the bupropion treatment options, and 12% of bupropion-treated patients lost substantial weight, versus 5% on aripiprazole. Thus, the small advantage in effectiveness for aripiprazole was balanced negatively by these weight considerations. In addition, it should be noted that the population was predominantly male. Most non-veteran depressed outpatients are female and may have different propensities to improve and have changes in weight from medications. Also, civilian depressions have much lower rates of comorbid PTSD. Bupropion has not shown efficacy versus placebo for PTSD,[155] but aripiprazole has some moderate evidence of usefulness in PTSD[156]— which may account for all of the advantage for aripiprazole found in the veteran population.

In view of the above, it is hard to differentiate among the treatment options for a third trial in depressed outpatients. Decisions should again be individualized, taking into account patient demographics, side-effect vulnerabilities, and personal preferences. We therefore propose basically the same options as in Node 4B, the second pharmacotherapy trial, and the patient should play a key role in helping make the selection after being apprised of the advantages and disadvantages of each. To these, we would add a few additional considerations.

Switch Options Two preferred choices here at Node 5B (third trial, no comorbidities, not atypical depression) would be venlafaxine again or a TCA (imipramine or nortriptyline). In STAR*D the remission rate with a switch to venlafaxine after the initial trial with citalopram was 25%, which was numerically higher than the 18% rate with a switch to another SSRI, sertraline.[16] The ARGOS study had similar findings.[157] In regard to TCAs, Thase and colleagues[158] reported that both the switch from sertraline to imipramine and the switch from imipramine to sertraline resulted in significant improvements in some patients with a history of treatment-resistant chronic depression. In STAR*D the switch to nortriptyline in the third trial, after two failed antidepressant trials, produced a remission rate of almost 20%, versus 12% for a switch to mirtazapine (nonsignificant).

Antidepressant Combination Option Another combination option to consider here at Node 5B (in addition to those mentioned in Node 4B) would be mirtazapine plus venlafaxine. In STAR*D this option was offered in Level 4 (i.e., after three failed trials), and it was numerically superior, with 14% remissions compared to the MAOI tranylcypromine, which produced 7% remissions (nonsignificant, because of small number of patients at this point). Another study (a randomized trial supported by the manufacturer of mirtazapine) found better results with this combination than with three other combinations.[159]

ECT remains the most effective type of treatment for patients who have not yet responded adequately to a number of medication trials.[160,161]

NODE 6: TRD WITH COMORBIDITIES

In Node 5 we considered additional medication choices in the case of patients with no significant comorbidities. The patient's treatment resistance might be due, however, to the presence of a comorbidity that was previously considered secondary in importance to the depression with the consequence that the initial treatment trials were directed toward the depression. As noted in Figure 1, you skip Node 5 and go directly to Node 6 if comorbidities could potentially be explaining the TRD; if the depression is potentially secondary to the comorbidity, treatment directed toward the comorbidity might produce a more satisfactory outcome for both the depression and the comorbidity itself. For the four comorbidities considered, the evidence-based approaches may be different from the recommended treatment for those who are depressed without the comorbidity: chronic pain, obsessive-compulsive disorder, attention-deficit/hyperactivity disorder (ADHD), and posttraumatic stress disorder (PTSD).

Chronic Pain

Chronic pain persisting for more than three months is a common complaint among patients with depression. It is predictive of a poor prognosis and is a major risk factor for suicidal behavior.[162] Many antidepressants have been evaluated for their ability to relieve pain from various causes in depressed patients. As mentioned in Node 4, however, a recent meta-analysis of 14 studies found them to be largely equivalent in effect (duloxetine, as noted earlier, had no greater benefit), and the effect sizes were small and strongly correlated with their antidepressant effects.[108] Other meta-analyses have evaluated the effect of psychotropic drugs, including antidepressants, for chronic pain syndromes in patients who were not necessarily depressed.[163] The findings of these reviews provide options to think about when chronic pain is present as a comorbid problem and the depression is not responding to antidepressants.

TCAs have the longest track record of any antidepressant class for the treatment of pain syndromes and depression with comorbid chronic pain.[164,165] The usual doses of TCAs for pain relief are typically lower than the doses typically used for treating depression. As discussed by Shembalkar and Anand,[166] clomipramine and amitriptyline have been the most widely used antidepressants in pain therapy. Amitriptyline has been preferred perhaps because primary care clinicians are less familiar with clomipramine. In the two direct comparisons of clomipramine and amitriptyline for pain syndromes, however, clomipramine had superior effectiveness.[163]

Several randomized, controlled studies have reported the efficacy of duloxetine over placebo.[167–170] Subsequently, duloxetine obtained FDA approval for fibromyalgia pain, diabetic peripheral neuropathic pain, and musculoskeletal pain. As noted earlier, however, a meta-analysis of five duloxetine trials involving 1448 patients concluded that the effect size was too small to be clinically meaningful (0.115 by Cohen's d) and that the manufacturer's claims are not supported by good evidence.

Anticonvulsants may also be useful for patients with depression and comorbid chronic pain. Carbamazepine is considered an effective treatment for trigeminal neuralgia. Pregabalin has FDA approvals for post-herpetic neuralgia, spinal injury neuropathic pain, fibromyalgia, and diabetic peripheral neuropathy.[171] Gabapentin, a similar compound, is FDA approved for post-herpetic neuralgia and has some evidence for use in peripheral neuropathic pain.[172,173]

Obsessive-Compulsive Disorder

SSRIs are the first-line treatment for obsessive-compulsive disorder. Notably, however, the effective dose of the SSRIs is often higher, and the duration of the SSRI trials may need to be longer, than when treating depression.[174,175] Some studies show that the separation from placebo does not begin until week 5 and then gradually increases up to week 10.[176]

In cases of unsatisfactory OCD response, treatment with the SSRI can be augmented with a second-generation antipsychotic, especially risperidone or aripiprazole.[177]

Attention-Deficit/Hyperactivity Disorder

Stimulants (e.g., dextroamphetamine, methylphenidate) are the first-line pharmacotherapy for adults with ADHD.[178] Stimulants may even be useful in some adult ADHD patients struggling with substance use disorders.[179] They were not found effective, however, for moderate to severe major depression as monotherapy or as augmentations of antidepressants.[180] Nevertheless, for patients with treatment-resistant depression and comorbid ADHD, stimulant treatments could be helpful, perhaps by addressing the emotional dysregulation that is frequently associated with ADHD and that can respond to stimulant therapy.[181]

Atomoxetine has also been shown to be an effective treatment for adults with ADHD, though effectiveness is probably less than with the stimulants, and it takes 5–10 weeks to reach maximum effectiveness.[182]

Randomized, controlled trials support the use of bupropion and desipramine as second-line (less effective) choices in treating ADHD.[183,184] Venlafaxine has also been reported to be effective in adult ADHD in open-label trials.[185,186] Some of these antidepressants may have already been tried at earlier points in the algorithm.

Posttraumatic Stress Disorder

SSRIs are the only FDA-approved medications for treating PTSD, and they would probably have been tried by this point.

Trauma-related nightmares, disturbed awakenings without nightmare recollection, and daytime hypervigilance and irritability are some of the most debilitating symptoms of PTSD, leading to impaired sleep, avoidant behavior, and secondary depression. It may be that the patient has a primary problem with PTSD. Doxazosin and prazosin are alpha-1 antagonists that can treat these symptoms by reducing noradrenergic activity.[187,188]

The effect size of the benefits on PTSD symptoms has been much greater with prazosin than with antidepressants, including SSRIs.[27]

HIGHLY TREATMENT-RESISTANT DEPRESSION

By this point (see Figure 1), the patient will have had four or more medication trials and perhaps ECT. We are beyond the end of STAR*D, and we have given due consideration to medical and psychiatric comorbidity and to psychosocial factors that may be fueling the condition. Some somatic therapy options are still potentially available in addition to the better-evidenced options discussed above but not yet tried. These options range from minimally evidenced, often novel psychopharmacology strategies to invasive, device-based or surgical techniques such as vagus nerve stimulation.[189] Decisions to employ these options are highly influenced by local interest, availability, and cost considerations. They seem to be beyond the scope of what seems reasonable to prioritize and include in an algorithm for general use.

COMPARISON WITH OTHER RECENT GUIDELINES AND ALGORITHMS

Many other guidelines and some algorithms have been published in recent years. We offer in Table 2 a brief comparison of key features of several of these and how the present algorithm differs in key recommendations.

Strengths of the present algorithm include simplifying the switching and augmentation options to those that have the best evidence for efficacy and the lowest risk of the more problematic side effects, and that are the most cost-effective. We also give more weight than other algorithms to patient preferences at key points where the evidence supporting what to do next is not that definitive. Finally, we consider the impact of severity, key specifiers, and important comorbidities on medication choice.

DISCUSSION

Some physicians do not welcome the appearance of medication treatment algorithms and are reluctant to follow them, no matter how evidence-supported and peer-reviewed the algorithms may be.[190] Such physicians have more faith in the quick, intuitive decision-making process generally known as the art of medicine. Faith in this art is part of the culture of medicine and has deep historical roots. This art is initially conveyed by more experienced mentors and is then refined by personal experience as the emerging practitioner makes his or her own mistakes. As Groupman[191] has noted, however, we do not want airline pilots to learn from their mistakes; we want them to make the right decision every time. Even the expert mentors, if we judge by studies in other fields (e.g., engineering), make more errors using their art and experience than would be made by following algorithms devised a priori by other experts in the field.[192,193] Unfortunately for patients, the health care system continues to be built on a foundation of mistakes

Table 2 | Comparison of Present Algorithm to Other Recent Algorithms and Guidelines for Unipolar Depression

Algorithm/guideline	Year	Other algorithms/guidelines	PAPHSS algorithm
Texas Medication Algorithm Project: Report of the Texas Consensus Conference Panel on Medication Treatment of Major Depressive Disorder[31]	1999	No distinction between inpatient and outpatient treatment of depression First-line options include SSRIs as a class, nefazodone, bupropion SR, venlafaxine XR, and mirtazapine If no response to treatment, recommendations include (1) augmentation with a different class medication among the choices listed above or with lithium, and (2) combination treatment with two medications from different classes (from the options mentioned above)	For inpatients with severe melancholic depression, we recommend venlafaxine, mirtazapine, or a TCA, whereas for outpatients we recommend sertraline, escitalopram, or bupropion first-line We do not recommend SNRIs, mirtazapine, or nefazodone first-line for outpatients because of greater side effects Augmentation options include, but are not limited to, nutraceutical agents, light therapy, a second-generation antipsychotic, bupropion, mirtazapine, lithium, or T3
World Federation of Societies of Biological Psychiatry (WFSBP) Guidelines for Biological Treatment of Unipolar Depressive Disorders, Part 1: Update 2013 on the Acute and Continuation Treatment of Unipolar Depressive Disorders[32]	2013	For initial treatment of depression: For mild and moderate depression, SSRIs as a class and escitalopram, sertraline, mirtazapine, and venlafaxine are recommended For severe depression, SSRIs, SNRIs, and TCAs are recommended (without stating preference of one agent over another within different classes) If no response to initial treatment, one of the recommendations is to augment with lithium, thyroid hormone, quetiapine or aripiprazole or olanzapine (in combination with fluoxetine), or St. John's wort	For inpatients with severe melancholic depression, we recommend venlafaxine, mirtazapine, or a TCA For outpatients, we recommend sertraline, escitalopram, or bupropion first-line We do not recommend SNRIs, TCAs, or mirtazapine first-line for outpatients because of greater side effects If no response to initial treatment, we offer more specific switches and augmentations: patient can switch to one of the initial options not previously tried, to a dual-action agent, to transcranial magnetic stimulation, or to S-adenosylmethionine/St. John's wort, or augment with selected evidenced nutrients such as L-methylfolate, light therapy, second-generation antipsychotics (aripiprazole, quetiapine, or risperidone), bupropion, mirtazapine, lithium, or T3 We do not recommend olanzapine or quetiapine, because of greater side effects (especially metabolic)

(continued)

Table 2 | Comparison of Present Algorithm to Other Recent Algorithms and Guidelines for Unipolar Depression (continued)

Algorithm/guideline	Year	Other algorithms/guidelines	PAPHSS algorithm
Canadian Network for Mood and Anxiety Treatments (CANMAT) 2016 Clinical Guidelines for the Management of Adults with Major Depressive Disorder[33]	2016	Based on CANMAT's criteria for the level of evidence and stated principles of pharmacotherapy management, the recommended first-line antidepressants include agomelatine, bupropion, citalopram, desvenlafaxine, duloxetine, escitalopram, fluoxetine, fluvoxamine, mianserin, milnacipran, mirtazapine, paroxetine, sertraline, venlafaxine, and vortioxetine If no response to initial treatment, the recommendations are to either switch or augment First-line augmenters are aripiprazole, quetiapine, and risperidone	For inpatients with severe melancholic depression, we recommend venlafaxine, mirtazapine, or a TCA For outpatients, we recommend sertraline, escitalopram, or bupropion first-line We do not recommend other agents as first-line for outpatients because of greater side effects, inferior performance in head-to-head comparisons, and in some cases, unavailability in the United States If no response to initial treatment, we offer more specific switches and augmentations: one can switch to one of the initial options not previously tried, to a dual action agent, to transcranial magnetic stimulation, or to S-adenosylmethionine/ St. John's wort, or augment with selected evidenced nutrients such as L-methylfolate, light therapy, second-generation antipsychotics (aripiprazole, quetiapine, or risperidone), bupropion, mirtazapine, lithium, or T3
Florida Best Practice Psychotherapeutic Medication Guidelines for Adults with Major Depressive Disorder[34]	2017	Do not distinguish between inpatient and outpatient treatment of depression For initial treatment of depression, recommend an SSRI (without stating preference of one agent over another within this class), an SNRI (without stating preference of one agent over another within this class), bupropion, mirtazapine, or vortioxetine	For inpatients with severe melancholic depression, we recommend venlafaxine, mirtazapine, or a TCA For outpatients, we recommend sertraline, escitalopram, or bupropion first-line We do not recommend SNRIs or mirtazapine first-line for outpatients because of greater side effects We do not recommend vortioxetine because of lack of robust evidence thus far We provide different recommendations for commonly seen comorbid conditions

PAPHSS, Psychopharmacology Algorithm Project at the Harvard South Shore Program; SNRI, serotonin-norepinephrine reuptake inhibitor; SSRI, selective serotonin reuptake inhibitor; T3, triiodothyronine; TCA, tricyclic antidepressant.

followed by "corrective action plans."[191] Following standardized care driven by evidence-supported algorithms, however, is a model that has produced superior and cost-effective outcomes with illnesses such as diabetes, pneumonia, and heart disease,[194] and the aggregate evidence of their use to improve depression outcomes seems comparable.[21,22,195] A more detailed review, by PAPHSS authors, of issues related to the value of following evidence-supported psychopharmacology algorithms has been published previously.[196]

A limitation in the value of the proposed medication treatment sequences is that the quantity and quality of evidence supporting each recommendation varies considerably. The funding sources may include industry (which adds potential bias in favor of the sponsor's product), government, or both in differing ratios.

It is important for prescribers to remember that all available antidepressants work by similar mechanisms. It is therefore not surprising that STAR*D found that after patients have failed a couple of trials, the odds of responding become much lower, and any remissions are likely to have a high risk of not being maintained. This algorithm offers an organized and efficient approach to early medication selection from among the best supported and safest options available, while also taking in account that medical and other comorbidities might be the primary problem (with the depression secondary).

Our mission as medical providers is to provide patients with an understanding of the existing evidence, including an analysis of risks and benefits, and to help them make an informed decision about what treatments to try. This noncommercial, evidence-informed informational heuristic, which includes specific opportunities for patients to contribute to decision making, can be used by clinicians to guide such discussions.

Declaration of interest: The authors report no conflicts of interest. The authors alone are responsible for the content and writing of the article.

We would like to thank Benjamin Gonzalez, MD, for work on an initial draft; Ronald Pies, MD, for his helpful review; and Rachel Meyen, MD, for researching the evidence on geriatric depression.

REFERENCES

1. World Health Organization. The global burden of disease: 2004 update. Geneva: WHO, 2008.
2. Kessler RC, Chiu WT, Demler O, Merikangas KR, Walters EE. Prevalence, severity, and comorbidity of 12-month DSM-IV disorders in the National Comorbidity Survey Replication. Arch Gen Psychiatry 2005;62:617–27.
3. Olfson M, Blanco C, Marcus SC. Treatment of adult depression in the United States. JAMA Intern Med 2016;176:1482–91.
4. Turner EH, Matthews AM, Linardatos E, Tell RA, Rosenthal R. Selective publication of antidepressant trials and its influence on apparent efficacy. N Engl J Med 2008;358:252–60.
5. Kirsch I. Antidepressant drugs 'work,' but they are not clinically effective. Br J Hosp Med (Lond) 2008;69:359.
6. Kirsch I, Johnson BT. Moving beyond depression: how full is the glass? BMJ 2008;336:629–30.
7. Fountoulakis KN, Moller HJ. Efficacy of antidepressants: a re-analysis and re-interpretation of the Kirsch data. Int J Neuropsychopharmacol 2011;14:405–12.
8. Moller HJ. Isn't the efficacy of antidepressants clinically relevant? A critical comment on the results of the metaanalysis by Kirsch et al. Eur Arch Psychiatry Clin Neurosci 2008;258:451–5.
9. Parker G. Antidepressants on trial: how valid is the evidence? Br J Psychiatry 2009;194:1–3.

10. Zimmerman M. The FDA's failure to address the lack of generalisability of antidepressant efficacy trials in product labelling. Br J Psychiatry 2016;208:512–4.

11. Denton WH, Carmody TJ, Rush AJ, et al. Dyadic discord at baseline is associated with lack of remission in the acute treatment of chronic depression. Psychol Med 2010;40:415–24.

12. Jain R, Maletic V, McIntyre RS. Diagnosing and treating patients with mixed features. J Clin Psychiatry 2017;78:1091–102.

13. Pacchiarotti I, Bond DJ, Baldessarini RJ, et al. The International Society for Bipolar Disorders (ISBD) task force report on antidepressant use in bipolar disorders. Am J Psychiatry 2013;170:1249–62.

14. Fava M, Rush AJ, Alpert JE, et al. Difference in treatment outcome in outpatients with anxious versus nonanxious depression: a STAR*D report. Am J Psychiatry 2008;165:342–51.

15. Davies SJ, Jackson PR, Potokar J, Nutt DJ. Treatment of anxiety and depressive disorders in patients with cardiovascular disease. BMJ 2004;328:939–43.

16. Rush AJ, Trivedi MH, Wisniewski SR, et al. Acute and longer- term outcomes in depressed outpatients requiring one or several treatment steps: a STAR*D report. Am J Psychiatry 2006;163:1905–17.

17. Zimmerman M, Thongy T. How often do SSRIs and other new-generation antidepressants lose their effect during continuation treatment? Evidence suggesting the rate of true tachyphylaxis during continuation treatment is low. J Clin Psychiatry 2007;68:1271–6.

18. O'Donnell M. A sceptic's medical dictionary. London: BMJ, 1997.

19. Osser DN, Patterson RD. Algorithms for the pharmacotherapy of depression, parts one and two. Dir Psychiatry 1998;18: 303–34.

20. Hripcsak G, Ryan PB, Duke JD, et al. Characterizing treatment pathways at scale using the OHDSI network. Proc Natl Acad Sci U S A 2016;113:7329–36.

21. Adli M, Wiethoff K, Baghai TC, et al. How effective is algorithm-guided treatment for depressed inpatients? Results from the randomized controlled multicenter German Algorithm Project 3 trial. Int J Neuropsychopharmacol 2017;20: 721–30.

22. Trivedi MH, Rush AJ, Crismon ML, et al. Clinical results for patients with major depressive disorder in the Texas Medication Algorithm Project. Arch Gen Psychiatry 2004;61:669–80.

23. Nakagawa A, Mitsuda D, Sado M, et al. Effectiveness of supplementary cognitive-behavioral therapy for pharmacotherapy-resistant depression: a randomized controlled trial. J Clin Psychiatry 2017;78:1126–35.

24. Davidson JR, Zhang W, Connor KM, et al. A psychopharmacological treatment algorithm for generalised anxiety disorder (GAD). J Psychopharmacol 2010;24:3–26.

25. Mohammad O, Osser DN. The psychopharmacology algorithm project at the Harvard South Shore Program: an algorithm for acute mania. Harv Rev Psychiatry 2014;22:274–94.

26. Ansari A, Osser DN. The psychopharmacology algorithm project at the Harvard South Shore Program: an update on bipolar depression. Harv Rev Psychiatry 2010;18:36–55.

27. Bajor LA, Ticlea AN, Osser DN. The Psychopharmacology Algorithm Project at the Harvard South Shore Program: an update on posttraumatic stress disorder. Harv Rev Psychiatry 2011;19:240–58.

28. Hamoda HM, Osser DN. The Psychopharmacology Algorithm Project at the Harvard South Shore Program: an update on psychotic depression. Harv Rev Psychiatry 2008;16:235–47.

29. Osser DN, Roudsari MJ, Manschreck T. The Psychopharmacology Algorithm Project at the Harvard South Shore Program: an update on schizophrenia. Harv Rev Psychiatry 2013;21:18–40.

30. Osser DN. A systematic approach to the classification and pharmacotherapy of nonpsychotic major depression and dysthymia. J Clin Psychopharmacol 1993;13:133–44.

31. Crismon ML, Trivedi M, Pigott TA, et al. The Texas Medication Algorithm Project: report of the Texas Consensus Conference Panel on Medication Treatment of Major Depressive Disorder. J Clin Psychiatry 1999;60:142–56.

32. Bauer M, Pfennig A, Severus E, et al. World Federation of Societies of Biological Psychiatry (WFSBP) guidelines for biological treatment of unipolar depressive disorders, part 1: update 2013 on the acute and continuation treatment of unipolar depressive disorders. World J Biol Psychiatry 2013;14:334–85.

33. Kennedy SH, Lam RW, McIntyre RS, et al. Canadian Network for Mood and Anxiety Treatments (CANMAT) 2016 clinical guidelines for the management of adults with major depressive disorder: section 3. Pharmacological treatments. Can J Psychiatry 2016;61:540–60.

34. McIntyre RS, Suppes T, Tandon R, Ostacher M. Florida Best Practice Psychotherapeutic Medication Guidelines for adults with major depressive disorder. J Clin Psychiatry 2017;78: 703–13.

35. American Psychiatric Association. Diagnostic and statistical manual of mental disorders. 5th ed. Arlington, VA: American Psychiatric Publishing, 2013.

36. Trivedi MH, Thase ME, Fava M, et al. Adjunctive aripiprazole in major depressive disorder: analysis of efficacy and safety in patients with anxious and atypical features. J Clin Psychiatry 2008;69:1928–36.

37. Carney RM, Freedland KE. Treatment-resistant depression and mortality after acute coronary syndrome. Am J Psychiatry 2009;166:410–7.

38. Glassman AH, O'Connor CM, Califf RM, et al. Sertraline treatment of major depression in patients with acute MI or unstable angina. JAMA 2002;288:701–9.

39. Kang HJ, Bae KY, Kim SW, et al. Associations between serotonergic genes and escitalopram treatment responses in patients with depressive disorder and acute coronary syndrome: the EsDEPACS Study. Psychiatry Investig 2016;13:157–60.

40. Walther CP, Shah AA, Winkelmayer WC. Treating depression in patients with advanced CKD: beyond the generalizability frontier. JAMA 2017;318:1873–4.

41. Thanacoody HK, Thomas SH. Tricyclic antidepressant poisoning: cardiovascular toxicity. Toxicol Rev 2005;24:205–14.

42. Vieweg WV, Hasnain M, Howland RH, et al. Citalopram, QTc interval prolongation, and torsade de pointes. How should we apply the recent FDA ruling? Am J Med 2012;125:859–68.

43. Paton C, Ferrier IN. SSRIs and gastrointestinal bleeding. BMJ 2005;331:529–30.

44. Na KS, Jung HY, Cho SJ, Cho SE. Can we recommend mirtazapine and bupropion for patients at risk for bleeding? A systematic review and meta-analysis. J Affect Disord 2018; 225:221–6.

45. Mead GE, Hsieh CF, Lee R, et al. Selective serotonin reuptake inhibitors (SSRIs) for stroke recovery. Cochrane Database Syst Rev 2012;11:CD009286.

46. Picker L, Van Den Eede F, Dumont G, Moorkens G, Sabbe BG. Antidepressants and the risk of hyponatremia: a class-by-class review of literature. Psychosomatics 2014;55:536–47.

47. Thorlund K, Druyts E, Wu P, Balijepalli C, Keohane D, Mills E. Comparative efficacy and safety of selective serotonin reuptake inhibitors and serotonin-norepinephrine reuptake inhibitors in older adults: a network meta-analysis. J Am Geriatr Soc 2015;63: 1002–9.

48. Naples JG, Kotlarczyk MP, Perera S, Greenspan SL, Hanlon JT. Non-tricyclic and non-selective serotonin reuptake inhibitor antidepressants and recurrent falls in frail older women. Am J Geriatr Psychiatry 2016;24:1221–7.

49. Kellner CH, Husain MM, Knapp RG, et al. Right unilateral ultrabrief pulse ECT in geriatric depression: phase 1 of the PRIDE study. Am J Psychiatry 2016;173:1101–9.

50. Fenske JN, Petersen K. Obsessive-compulsive disorder: diagnosis and management. Am Fam Physician 2015;92:896–903.

51. Lavretsky H, Reinlieb M, St Cyr N, Siddarth P, Ercoli LM, Senturk D. Citalopram, methylphenidate, or their combination in geriatric depression: a randomized, double-blind, placebo-controlled trial. Am J Psychiatry 2015;172:561–9.

52. Bennett HA, Einarson A, Taddio A, Koren G, Einarson TR. Prevalence of depression during pregnancy: systematic review. Obstet Gynecol 2004;103:698–709.

53. Cohen LS, Altshuler LL, Harlow BL, et al. Relapse of major depression during pregnancy in women who maintain or discontinue antidepressant treatment. JAMA 2006;295: 499–507.

54. Addis A, Koren G. Safety of fluoxetine during the first trimester of pregnancy: a meta-analytical review of epidemiological studies. Psychol Med 2000;30:89–94.

55. Kieler H, Artama M, Engeland A, et al. Selective serotonin reuptake inhibitors during pregnancy and risk of persistent pulmonary hypertension in the newborn: population based cohort study from the five Nordic countries. BMJ 2012;344:d8012.

56. Brown AS, Gyllenberg D, Malm H, et al. Association of selective serotonin reuptake inhibitor exposure during pregnancy with speech, scholastic, and motor disorders in offspring. JAMA Psychiatry 2016;73:1163–70.

57. Reefhuis J, Devine O, Friedman JM, Louik C, Honein MA; National Birth Defects Prevention Study. Specific SSRIs and birth defects: Bayesian analysis to interpret new data in the context of previous reports. BMJ 2015;351:h3190.

58. Coryell W. A medication for depression with mixed features. Am J Psychiatry 2016;173:315–6.

59. Suppes T, Silva R, Cucchiaro J, et al. Lurasidone for the treatment of major depressive disorder with mixed features: a randomized, double-blind, placebo-controlled study. Am J Psychiatry 2016;173:400–7.

60. Thase ME, Demyttenaere K, Earley WR, Gustafsson U, Udd M, Eriksson H. Extended release quetiapine fumarate in major depressive disorder: analysis in patients with anxious depression. Depress Anxiety 2012;29:574–86.

61. Pringsheim T, Gardner D, Patten SB. Adjunctive treatment with quetiapine for major depressive disorder: are the benefits of treatment worth the risks? BMJ 2015;350:h569.

62. Anderson IM. SSRIs versus tricyclic antidepressants in depressed inpatients: a meta-analysis of efficacy and tolerability. Depress Anxiety 1998;7 suppl 1:11–7.

63. Guelfi JD, Ansseau M, Timmerman L, Kørsgaard S; MirtazapineVenlafaxine Study Group. Mirtazapine versus venlafaxine in hospitalized severely depressed patients with melancholic features. J Clin Psychopharmacol 2001;21:425–31.

64. Husain MM, Rush AJ, Fink M, et al. Speed of response and remission in major depressive disorder with acute electroconvulsive therapy (ECT): a Consortium for Research in ECT (CORE) report. J Clin Psychiatry 2004;65:485–91.

65. Schulze-Rauschenbach SC, Harms U, Schlaepfer TE, Maier W, Falkai P, Wagner M. Distinctive neurocognitive effects of repetitive transcranial magnetic stimulation and electroconvulsive therapy in major depression. Br J Psychiatry 2005;186: 410–6.

66. Sackeim HA, Prudic J, Devanand DP, et al. A prospective, randomized, double-blind comparison of bilateral and right unilateral electroconvulsive therapy at different stimulus intensities. Arch Gen Psychiatry 2000;57:425–34.

67. McCall WV, Reboussin DM, Weiner RD, Sackeim HA. Titrated moderately suprathreshold vs. fixed high-dose right unilateral electroconvulsive therapy: acute antidepressant and cognitive effects. Arch Gen Psychiatry 2000;57:438–44.

68. Kho KH, Zwinderman AH, Blansjaar BA. Predictors for the efficacy of electroconvulsive therapy: chart review of a naturalistic study. J Clin Psychiatry 2005;66:894–9.

69. Sanacora G, Frye MA, McDonald W, et al. A consensus statement on the use of ketamine in the treatment of mood disorders. JAMA Psychiatry 2017;74:399–405.

70. Wilkinson ST, Sanacora G. Considerations on the off-label use of ketamine asa treatment for mood disorders. JAMA 2017;318: 793–4.

71. Wilkinson ST, Toprak M, Turner MS, Levine SP, Katz RB, Sanacora G. A survey of the clinical, off-label use of ketamine as a treatment for psychiatric disorders. Am J Psychiatry 2017;174:695–6.

72. Bjerre J, Fontenay C. Ketamine in melancholic depression. Ugeskr Laeger 2010;172:460–1.

73. Marder SR, Gitlin MJ. A cruel irony for clinicians who treat depression. Am J Psychiatry 2017;174:409–10.

74. White N, Litovitz T, Clancy C. Suicidal antidepressant overdoses: a comparative analysis by antidepressant type. J Med Toxicol 2008;4:238–50.

75. Benkert O, Grunder G, Wetzel H, Hackett D. A randomized, double-blind comparison of a rapidly escalating dose of venlafaxine and imipramine in inpatients with major depression and melancholia. J Psychiatr Res 1996;30:441–51.

76. Guelfi JD, White C, Hackett D, Guichoux JY, Magni G. Effectiveness of venlafaxine in patients hospitalized for major depression and melancholia. J Clin Psychiatry 1995;56: 450–8.

77. Connolly KR, Thase ME. If at first you don't succeed: a review of the evidence for antidepressant augmentation, combination and switching strategies. Drugs 2011;71:43–64.

78. Crossley NA, Bauer M. Acceleration and augmentation of antidepressants with lithium for depressive disorders: two meta-analyses of randomized, placebo-controlled trials. J Clin Psychiatry 2007;68:935–40.

79. Aronson R, Offman HJ, Joffe RT, Naylor CD. Triiodothyronine augmentation in the treatment of refractory depression. A meta-analysis. Arch Gen Psychiatry 1996;53:842–8.

80. Altshuler LL, Bauer M, Frye MA, et al. Does thyroid supplementation accelerate tricyclic antidepressant response? A review and meta-analysis of the literature. Am J Psychiatry 2001;158:1617–22.

81. Nierenberg AA, Fava M, Trivedi MH, et al. A comparison of lithium and T(3) augmentation following two failed medication treatments for depression: a STAR*D report. Am J Psychiatry 2006;163:1519–30; quiz 665.

82. Carvalho AF, Cavalcante JL, Castelo MS, Lima MC. Augmentation strategies for treatment-resistant depression: a literature review. J Clin Pharm Ther 2007;32:415–28.

83. Kirino E. Escitalopram for the management of major depressive disorder: a review of its efficacy, safety, and patient acceptability. Patient Prefer Adherence 2012;6:853–61.

84. Carlat D. Evidence-based somatic treatment of depression in adults. Psychiatr Clin North Am 2012;35:131–42.

85. Garnock-Jones KP, McCormack PL. Escitalopram: a review of its use in the management of major depressive disorder in adults. CNS Drugs 2010;24:769–96.

86. Sanchez C, Reines EH, Montgomery SA. A comparative review of escitalopram, paroxetine, and sertraline: are they all alike? Int Clin Psychopharmacol 2014;29:185–96.

87. Rosenbluth M, Macqueen G, McIntyre RS, et al. The Canadian Network for Mood and Anxiety Treatments (CANMAT) task force recommendations for the management of patients with mood disorders and comorbid personality disorders. Ann Clin Psychiatry 2012;24:56–68.

88. McIntyre RS, Alsuwaidan M, Goldstein BI, et al. The Canadian Network for Mood and Anxiety Treatments (CANMAT) task force recommendations for the management of patients with mood disorders and comorbid metabolic disorders. Ann Clin Psychiatry 2012;24:69–81.

89. Ramasubbu R, Taylor VH, Samaan Z, et al. The Canadian Network for Mood and Anxiety Treatments (CANMAT) task force recommendations for the management of patients with mood disorders and select comorbid medical conditions. Ann Clin Psychiatry 2012;24:91–109.

90. Cleare A, Pariante CM, Young AH, et al. Evidence-based guidelines for treating depressive disorders with antidepressants: a revision of the 2008 British Association for Psychopharmacology guidelines. J Psychopharmacol 2015;29:459–525.

91. Cipriani A, Furukawa TA, Salanti G, et al. Comparative efficacy and acceptability of 12 new-generation antidepressants: a multiple-treatments meta-analysis. Lancet 2009;373:746–58.

92. Cipriani A, Furukawa TA, Salanti G, et al. Comparative efficacy and acceptability of 21 antidepressant drugs for the acute treatment of adults with major depressive disorder: a systematic review and network meta-analysis. Lancet 2018;391:1357–66.

93. Sung SC, Haley CL, Wisniewski SR, et al. The impact of chronic depression on acute and long-term outcomes in a randomized trial comparing selective serotonin reuptake inhibitor monotherapy versus each of 2 different antidepressant medication combinations. J Clin Psychiatry 2012;73:967–76.

94. Anderson IM, Ferrier IN, Baldwin RC, et al. Evidence-based guidelines for treating depressive disorders with antidepressants: a revision of the 2000 British Association for Psychopharmacology guidelines. J Psychopharmacol 2008;22:343–96.

95. Zimmerman M, Posternak MA, Attiullah N, et al. Why isn't bupropion the most frequently prescribed antidepressant? J Clin Psychiatry 2005;66:603–10.

96. Trivedi MH, Rush AJ, Carmody TJ, et al. Do bupropion SR and sertraline differ in their effects on anxiety in depressed patients? J Clin Psychiatry 2001;62:776–81.

97. Dunner DL, Zisook S, Billow AA, Batey SR, Johnston JA, Ascher JA. A prospective safety surveillance study for bupropion sustained-release in the treatment of depression. J Clin Psychiatry 1998;59:366–73.

98. Tripp AC. Bupropion, a brief history of seizure risk. Gen Hosp Psychiatry 2010;32:216–7.

99. Mohamed S, Johnson GR, Chen P, et al. Effect of antidepressant switching vs. augmentation on remission among patients with major depressive disorder unresponsive to antidepressant treatment: the VAST-D randomized clinical trial. JAMA 2017; 318:132–45.

100. Gandhi TK, Weingart SN, Borus J, et al. Adverse drug events in ambulatory care. N Engl J Med 2003;348:1556–64.

101. Serretti A, Chiesa A. Treatment-emergent sexual dysfunction related to antidepressants: a meta-analysis. J Clin Psychopharmacol 2009;29:259–66.

102. Montejo AL, Llorca G, Izquierdo JA, Rico-Villademoros F. Incidence of sexual dysfunction associated with antidepressant agents: a prospective multicenter study of 1022 outpatients. Spanish Working Group for the Study of Psychotropic-Related Sexual Dysfunction. J Clin Psychiatry 2001;62 suppl 3:10–21.

103. Fava M, Nurnberg HG, Seidman SN, et al. Efficacy and safety of sildenafil in men with serotonergic antidepressant-associated erectile dysfunction: results from a randomized, double-blind, placebo-controlled trial. J Clin Psychiatry 2006;67:240–6.

104. Moon CA, Laws D, Stott PC, Hayes G. Efficacy and tolerability of controlled-release trazodone in depression: a large multicentre study in general practice. Curr Med Res Opin 1990;12:160–8.

105. Frampton JE. Vortioxetine: a review in cognitive dysfunction in depression. Drugs 2016;76:1675–82.

106. McIntyre RS, Florea I, Tonnoir B, Loft H, Lam RW, Christensen MC. Efficacy of vortioxetine on cognitive functioning in working patients with major depressive disorder. J Clin Psychiatry 2017;78:115–21.

107. Spielmans GI. Duloxetine does not relieve painful physical symptoms in depression: a meta-analysis. Psychother Psychosom 2008;77:12–6.

108. Gebhardt S, Heinzel-Gutenbrunner M, Konig U. Pain relief in depressive disorders: a meta-analysis of the effects of antidepressants. J Clin Psychopharmacol 2016;36:658–68.

109. Leong C, Alessi-Severini S, Enns MW, et al. Cerebrovascular, cardiovascular, and mortality events in new users of selective serotonin reuptake inhibitors and serotonin norepinephrine reuptake inhibitors: a propensity score-matched population-based study. J Clin Psychopharmacol 2017;37:332–40.

110. Safer DJ. Raising the minimum effective dose of serotonin reuptake inhibitor antidepressants: adverse drug events. J Clin Psychopharmacol 2016;36:483–91.

111. Uher R, Mors O, Rietschel M, et al. Early and delayed onset of response to antidepressants in individual trajectories of change during treatment of major depression: a secondary analysis of data from the Genome-Based Therapeutic Drugs for Depression (GENDEP) study. J Clin Psychiatry 2011;72:1478–84.

112. Nelson JC. Treatment of antidepressant nonresponders: augmentation or switch? J Clin Psychiatry 1998;59 suppl 15: 35–41.

113. Gaynes BN, Dusetzina SB, Ellis AR, et al. Treating depression after initial treatment failure: directly comparing switch and augmenting strategies in STAR*D. J Clin Psychopharmacol 2012;32:114–9.

114. Quitkin FM, McGrath PJ, Stewart JW, et al. Remission rates with 3 consecutive antidepressant trials: effectiveness for depressed outpatients. J Clin Psychiatry 2005;66:670–6.

115. Papakostas GI, Fava M, Thase ME. Treatment of SSRI- resistant depression: a meta-analysis comparing within- versus across-class switches. Biol Psychiatry 2008;63:699–704.

116. Ruhe HG, Huyser J, Swinkels JA, Schene AH. Switching antidepressants after a first selective serotonin reuptake inhibitor in major depressive disorder: a systematic review. J Clin Psychiatry 2006;67:1836–55.

117. Souery D, Serretti A, Calati R, et al. Switching antidepressant class does not improve response or remission in treatmentresistant depression. J Clin Psychopharmacol 2011;31:512–6.

118. Bschor T, Baethge C. No evidence for switching the antidepressant: systematic review and meta-analysis of RCTs of a common therapeutic strategy. Acta Psychiatr Scand 2010;121:174–9.

119. Bauer M, Tharmanathan P, Volz HP, Moeller HJ, Freemantle N. The effect of venlafaxine compared with other antidepressants and placebo in the treatment of major depression: a metaanalysis. Eur Arch Psychiatry Clin Neurosci 2009;259:172–85.

120. Smith D, Dempster C, Glanville J, Freemantle N, Anderson I. Efficacy and tolerability of venlafax-ine compared with selective serotonin reuptake inhibitors and other antidepressants: a meta-analysis. Br J Psychiatry 2002;180:396–404.

121. Rudolph RL, Feiger AD. A double-blind, randomized, placebo-controlled trial of once-daily venlafaxine extended release (XR) and fluoxetine for the treatment of depression. J Affect Disord 1999;56:171–81.

122. Leinonen E, Skarstein J, Behnke K, Agren H, Helsdingen JT. Efficacy and tolerability of mirtazapine versus citalopram: a double-blind, randomized study in patients with major depressive disorder. Nordic Antidepressant Study Group. Int Clin Psychopharmacol 1999;14:329–37.

123. Watanabe N, Omori IM, Nakagawa A, et al. Mirtazapine versus other antidepressants in the acute-phase treatment of adults with major depression: systematic review and meta-analysis. J Clin Psychiatry 2008;69:1404–15.

124. Schutter DJ, van Honk J. A framework for targeting alternative brain regions with repetitive transcranial magnetic stimulation in the treatment of depression. J Psychiatry Neurosci 2005;30: 91–7.

125. Seminowicz DA, Mayberg HS, McIntosh AR, et al. Limbic- frontal circuitry in major depression: a path modeling metanalysis. Neuroimage 2004;22:409–18.

126. Eranti S, Mogg A, Pluck G, et al. A randomized, controlled trial with 6-month follow-up of repetitive transcranial magnetic stimulation and electroconvulsive therapy for severe depression. Am J Psychiatry 2007;164:73–81.

127. O'Reardon JP, Cristancho P, Pilania P, Bapatla KB, Chuai S, Peshek AD. Patients with a major depres-sive episode responding to treatment with repetitive transcranial magnetic stimulation (rTMS) are resis-tant to the effects of rapid tryptophan depletion. Depress Anxiety 2007;24:537–44.

128. Sharma A, Gerbarg P, Bottiglieri T, et al. S-adenosylmethionine (SAMe) for neuropsychiatric disorders: a clinician-oriented review of research. J Clin Psychiatry 2017;78:e656-e67.

129. Linde K, Berner MM, Kriston L. St John's wort for major depression. Cochrane Database Syst Rev 2008;(4):CD000448.

130. Papakostas GI, Shelton RC, Zajecka JM, et al. L-methylfolate as adjunctive therapy for SSRI-resistant major depression: results of two randomized, double-blind, parallel-sequential trials. Am J Psychiatry 2012;169:1267–74.

131. Berk M, Dean OM, Cotton SM, et al. The efficacy of adjunctive N-acetylcysteine in major depressive disorder: a double-blind, randomized, placebo-controlled trial. J Clin Psychiatry 2014;75:628–36.

132. Gertsik L, Poland RE, Bresee C, Rapaport MH. Omega-3 fatty acid augmentation of citalopram treat-ment for patients with major depressive disorder. J Clin Psychopharmacol 2012;32:61–4.

133. Perera S, Eisen R, Bhatt M, et al. Light therapy for nonseasonal depression: systematic review and meta-analysis. BJPsych Open 2016;2:116–26.

134. Sarris J, Murphy J, Mischoulon D, et al. Adjunctive nutraceuticals for depression: a systematic review and meta-analyses. Am J Psychiatry 2016;173:575–87.

135. Jefferson JW. Folate for depression: fabulous facilitator or fantastic flop? Psychopharm Rev 2007;42:75–82.

136. Lam RW, Levitt AJ, Levitan RD, et al. Efficacy of bright light treatment, fluoxetine, and the combina-tion in patients with nonseasonal major depressive disorder: a randomized clinical trial. JAMA Psychia-try 2016;73:56–63.

137. Ostroff RB, Nelson JC. Risperidone augmentation of selective serotonin reuptake inhibitors in major depression. J Clin Psychiatry 1999;60:256–9.

138. Nelson JC, Papakostas GI. Atypical antipsychotic augmentation in major depressive disorder: a meta-analysis of placebocontrolled randomized trials. Am J Psychiatry 2009;166: 980–91.

139. Spielmans GI, Berman MI, Linardatos E, Rosenlicht NZ, Perry A, Tsai AC. Adjunctive atypical antipsy-chotic treatment for major depressive disorder: a meta-analysis of depression, quality of life, and safety outcomes. PLoS Med 2013;10: e1001403.

140. Fava M, Rush AJ, Trivedi MH, et al. Background and rationale for the Sequenced Treatment Alterna-tives to Relieve Depression (STAR*D) study. Psychiatr Clin North Am 2003;26: 457–94, x.

141. Carpenter LL, Yasmin S, Price LH. A double-blind, placebo- controlled study of antidepressant augmentation with mirtazapine. Biol Psychiatry 2002;51:183–8.

142. Carpenter LL, Jocic Z, Hall JM, Rasmussen SA, Price LH. Mirtazapine augmentation in the treatment of refractory depression. J Clin Psychiatry 1999;60:45–9.

143. Atmaca M, Korkmaz S, Topuz M, Mermi O. Mirtazapine augmentation for selective serotonin reuptake inhibitor-induced sexual dysfunction: a retrospective investigation. Psychiatry Investig 2011;8:55–7.

144. Ivanova JI, Birnbaum HG, Kidolezi Y, Subramanian G, Khan SA, Stensland MD. Direct and indirect costs of employees with treatment-resistant and non-treatment-resistant major depressive disorder. Curr Med Res Opin 2010;26:2475–84.

145. Pae CU, Tharwani H, Marks DM, Masand PS, Patkar AA. Atypical depression: a comprehensive review. CNS Drugs 2009;23:1023–37.

146. Joyce PR, Mulder RT, Luty SE, et al. Patterns and predictors of remission, response and recovery in major depression treated with fluoxetine or nortriptyline. Aust N Z J Psychiatry 2002; 36:384–91.

147. Sogaard J, Lane R, Latimer P, et al. A 12-week study comparing moclobemide and sertraline in the treatment of outpatients with atypical depression. J Psychopharmacol 1999; 13:406–14.

148. Henkel V, Mergl R, Allgaier AK, Kohnen R, Moller HJ, Hegerl U. Treatment of depression with atypical features: a meta-analytic approach. Psychiatry Res 2006;141:89–101.

149. Stewart JW, Tricamo E, McGrath PJ, Quitkin FM. Prophylactic efficacy of phenelzine and imipramine in chronic atypical depression: likelihood of recurrence on discontinuation after 6 months' remission. Am J Psychiatry 1997;154:31–6.

150. Rabkin J, Quitkin F, Harrison W, Tricamo E, McGrath P. Adverse reactions to monoamine oxidase inhibitors. Part I. A comparative study. J Clin Psychopharmacol 1984;4:270–8.

151. Patkar AA, Pae CU, Masand PS. Transdermal selegiline: the new generation of monoamine oxidase inhibitors. CNS Spectr 2006;11:363–75.

152. Rapaport MH, Thase ME. Translating the evidence on atypical depression into clinical practice. J Clin Psychiatry 2007; 68:e11.

153. Stahl SM. Prescriber's guide: Stahl's essential psychopharmacology. 6th ed. Cambridge: Cambridge University Press, 2017:663.

154. Asnis GM, Henderson MA. EMSAM (deprenyl patch): how a promising antidepressant was underutilized. Neuropsychiatr Dis Treat 2014;10:1911–23.

155. Becker ME, Hertzberg MA, Moore SD, Dennis MF, Bukenya DS, Beckham JC. A placebo-controlled trial of bupropion SR in the treatment of chronic posttraumatic stress disorder. J Clin Psychopharmacol 2007;27:193–7.

156. Fava M. Lessons learned from the VA Augmentation and Switching Treatments for Improving Depression Outcomes (VAST-D) study. JAMA 2017;318:126–8.

157. Baldomero EB, Ubago JG, Cercos CL, Ruiloba JV, Calvo CG, Lopez RP. Venlafaxine extended release versus conventional antidepressants in the remission of depressive disorders after previous antidepressant failure: ARGOS study. Depress Anxiety 2005;22:68–76.

158. Thase ME, Rush AJ, Howland RH, et al. Double-blind switch study of imipramine or sertraline treatment of antidepressant resistant chronic depression. Arch Gen Psychiatry 2002;59: 233–9.

159. Blier P, Ward HE, Tremblay P, Laberge L, Hebert C, Bergeron R. Combination of antidepressant medications from treatment initiation for major depressive disorder: a double-blind randomized study. Am J Psychiatry 2010;167:281–8.

160. Rasmussen KG, Mueller M, Knapp RG, et al. Antidepressant medication treatment failure does not predict lower remission with ECT for major depressive disorder: a report from the Consortium for Research in Electroconvulsive Therapy. J Clin Psychiatry 2007;68:1701–6.

161. Dombrovski AY, Mulsant BH, Haskett RF, Prudic J, Begley AE, Sackeim HA. Predictors of remission after electroconvulsive therapy in unipolar major depression. J Clin Psychiatry 2005;66:1043–9.

162. Briley M, Moret C. Treatment of comorbid pain with serotonin norepinephrine reuptake inhibitors. CNS Spectr 2008;13: 22–6.

163. Philipp M, Fickinger M. Psychotropic drugs in the management of chronic pain syndromes. Pharmacopsychiatry 1993;26: 221–34.

164. Rintala DH, Holmes SA, Courtade D, Fiess RN, Tastard LV, Loubser PG. Comparison of the effectiveness of amitriptyline and gabapentin on chronic neuropathic pain in persons with spinal cord injury. Arch Phys Med Rehabil 2007;88:1547–60.

165. Finnerup NB, Otto M, McQuay HJ, Jensen TS, Sindrup SH. Algorithm for neuropathic pain treatment: an evidence-based proposal. Pain 2005;118:289–305.

166. Bech P, Gormsen L, Loldrup D, Lunde M. The clinical effect of clomipramine in chronic idiopathic pain disorder revisited using the Spielberger State Anxiety Symptom Scale (SSASS) as outcome scale. J Affect Disord 2009;119:43–51.

167. Perahia DG, Pritchett YL, Desaiah D, Raskin J. Efficacy of duloxetine in painful symptoms: an analgesic or antidepressant effect? Int Clin Psychopharmacol 2006;21:311–7.

168. Raskin J, Pritchett YL, Wang F, et al. A double-blind, randomized multicenter trial comparing duloxetine with placebo in the management of diabetic peripheral neuropathic pain. Pain Med 2005;6:346–56.

169. Arnold LM, Pritchett YL, D'Souza DN, Kajdasz DK, Iyengar S, Wernicke JF. Duloxetine for the treatment of fibromyalgia in women: pooled results from two randomized, placebo-controlled clinical trials. J Womens Health (Larchmt) 2007;16:1145–56.

170. Brecht S, Courtecuisse C, Debieuvre C, et al. Efficacy and safety of duloxetine 60 mg once daily in the treatment of pain in patients with major depressive disorder and at least moderate pain of unknown etiology: a randomized controlled trial. J Clin Psychiatry 2007;68:1707–16.

171. Freeman R, Durso-Decruz E, Emir B. Efficacy, safety, and tolerability of pregabalin treatment for painful diabetic peripheral neuropathy: findings from seven randomized, controlled trials across a range of doses. Diabetes Care 2008;31: 1448–54.

172. Wiffen PJ, McQuay HJ, Edwards JE, Moore RA. Gabapentin for acute and chronic pain. Cochrane Database Syst Rev 2011;(3):CD005452.

173. Moore RA, Wiffen PJ, Derry S, McQuay HJ. Gabapentin for chronic neuropathic pain and fibromyalgia in adults. Cochrane Database Syst Rev 2011;(3):CD007938.

174. Bloch MH, McGuire J, Landeros-Weisenberger A, Leckman JF, Pittenger C. Meta-analysis of the dose-response relationship of SSRI in obsessive-compulsive disorder. Mol Psychiatry 2010;15: 850–5.

175. Dougherty DD, Rauch SL, Jenike MA. Pharmacotherapy for obsessive-compulsive disorder. J Clin Psychol 2004;60: 1195–202.

176. Tollefson GD, Rampey AHJr, Potvin JH, et al. A multicenter investigation of fixed-dose fluoxetine in the treatment of obsessive-compulsive disorder. Arch Gen Psychiatry 1994;51: 559–67.

177. Veale D, Miles S, Smallcombe N, Ghezai H, Goldacre B, Hodsoll J. Atypical antipsychotic augmentation in SSRI treatment refractory obsessive-compulsive disorder: a systematic review and meta-analysis. BMC Psychiatry 2014;14:317.

178. Wilens TE, Morrison NR, Prince J. An update on the pharmacotherapy of attention-deficit/hyperactivity disorder in adults. Expert Rev Neurother 2011;11:1443–65.

179. Nuijten M, Blanken P, van de Wetering B, Nuijen B, van den Brink W, Hendriks VM. Sustained-release dexamfetamine in the treatment of chronic cocaine-dependent patients on heroin-assisted treatment: a randomised, double-blind, placebo- controlled trial. Lancet 2016;387:2226–34.

180. McIntyre RS, Lee Y, Zhou AJ, et al. The efficacy of psychostimulants in major depressive episodes: a systematic review and meta-analysis. J Clin Psychopharmacol 2017;37:412–8.

181. Rosler M, Retz W, Fischer R, et al. Twenty-four-week treatment with extended release methylphenidate improves emotional symptoms in adult ADHD. World J Biol Psychiatry 2010;11:709–18.

182. Wernicke JF, Adler L, Spencer T, et al. Changes in symptoms and adverse events after discontinuation of atomoxetine in children and adults with attention deficit/hyperactivity disorder: a prospective, placebo-controlled assessment. J Clin Psychopharmacol 2004;24:30–5.

183. Wilens TE, Haight BR, Horrigan JP, et al. Bupropion XL in adults with attention-deficit/hyperactivity disorder: a randomized, placebo-controlled study. Biol Psychiatry 2005;57: 793–801.

184. Wilens TE, Biederman J, Mick E, Spencer TJ. A systematic assessment of tricyclic antidepressants in the treatment of adult attention-deficit hyperactivity disorder. J Nerv Ment Dis 1995;183:48–50.
185. Hornig-Rohan M, Amsterdam JD. Venlafaxine versus stimulant therapy in patients with dual diagnosis ADD and depression. Prog Neuropsychopharmacol Biol Psychiatry 2002;26: 585–9.
186. Adler LA, Resnick S, Kunz M, Devinsky O. Open-label trial of venlafaxine in adults with attention deficit disorder. Psychopharmacol Bull 1995;31:785–8.
187. Raskind MA, Peterson K, Williams T, et al. A trial of prazosin for combat trauma PTSD with nightmares in active-duty soldiers returned from Iraq and Afghanistan. Am J Psychiatry 192. 2013;170:1003–10.
188. De Jong J, Wauben P, Huijbrechts I, Oolders H, Haffmans J. 193. Doxazosin treatment for posttraumatic stress disorder. J Clin Psychopharmacol 2010;30:84–5.
189. Aaronson ST, Sears P, Ruvuna F, et al. A 5-year observational study of patients with treatment-resistant depression treated 194. with vagus nerve stimulation or treatment as usual: comparison of response, remission, and suicidality. Am J Psychiatry 195. 2017;174:640–8.
190. Avorn J. The psychology of clinical decision making—implications for medication use. N Engl J Med 2018;378:689–91.
191. Groopman J. How doctors think. Boston: Houghton Mifflin, 2007.
192. Dawes RM, Faust D, Meehl PE. Clinical versus actuarial judgment. Science 1989;243:1668–74.
193. Dawes RM. The robust beauty of improper linear models in decision making. In: Kahneman D, Slovic P, Tversky A, eds. Judgment under uncertainty: heuristics and biases. New York: Cambridge University Press, 1983:391–407.
194. Mullaney TJ. Doctors wielding data. Bus Week 2005;21 Nov: 94,98.
195. Adli M, Bauer M, Rush AJ. Algorithms and collaborative-care systems for depression: are they effective and why? A systematic review. Biol Psychiatry 2006;59:1029–38.
196. Osser D, Patterson R. On the value of evidence-based psychopharmacology algorithms. Bull Clin Psychopharmacol 2013;23: 1–5.

NOTE: There have been a few changes in this text that corrected errors in the original publication. The changes can be obtained from the author upon request.

UPDATE
MAJOR DEPRESSION

The major depression algorithm was published less than 1 year ago, and there have not been significant changes in the recommendations, although there have been some new studies that add to the evidence base supporting basic and specific recommendations. There have also been developments with ketamine and particularly its S-enantiomer "esketamine" that require discussion. The published algorithm did propose a role for intravenous ketamine for severely ill inpatients with melancholia if electroconvulsive therapy (ECT) is ineffective or refused. Another development is the release and marketing of the ™GeneSight genetic test for predicting antidepressant response.

Esketamine for Treatment-Resistant Depression?

Esketamine in the form of a nasal spray was approved by the U.S. Food and Drug Administration (FDA) as an augmentation of antidepressants for treatment-resistant depression (TRD) in June of 2019. It is expensive, with a retail price of $7000–$10,600 for the labeled initial 2-month treatment course.[1] The history of studies leading to this approval is complicated.[2] There was a need to balance concerns about potential harms, including abuse potential (ketamine was known on the street as "Special K" because of its dissociative effects), hypertension (transient increases of 40 mm Hg can occur), risk of suicide, and sedation. The FDA approved it with a Risk Evaluation and Mitigation Strategy (REMS) requiring that it be given only in major clinical centers where the patient can be observed for 2 hours after each administration. It was tested and approved as an augmentation of an antidepressant, because it was considered unethical to treat patients with a serious illness like TRD without a potentially effective treatment on board. TRD has many definitions. In our algorithm, it is defined as failure to respond satisfactorily to two adequate trials of antidepressant therapy (either successive monotherapies or a single antidepressant followed by an evidence-supported augmentation trial). In the esketamine studies, TRD was defined as two adequate trials (one of those was observed prospectively). There were many exclusion criteria: psychosis, bipolar disorder, personality disorders, moderate or severe substance use disorders within the past 6 months or a positive recent screen, and obsessive-compulsive disorder. Some of the excluded depressed patients could be covered by the algorithms in this book for bipolar depression and psychotic depression.

A commentary on the esketamine studies leading to FDA approval by Alan Schatzberg in the *American Journal of Psychiatry* is telling and had more questions than answers.[3] Although easier to administer than intravenous ketamine, the efficacy of esketamine in some of the studies was marginal. It was unclear how long it should be prescribed (in addition to the antidepressant) and what to do if effectiveness was lost. There were some suggestions that patients can relapse rapidly, and might become suicidal. Significant concern was also expressed about the mechanism of action: Is it an opiate receptor-mediated effect and will abusability issues become more and more evident as we gain more experience with esketamine?[4] The 12-week maintenance followed by discontinuation trial recently published was somewhat reassuring in that regard,[5] but the patients enrolled mostly had only one or two previous antidepressant trials, and the antidepressants to which the esketamine was added were suboptimally dosed. Thus, it is not clear if a higher dose of the antidepressants or another augmentation strategy would have been as effective, according to a comment by Steven Dubovsky in the *New England Journal of Medicine Journal Watch Psychiatry* newsletter, December 2019.

Another concern regarding abuse potential is whether depressed patients, when they no longer have access to ketamine or esketamine, might turn to opiates or other abusable drugs or illegal ketamine.[6] Evidently, the registries that have been set up do not capture this information.

In conclusion, regarding esketamine, it does not appear to be ready to replace any of our favored switches or augmentations for the second or even the third trial in the algorithm. The evidence-base is rapidly evolving and should be followed closely, but at this time esketamine seems to belong in the algorithm only at the end after at least several reasonably conducted antidepressant trials have been completed.

Table 1: Comorbidities and other features in major depression and how they affect the algorithm

The last item in this table is depression with anxious distress. We noted that in STAR*D and other studies, this is a common comorbidity and it is associated with poorer response to antidepressants and most augmenters. Sedating second-generation or "atypical" antipsychotics such as quetiapine can be effective as augmenters in this diagnostic situation, but they bring a significant side-effect burden. Aripiprazole, which is less sedating, is another option. We failed to mention the option of adding a benzodiazepine. They have their own burden of side effects of course, and they were not utilized in STAR*D, but there is an older literature suggesting that they may enhance depression outcome in some patients. In a meta-analysis published in 2001, of 9 studies involving 697 subjects,[7] the rate of response of depression (response = 50% reduction in rating scale scores) with an added benzodiazepine was 63% versus 38% with the antidepressant alone. Number needed to treat (NNT) was 4. These were all short-term studies of 4–8 weeks so the long-term risks of the combination could not be known, but they certainly might include dependence on the benzodiazepine and accident proneness.

Node 4B: If Response to the First Antidepressant Trial Is Unsatisfactory, Try One of These

Four options for switching and four options for augmenting were offered. No clear differences in efficacy could be discerned from the evidence base, so the choice would be heavily influenced by what side effects and costs would be involved for the individual patient. Patient preference has always been important, but was even more so at this step in the algorithm. To reiterate, the switching choices were (1) to a different agent from the Node 4 first-line choices (sertraline, escitalopram, or bupropion); (2) to a dual-action agent (venlafaxine or mirtazapine); (3) to repetitive transcranial magnetic stimulation (rTMS); or (4) to S-adenosylmethionine or St. John's wort. The augmentation options were (1) omega-3 fatty acid, L-methylfolate, N-acetylcysteine, or bright light therapy; (2) aripiprazole, quetiapine, or risperidone; (3) an antidepressant (bupropion or mirtazapine); or (4) lithium or triiodothyronine (T3).

A new study compared two augmentations head-to-head in a fairly large open-label trial. A total of 104 patients with severe (Hamilton Depression Rating of 24 or more) major depression (16% inpatients) who had failed to respond to a 10-week trial of imipramine at therapeutic levels were randomized to add-on lithium versus addition of citalopram.[8] About 21% remitted with the lithium compared with 40% with the citalopram over the next 10 weeks, which was a significant difference and had an NNT of 5. Although the order of combining the imipramine and citalopram is reversed from what it would be if one were following the algorithm, the study does suggest that the combination of a selective serotonin reuptake inhibitor (SSRI) and a tricyclic antidepressant is an evidenced option (superior to lithium addition in this study, even though lithium augmentation of tricyclic antidepressants is reasonably evidenced[9]) and could be a third choice added to the bupropion and mirtazapine group. Tricyclics do, however, introduce more side effects than the other two antidepressants.

Node 5B: TRD Without Comorbidities and Without Atypical Features

At this point in the algorithm, the patient has had two adequate antidepressant trials. It was proposed that the prescriber consider some of the eight options for switches and augmentations not yet tried that were offered for the second trial at Node 4B (plus, a few other choices were added). As noted earlier, one of those eight options was rTMS, which is FDA approved after one failed antidepressant trial but not after two failed trials. Many clinicians think rTMS is an evidenced treatment for TRD, but actually the evidence of success with it after two or more failed trials is mostly uncontrolled. There is one large study in civilian patients with a moderate level of treatment resistance (1–4 previous trials, mean of 1.5 trials), which found that 14% receiving rTMS remitted compared to 5% getting sham treatment (statistically significant, NNT of 11).[10] Therefore, although not a particularly impressive option, rTMS was left in the algorithm as an option to consider at Node 5B. However, a new large study of rTMS in U.S. veterans with about the same moderate level of TRD (at least two failed trials) did not find an advantage of rTMS over sham. A total of 164 participants were randomized and

41% remitted with rTMS and 37% with sham (NNT = 25).[11] The reasons for the overall higher rate of remission in the veteran population are difficult to explain; perhaps the complex procedures in both groups had a high placebo effect in this group. Nevertheless, it seemed that the rTMS had at best a very minor impact on their TRD. The authors speculated that advances in the techniques of administering rTMS could have produced better results if the study was to be repeated with those techniques, but a letter to the editor sharply disagreed with concluding the article with that speculation.[1] Further study is needed before giving TMS greater prominence in the algorithm.

It was noted earlier that, in addition to reconsidering the eight switch and augmentation options offered after failure on the first trial, several additional options were added at this point. They were switching to a tricyclic antidepressant, using a combination of venlafaxine and mirtazapine, and ECT. A newly published study from Barcelona, Spain, enhances the evidence for a switch to a tricyclic. Navarro and colleagues developed a sample of 112 patients (90% outpatients) with moderate treatment resistance but with significant severity (Hamilton Depression Ratings of 21 or more) whose last trial was with venlafaxine 225–300 mg daily for 10 weeks.[13] These subjects were randomized (open label) to have mirtazapine added to their venlafaxine versus switching to imipramine with dose adjusted with plasma levels. A total of 71% responded to the imipramine, whereas 39% responded to the mirtazapine addition (NNT = 3 favoring imipramine).

The GeneSight Genetic Test and Other Pharmacogenomic Testing Strategies

In a multicenter randomized trial of this amalgam of 59 genetic tests related to the pharmacogenetics of drug metabolism and pharmacodynamics of 38 medications, the use of the test to select treatment was compared with "treatment as usual" by primary care and psychiatric clinicians.[14] A total of 1541 patients participated. There was no difference in rating scale measures of depression (the primary outcome measure) but secondary outcomes of improvement and remission slightly favored the GeneSight group (NNT of 16 for improvement, 20 for remission). These are differences that are not clinically meaningful. Also, clinicians were not blinded and could have communicated group assignments some of the time, and the study was funded by GeneSight. With all due respect for the clinical acumen and experience of the practitioners in the study, their treatment as usual may not necessarily be evidence supported. These genomic products need to compare their results with the results by clinicians endeavoring to utilize the evidence base as closely as possible, employing algorithms based on the evidence such as the one in this book.[15] None of the studies have done that. Another difficulty is the lack of transparency in these genomic products. There is no reasoning offered for why the test is predicting a particular drug. Indeed, their algorithm of how the computer mixes and matches the gene results to make a prediction is proprietary and a secret. It would seem that clinicians should not cease efforts to stay up-to-date and to practice in accord with the best evidence rather than letting the decisions be made by reasoning that is blinded to the prescriber and patient using costly tests like GeneSight.

REFERENCES

1. Wilkinson ST, Howard DH, Busch SH. Psychiatric practice patterns and barriers to the adoption of esketamine. JAMA 2019;322:1039–40.
2. Kim J, Farchione T, Potter A, Chen Q, Temple R. Esketamine for treatment-resistant depression—first FDA-approved antidepressant in a new class. N Engl J Med 2019;381:1–4.
3. Schatzberg AF. A word to the wise about intranasal esketamine. Am J Psychiatry 2019;176:422–4.
4. George MS. Is there really nothing new under the sun? Is low-dose ketamine a fast-acting antidepressant simply because it is an opioid? Am J Psychiatry 2018;175:1157–8.
5. Daly EJ, Trivedi MH, Janik A, et al. Efficacy of esketamine nasal spray plus oral antidepressant treatment for relapse prevention in patients with treatment-resistant depression: a randomized clinical trial. JAMA Psychiatry 2019;76:893–903.
6. McShane R, Baldwin DS, McAllister-Williams RH, et al. Esketamine and the need for a new type of registry for drugs with abuse potential. Am J Psychiatry 2019;176:966.
7. Furukawa TA, Streiner DL, Young LT. Is antidepressant-benzodiazepine combination therapy clinically more useful? A meta-analytic study. J Affect Disord 2001;65:173–7.
8. Navarro V, Boulahfa I, Obach A, et al. Lithium augmentation versus citalopram combination in imipramine-resistant major depression: a 10-week randomized open-label study. J Clin Psychopharmacol 2019;39:254–7.
9. Thase ME. Therapeutic alternatives for difficult-to-treat depression: a narrative review of the state of the evidence. CNS Spectr 2004;9:808–16, 18–21.
10. George MS, Lisanby SH, Avery D, et al. Daily left prefrontal transcranial magnetic stimulation therapy for major depressive disorder: a sham-controlled randomized trial. Arch Gen Psychiatry 2010;67:507–16.
11. Yesavage JA, Fairchild JK, Mi Z, et al. Effect of repetitive transcranial magnetic stimulation on treatment-resistant major depression in US veterans: a randomized clinical trial. JAMA Psychiatry 2018;75:884–93.
12. Chow ZR. Sham treatment is as effective for treatment-resistant depression as repetitive transcranial magnetic stimulation. JAMA Psychiatry 2019;76:99.
13. Navarro V, Boulahfa I, Obach A, et al. Switching to imipramine versus add-on mirtazapine in venlafaxine-resistant major depression: a 10-week randomized open study. J Clin Psychopharmacol 2019;39:63–6.
14. Greden JF, Parikh SV, Rothschild AJ, et al. Impact of pharmacogenomics on clinical outcomes in major depressive disorder in the GUIDED trial: a large, patient- and rater-blinded, randomized, controlled study. J Psychiatr Res 2019;111:59–67.
15. Zubenko GS, Sommer BR, Cohen BM. On the marketing and use of pharmacogenetic tests for psychiatric treatment. JAMA Psychiatry 2018;75:769–70.

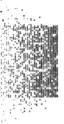

The Psychopharmacology Algorithm Project at the Harvard South Shore Program: 2012 Update on Psychotic Depression

Michael Tang, DO[1] and David N. Osser, MD[2]

Abstract: *The Psychopharmacology Algorithm Project at the Harvard South Shore Program: 2012 Update on Psychotic Depression*

Background: *The Psychopharmacology Algorithm Project at the Harvard South Shore Program (PAPHSS) has published evidence-supported algorithms for the pharmacological treatment of major depressive disorder with psychotic features (psychotic depression) in 1998 and 2008. This article is an update for the 2008 algorithm.*

Method: *Using similar methodology as with the 2008 update, PubMed and EMBASE searches were conducted to identity relevant literature in the English language from November 2007 through July 2012. Articles were evaluated for quality of the data and for whether they provided additional evidence support for previous recommendations or prompted changes to the prior algorithm.*

Results: *Minor changes were made to the algorithm: most prior recommendations were upheld. The most effective treatment for hospitalized, severe psychotic depression patients remains electroconvulsive therapy (ECT). The combination of an antidepressant (tricyclic [TCA], selective serotonin reuptake inhibitor [SSRI], or serotonin-norepinephrine reuptake inhibitor [SNRI]) plus an antipsychotic continues to be the preferred pharmacological modality when ECT is an unavailable/deferred option. Since the last update, new evidence tends to support using venlafaxine ER, a SNRI, as the first choice antidepressant. Regarding the antipsychotic, both olanzapine and quetiapine have new data demonstrating efficacy. Nevertheless, it is suggested that it may be reasonable to try other atypical antipsychotics with more benign safety profiles (e.g. ziprasidone, aripiprazole) as the first choice antipsychotic. New data also suggest at least four months of maintenance therapy is effective. If the first antidepressant-antipsychotic combination produces an unsatisfactory outcome, and ECT is still not acceptable or appropriate, the second pharmacotherapy trial can be with a change in the antidepressant, as was recommended in the 2008 algorithm. After two trials of combination therapy have failed (and, again, ECT is not an option), the algorithm continues to recommend augmentation with lithium. Limited evidence also suggests*

[1]DO, Harvard Medical School; VA Boston Healthcare System, Brockton Division, Brockton, MA
[2]MD, Harvard Medical School; VA Boston Healthcare System, Brockton Division, Brockton, MA
Address reprint requests to: David N. Osser, MD, VA Boston Healthcare System, Brockton Division, 940 Belmont Street, Brockton, MA 02301
Phone: 774-826-1650
Fax: 774-826-1655
E-mail address: David.Osser@va.gov
Date of acceptance: 9 Aralık 2012 / December 9, 2012
Declaration of interest:
M.T., D.N.O.: The authors reported no conflict of interest related to this article.

consideration of a switch to clozapine monotherapy. Augmentation with methylphenidate is a newly mentioned possible option based on very small evidence. When combination therapy is deferred, evidence suggests monotherapy with a TCA may be more effective than an SNRI or SSRI. However, safety issues and possible increased risk of psychosis exacerbation are unfavorable factors for TCA monotherapy. ECT or addition of an antipsychotic should be reconsidered if antidepressant monotherapy failed.

Conclusion: *This heuristic further refines the previous PAPHSS analysis of the available evidence for pharmacological treatment of psychotic depression. The validity of the conclusions is limited by the quality and quantity of the literature available: the number of head-to-head prospective trials in psychotic depression is still relatively small. However, this algorithm may serve as a guide for clinicians in the management of psychotic depression.*

Key words: affective disorders, psychotic, psychotic depression, delusional depression, pharmacological treatment, psychopharmacology

INTRODUCTION

The pharmacological management of psychotic depression has varied among clinicians, and debate regarding the optimum approach is ongoing. The Psychopharmacology Algorithm Project at the Harvard South Shore Program (PAPHSS) created and published evidence-supported heuristics for the use of medication in psychotic depression in 1998 and 2008 (1,2). This article serves as an update to the 2008 algorithm.

It is estimated that psychotic depression occurs in 14%–18% of all patients with depressive episodes (3,4), and in approximately 25% of patients hospitalized for major depressive disorder (5). However, there is evidence of diagnostic instability when patients are followed longitudinally. In a 10-year prospective study by Ruggero and colleagues (6), 80 subjects initially diagnosed with psychotic depression by the DSM-IV criteria were followed. Only 36 (45%) retained the original diagnosis at year 10, while 11 (14%) were diagnosed with bipolar disorder and 33 (41%) had a non-mood disorder at year 10. In another study, Tohen and colleagues conducted a two-year follow up of 56 patients with first-episode psychotic depression (7). Seven dropped out of the study, 29 (59%) retained their initial diagnosis, and the other 20 changed to a diagnosis of either bipolar disorder (14/20) or schizoaffective disorder (6/20). Given such statistics, clinicians should remember that initial diagnosis is only provisional, and the subsequent course may result in a change in diagnosis and in the indicated psychopharmacology.

METHODS

This algorithm update is one of several recently published by the PAPHSS (1, 8-11) and available in condensed format for access on smart phone devices on the website www.psychopharm.mobi. The methods of producing these algorithms have been described in the previous publications. For this psychotic depression update, the authors utilized similar methodology to the 2008 update, in which PubMed and EMBASE searches were conducted to identify relevant studies, meta-analyses, practice guidelines, and reviews in English from November 2007 through July, 2012. Articles were evaluated for the quality of the evidence, and whether they either added support for previous conclusions of the PAPHSS algorithm or called for reconsideration or change of recommendations.

The algorithm is depicted in Figure 1. It focuses on psychopharmacological treatment of psychotic depression and does not address psychotherapy treatment options. Arabic numerals refer to "nodes" in the algorithm flowchart, and each node is reviewed below with discussion of the pertinent evidence and its limitations.

NODE 1: IF SEVERELY ILL, HAVE YOU CONSIDERED ELECTROCONVULSIVE THERAPY?

The algorithm starts with questioning the patient's appropriateness for electroconvulsive therapy (ECT) as the initial treatment. Consistent with the 2008 algorithm, ECT is still to be considered for hospitalized, severely ill patients, as it may be the most effective treatment for psychotic depression. However, the supporting data are all from uncontrolled studies. In an observational study by Petrides and colleagues, 77 subjects with psychotic depression receiving bilateral ECT achieved a remission rate of 95%, based on the 24-item Hamilton Depression Rating Scale (HAM-D-24) versus 83% in nonpsychotic depressed patients; (n=176), $p < .01$ (12). In a chart review comparing 14 patients receiving ECT and 12 unmatched patients receiving antidepressant plus antipsychotic combination, 86% of ECT patients received a favorable overall response as compared to 42% of patients in the combination group ($p < 0.05$) (13). This study had a small sample size, and ECT was compared to different combinations with varying doses and treatment periods.

Other uncontrolled studies found ECT to have better response rates than pharmacological management. Olfson and colleagues found that ECT is more rapidly effective than pharmacotherapy, shortens hospital stays, and reduces treatment costs if initiated within five days of admission (14).

However, ECT still remains to be compared randomly and prospectively in acute treatment with any medication regimen, and the duration of ECT effect still remains unclear (15).

Although this algorithm mainly focuses on acute management of psychotic depression, it is worth noting a new maintenance treatment study by Navarro and colleagues that reflects positively on the role of ECT (16). It was a 2-year randomized, single-blind study of patients age 60 or greater initially treated with ECT and nortriptyline, followed by either nortriptyline monotherapy (n=16) or ECT plus nortriptyline (n=17). The nortriptyline monotherapy group also was given 6 weeks of risperidone up to 2 mg daily. Results showed 5/17 patients on nortriptyline monotherapy did not have a recurrence, as compared to 11/16 in the ECT plus nortriptyline group ($p=0.009$). Both groups had 4 dropouts. Limitations to the study included its small sample size and the inclusion of only older subjects. Also, it would have been of interest to have a comparison group of patients maintained on combined antidepressant plus antipsychotic.

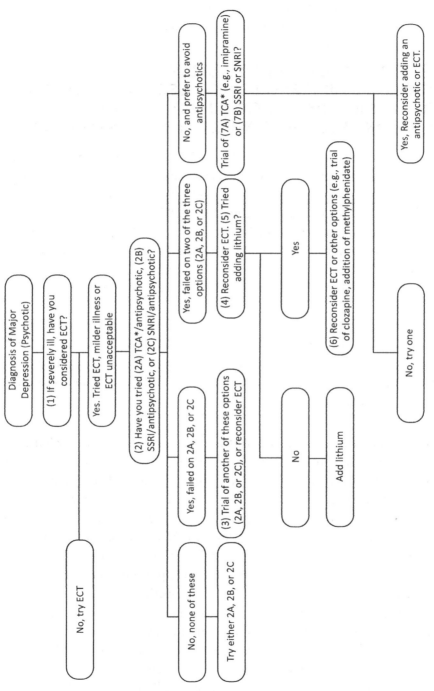

Figure 1: Flowchart of the Algorithm for Psychotic Depression

ECT: Therapy; SSRI: Selective Serotonin Reuptake Inhibitor; SNRI: Serotonin Norepinephrine Reuptake Inhibitor; TCA: Tricyclic Antidepressant. *Patients with psychotic depression are at a higher risk of suicide/overdose

Despite its apparent effectiveness, ECT has several problems including its limited availability and its side effects, most notably memory impairment. Also, some studies have also reported a high relapse rate in psychotic depression after a good response to ECT (17,18). In addition, patients and families may refuse ECT treatment, or patients may not be good candidates because of comorbid medical conditions.

NODE 2: HAVE YOU TRIED (2A) TRICYCLIC ANTIDEPRESSANT PLUS ANTIPSYCHOTIC, (2B) SELECTIVE SEROTONIN REUPTAKE INHIBITOR PLUS ANTIPSYCHOTIC, OR (2C) SEROTONIN NOREPINEPHRINE REUPTAKE INHIBITOR PLUS ANTIPSYCHOTIC?

When the patient has a milder presentation, refuses ECT, or is not a suitable candidate for ECT, pharmacological management is recommended by the 2010 American Psychiatric Association (APA) Practice Guideline (19) and the 2009 British National Institute for Clinical Excellence (NICE) guideline (20). The 2008 PAPHSS algorithm (1), the APA practice guideline, and a recent meta-analysis by Farahani et al (21) suggest that psychotic depression typically responds better to combination therapy with an antidepressant plus an antipsychotic than to monotherapy with either antidepressant or antipsychotic. The most recent update (2009) of the Cochrane collaboration meta-analysis on psychotic depression (22), however, continues to suggest that antidepressant monotherapy should be the initial offering and then combination antidepressant/antipsychotic therapy if the patient is not responding to antidepressant alone. They emphasize the potential for adverse effects associated with combination therapy. In this algorithm update, combination therapy still continues to be the first-line recommendation. We will evaluate the evidence related to these different opinions.

Node 2A: The Combination of a Tricyclic Antidepressant and an Antipsychotic As described in the 2008 version of the PAPHSS algorithm (1), below are some key studies pertinent to the issue of whether tricyclic antidepressant (TCA) and antipsychotic combination has a better treatment response as compared with TCA monotherapy.

In 1985, Spiker and colleagues conducted what may be considered the landmark pharmacotherapy study for psychotic depression with 51 delusional depression patients (23). Delusional depression is somewhat different from the current DSM-IV concept of psychotic depression, as was described in the previous algorithm paper (1). Patients were randomized for six weeks to either amitriptyline plus perphenazine combination therapy (n=18), amitriptyline monotherapy (n=17), or perphenazine monotherapy (n=16). Results showed combination therapy to have a 78% response rate as determined by the 17-item Hamilton Depression Rating Scale (HAM-D-17), as compared to 41% for amitriptyline monotherapy and 19% for perphenazine monotherapy (p<0.01). Limitations to the study included small sample size, the absence of a placebo group, and the fact that after taking into account several dropouts, the intent-to-treat analysis did not show a statistically significant benefit of combination therapy over antidepressant alone.

Anton and Burch (24) studied a similar comparison employing 38 inpatient subjects given either amitriptyline plus perphenazine or amoxapine alone for a 4-week period. Response rates (defined as >50% reduction in HAM-D-17) were 81% for combination therapy and 71% for monotherapy, a non-significant difference. 76% of patients on amitriptyline plus perphenazine had an improvement on the Brief Psychiatric Rating Scale (BPRS) of more than 50%, compared to 59% of the patients on amoxapine. This difference was also non-significant. Limitations to the study included its single-blind design, small sample size, and lack of placebo control. Importantly, the failure of combination therapy to produce more than a slight numerical advantage over amoxapine could be because amoxapine is actually a combination treatment: its main metabolite has dopamine receptor blocking properties and is probably an antipsychotic (1).

In another study with 35 delusionally depressed patients given desipramine plus perphenazine or plus haloperidol, Nelson and colleagues concluded from their results that both the TCA and the antipsychotic contributed independently to the clinical benefit (25). Responders had an average haloperidol dose of 12 mg/d versus nonresponders having a daily dose of 6 mg (p<.04). Perphenazine responders had an average dose over 48 mg daily. The number of responders when desipramine plasma levels were less than 100 ng/ml was 1 of 8 patients, compared to 15 of 23 patients when the levels were over 100 ng/ml (p<.05).

In a randomized double-blind trial by Mulsant and colleagues (26), 52 elderly patients (mean age=72) were initially started on nortriptyline monotherapy for a two week period This was followed by addition of either perphenazine (n=17) or placebo (n=19) for two more weeks. Response was defined as a HAM-D-17 score of less than 10 and remission of psychotic symptoms on the BPRS. Results showed 44% responding during initial nortriptyline monotherapy treatment. In the remaining period (with each group having 3 dropouts), response was seen in 50% (n=7) of the nortriptyline plus perphenazine group, and 44% (n=7) in the nortriptyline plus placebo group—a nonsignificant difference. Limitations of the study included small sample size and a population of elderly and demented patients that might have reduced response rates.

In their meta-analysis of the question of combination therapy versus TCA monotherapy, the Cochrane review considered only two of these four studies: Spiker et al and Mulsant et al. They found no significant advantage for the combination (relative risk ratio = 1.44; 95% confidence interval, 0.86–2.41; p=0.16). However, these two studies had small sample sizes, dissimilar patient populations (average age of 72 versus average age of 44), and different methodologies (e.g. – timing of initiating combination therapy). In the 2008 PAPHSS algorithm, it was noted that even with the limitation to these two studies, the numerical advantage for combination treatment appeared large enough to be clinically significant.

Node 2B: The Combination of a Selective Serotonin Reuptake Inhibitor and an Antipsychotic

Selective serotonin reuptake inhibitors (SSRIs) have displaced TCAs in the treatment of depression in usual practice because of their greater safety. However, some evidence supports the notion that TCAs are superior in efficacy, especially in men and in patients with more severe depression (27,28). In psychotic depression, unfortunately, head-to-head prospective comparisons between an SSRI plus an antipsychotic versus a TCA plus an antipsychotic still have not been done. Below, we briefly review some studies indirectly pertinent to these issues that were discussed in the 2008 algorithm and one new clinical trial.

SSRIs have been combined with both typical and atypical antipsychotics so we will discuss these combinations separately.

SSRIs and typical antipsychotics   Two small studies examined the combination of an SSRI and a typical antipsychotic.

The first was conducted by Rothschild and colleagues and included 30 patients (meeting DSM-III-R criteria for psychotic depression) treated with a combination of fluoxetine and perphenazine (29). 73% of the patients (23/30) had a reduction of HAM-D-17 and BPRS scores of 50% or more after five weeks. Study limitations include open-label design, small sample size, and lack of a placebo control group. Of note, 7/30 of patients carried bipolar diagnoses. The second study was conducted by Wolfersdorf and colleagues with 14 patients treated with paroxetine and either zotepine or haloperidol, or both (30). 3/4 patients receiving combined paroxetine plus haloperidol had a 50% or more reduction in HAM-D-24. Limitations to the study were its tiny sample size, non-blind design, lack of placebo control, and short 3-week treatment period.

SSRIs and atypical antipsychotics   Rothschild and colleagues (31) evaluated fluoxetine and olanzapine in two multisite, double-blind, randomized controlled trials (RCTs), with 124 inpatients in trial 1, and 125 inpatients in trial 2. Patients diagnosed with psychotic depression (meeting DSM-IV criteria) were randomized into three groups (placebo, olanzapine plus placebo, and olanzapine plus fluoxetine) and treated for an eight-week period. Response was defined as ≥50% decrease from baseline HAM-D-24. Results from trial 1 showed the combination group (n=22) having a significantly higher response rate (64%) than the placebo (28%: n=50; p=.004) or olanzapine (35%: n=43; p=.027) groups. However, trial 2 showed no significant differences in response among treatment groups (combination 48%; n=23, placebo 32%; n=44: p=.20, and olanzapine 36%; n=47: p=.35). Notably, olanzapine alone was not different from placebo in either study, but the 36% response rate seems higher than the 19% response rate to perphenazine monotherapy in the landmark Spiker et al study (23). This may be attributed to the possibility that less ill patients would be admitted to the Rothchild et al studies that had a placebo control than to one with all active treatment arms. A limitation of the study was its lack of a fluoxetine monotherapy group. Hence, it did not offer an opportunity to evaluate combination therapy vs. SSRI monotherapy (See Node 7).

Although it did not duplicate the results in trial 1, trial 2 actually had a trend that was possibly clinically significant in favor of combination treatment. The small sample sizes in the combination groups were due to the randomization schedule: the investigators only intended to use the combination group as an "exploratory pilot arm." The primary goal in these industry-sponsored trials was to evaluate olanzapine monotherapy for psychotic depression, and in that respect the results were disappointing.

Since the 2008 update, Meyers, Rothschild, and others published the "STOP-PD" study, a 12 week, double-blind RCT comparing olanzapine (15-20 mg/d) plus sertraline (150-200 mg/d) versus olanzapine plus placebo for psychotic depression (32). 259 patients were followed with remission as the primary outcome measure. Patients were evaluated weekly for the first 6 weeks, followed by every other week until week 12. Remission was defined as a HAM-D-24 score $\leq$ 10 at 2 consecutive assessments and absence of delusions at the second assessment. Results showed the combination produced significantly more remissions (odds ratio 1.28, 95% CI 1.12-1.47, p<0.001) than olanzapine alone. 41.9% (54/129) of patients with combination therapy were in remission during their last assessment compared with 23.9% (31/130) in patients on olanzapine (p=0.002). As in Rothschild and colleagues' earlier study with olanzapine, this study again lacked an antidepressant monotherapy arm, and it had a high attrition rate (42%).

Recently, the authors of this study published an evaluation of the impact of previous medication treatment before study entry (33). They found that if the patient had a prior failed adequate antidepressant monotherapy trial (n=35) and then received combination therapy in the trial, only 20% responded. By contrast, the 19 patients with no previous treatment who were put on the combination had a 63% response (12/19) vs. 33% response (4/12) if they were put on olanzapine alone. This suggests, despite the small numbers, that in this patient population failure to respond to SSRI monotherapy was associated with a guarded prognosis for adding an antipsychotic. For the treatment-naïve patients, the combination was superior.

In summary regarding the use of SSRIs, the combination of an SSRI plus a typical or an atypical antipsychotic is clearly effective compared with placebo or antipsychotic monotherapy, but there have been no direct comparisons of the combination with SSRI monotherapy. Thus, if an SSRI is chosen as the antidepressant, confidence that combination therapy will be superior to antidepressant monotherapy may be somewhat less than if a TCA is chosen.

Node 2C: The Combination of a Serotonin-Norepinephrine Reuptake Inhibitor and an Antipsychotic

Since the 2008 update, the first double-blind RCT involving a serotonin-norepinephrine reuptake inhibitor (SNRI) antidepressant (venlafaxine ER) has been published. In this trial, a TCA (imipramine), venlafaxine ER, and a combination of venlafaxine ER plus quetiapine were compared (34). 122 patients were randomized for a 7 week period. Venlafaxine ER dose was 375 mg daily, imipramine was dosed to produce a plasma level of 200- 300 ng/ml of imipramine + desipramine, and the combination involved venlafaxine ER at 375 mg daily and quetiapine at 600 mg daily. Response was defined as greater than a 50% decrease in the HAM-D-17 score and a final score of less than 15. Remission rates (HAM-D-17 < 8) were also examined. The results showed a 66% (27/41) response rate to the combination, 52% (22/42) in the imipramine group, and 33% (13/39) in the venlafaxine ER group. Combination therapy was shown to be more effective than venlafaxine alone (with adjusted odds ratio of 4.02, 95% confidence interval at 1.56-10.32), but there was no significant difference in response when compared with the imipramine group (adjusted odds ratio at 1.76, 95% CI 0.72-4.30). In remission comparisons, 42% (17/41) occurred in the combination group, 21% (9/42) in imipramine monotherapy, and 28% (11/39) in venlafaxine monotherapy. The combination was statistically superior only to the imipramine. In linear mixed models analysis, the mean score decrease of HAM-D was numerically (but not statistically significantly) greater with imipramine compared to venlafaxine.

Limitations to the study included lack of a placebo group, remission comparisons done as a post hoc secondary outcome measure, and small sample size. Nevertheless, this study suggests that an SNRI plus antipsychotic combination can be more effective than an SNRI or TCA alone. The study did not provide data on how an SNRI plus an antipsychotic would compare to a TCA or an SSRI plus an antipsychotic.

Nodes 2A, 2B, & 2C: Conclusions   Despite the limitations of the data, the authors still find sufficient support to conclude that the combination of an antidepressant and antipsychotic is the first-line psychopharmacological treatment for psychotic depression. However: which antidepressants are preferred?

Antidepressant preference: TCA, SSRI, or SNRI?   As noted, there are still no head-to-head comparisons of a TCA, SSRI, and SNRI in combination therapy. In our prior update, we presented a detailed effort to make a comparison based on indirect evidence and concluded there was a slight basis for preferring a TCA over an SSRI for effectiveness but a stronger basis to prefer an SSRI for safety including overdose risk (1). We now have some data with an SNRI (venlafaxine ER) in psychotic depression (34). It worked well in combination with an antipsychotic, separating from monotherapy with a TCA and an SNRI on either response or remission. When compared in monotherapy with a TCA, the different trends on response and (secondarily) remission made it difficult to have a preference. Safety concerns would favor venlafaxine over a TCA. In conclusion, venlafaxine has become our first choice for the antidepressant to be used in combination therapy.

There is no evidence to support the favoring of other antidepressant types (e.g. bupropion, mirtazapine, monoamine oxidase inhibitors) in psychotic depression.

Antipsychotic preference   No direct comparisons are available to test the relative efficacy and safety of different typical and atypical antipsychotics. Our previous analysis of the indirect evidence failed to find any basis for any preference based on effectiveness (1). Since the previous update, as we have noted, quetiapine and olanzapine have new RCTs and both were shown to be effective choices for combination therapy. Quetiapine has more efficacy than olanzapine and other atypical antipsychotics for some other depressive disorders such as bipolar depression (8). This suggests it might be favored (for effectiveness) for psychotic depression.

Regarding safety issues, typical antipsychotics have an increased risk of tardive dyskinesia when compared to atypical antipsychotics especially in mood-disordered psychotic patients (35). Atypical antipsychotics often produce weight gain and related metabolic problems, particularly olanzapine (36). Interestingly, Rothschild's group (37) evaluated the weight gain of 118 patients from their olanzapine and sertraline STOP-PD study, looking for risk factors. Age had a significant negative association with weight gain ($p=0.01$) even after controlling for differences in cumulative olanzapine dose and baseline body mass index. Each 10-year increase in age was associated with a decrease in mean weight gain over 12 weeks of approximately 0.6 kg ($p=0.01$). The results suggest that olanzapine-induced weight gain is more of a concern in younger patients.

Quetiapine causes weight gain as well, second only to olanzapine in a study in antipsychotic-naïve young patients (38). It also has a new package insert warning in 2011 regarding QTc prolongation and now must receive extra safety monitoring for this and may not be combined with at least 12 specified medications (to which should be added citalopram which has had a similar warning since September, 2011)

Given that olanzapine and quetiapine are both effective in psychotic depression combination treatment despite their different pharmacodynamic properties (e.g. olanzapine is strongly bound to the dopamine type 2 receptor and quetiapine is loosely bound), it may be reasonable to consider other atypical antipsychotics with a more benign safety profile even if their efficacy has not been as well-demonstrated. Ziprasidone (40-160 mg/d) was combined with sertraline (100 -200 mg/d) in 19 psychotic depression patients open-label for 4 weeks. 17 completed the study. Patients improved significantly on the HAM-D-21, BPRS, and other rating scales (39). There was no weight gain or prolactin increase, but QTc increased by a mean of 15 ms ($p=0.04$). Aripiprazole was combined with escitalopram in an open-label, 7-week trial (40). Response rate on the 13 completers was 63% with response defined as a 50% drop in the HAM-D-17 and no psychosis. Risperidone was combined with an antidepressant in 11 patients as part of an investigation in a heterogeneous population most of whom had psychotic depression and the results seemed promising (41).

Continuation of combination therapy after the acute phase Wijkstra and colleagues recently addressed this question in a 4-month follow up study of their comparison of acute treatment with venlafaxine, imipramine, and combined venlafaxine and quetiapine (42). 59 responders (20 patients from imipramine group, 13 from the venlafaxine group, and 26 from the combination group) had their HAM-D-17 measured during open-label follow-up for 4 months. Six dropped out, but 86% (51 of 59) maintained their response: 16/17 (94%) of imipramine patients, 12/12 (100%) on venlafaxine, and 23/24 (96%) on the combination ($p=1.0$). This study suggests that continuation of treatment with an initially effective medication regimen for at least 4 months is highly recommended.

In an older naturalistic follow-up study, 78 patients who had remitted on combination therapy had a high rate of relapse if they went off their antipsychotics (43). Patients were on the antipsychotics for a mean of 5.0 months but relapsed in a mean of 2.0 months after antipsychotic dosage reduction or discontinuation. Another study in older patients, however, found no differences in relapse rate with antipsychotic discontinuation (17). During a 6-month observation period, 7 of 28 subjects relapsed: 5 of 15 while on combination therapy compared with 2 of 13 on monotherapy ($p=0.4$). A recent two-year follow-up study of patients receiving naturalistic treatment after their first diagnosis of psychotic depression found that 45% experienced new episodes (7). It is unclear if this is because suboptimal treatment was prescribed, patients became non-adherent, or because of confounding changes in diagnosis over time.

In conclusion, this algorithm addresses acute management, and maintenance therapy data are limited. However, the most recent study suggests at least 4 months of maintenance is effective. One should particularly consider the long-term metabolic side effects associated with maintaining the antipsychotic that has received the most study, i.e. olanzapine. If metabolic side effects are significant, it may be worth trying to change to a different antipsychotic or seeing if it can be discontinued.

NODE 3: HAVE YOU TRIED SWITCHING THE ANTIDEPRESSANT IF A FIRST COMBINATION TRIAL HAS FAILED?

If the patient has had, and failed, an SSRI plus antipsychotic combination, one may consider switching the antidepressant to venlafaxine ER or to a TCA. As noted, this is based on very limited evidence – but it seems there is a little more rationale for this compared with the other option of switching the antipsychotic. If the patient initially failed on venlafaxine plus antipsychotic, close consideration of the conflicting monotherapy data from the Wijkstra et al study (34) suggests it is possible that they might do better on a TCA.

If the patient's initial treatment happened to have been with a TCA plus antipsychotic, there is minor evidence to suggest that a switch to an SSRI or SNRI as the antidepressant might be advantageous. In one study, eight patients with prior failure on full-dose TCA and typical antipsychotic combination therapy showed a 62% (5/8) response rate after being switched to SSRI plus antipsychotic therapy (29). Blumberger et al found that even after failure on an adequate trial of various (unspecified) combinations of antidepressants and antipsychotics (n=13), 25% then responded to the combination of sertraline plus olanzapine, and (surprisingly) 40% of 11 patients responded when assigned to olanzapine monotherapy even though that was not a good treatment for treatment-naïve patients in their study (33). Possibly the diagnoses of these 11 patients were incorrect and they actually had a primary psychotic disorder (6,7).

Thus, though this evidence is very limited, switching antidepressants seems to have some chance of success and it is proposed that this be the next intervention in Node 3.

Reconsideration of ECT should also occur here given its effectiveness in non-responsive patients (44).

NODE 4: IF TWO COMBINATION TRIALS FAILED, AGAIN RECONSIDER ECT

ECT is probably the treatment of choice after two failed combination trials with different antidepressants. As noted earlier, Blumberger and colleagues found that prior failure to respond to adequate antidepressant courses is associated with poor outcomes with olanzapine and sertraline combination therapy even under research conditions (33). In a study with 15 inpatients with psychotic depression (DSM-III criteria), 8/9 patients who were not responsive to TCA plus antipsychotic combination showed excellent clinical response after ECT (45). In Spiker and colleagues' 1985 study, all six patients failing combination therapy responded well with ECT (23).

NODE 5: DID TWO COMBINATIONS AND ECT ALL FAIL OR WAS ECT UNAVAILABLE OR UNACCEPTABLE?

Some evidence is available to support augmentation therapy with lithium in this situation. Lithium was used to augment a TCA plus antipsychotic combination in a 20-patient case series, and 40% had partial or marked response (46). In another augmentation series with 6 unresponsive patients to TCA plus antipsychotic combination, 3/6 had dramatic response and 2/6 had gradual response with lithium (47). Rothschild et al's early study had 3/8 patients responding to lithium augmentation after failing fluoxetine and perphenazine (29). Finally, since the last algorithm update, Birkenhager and colleagues reported on the open-label addition of lithium for 4 weeks to 15 non-responding patients from their venlafaxine/imipramine/quetiapine study (48). They were kept on their blinded initial medications. Nine patients (60%) had sustained remission. Five of the 15 patients were on combination therapy but unfortunately their results were not reported separately.

NODE 6: DID TWO COMBINATIONS AND LITHIUM AUGMENTATION FAIL?

ECT is still considered the best option at the point if not yet tried.

Clozapine may be considered based on evidence derived from case series and case reports. Three patients with refractory psychotic depression, not responding to ECT, had clozapine initiated (49). There was improvement in both psychotic and mood symptoms (response was delayed for 1 patient), and no relapses occurred over a 4-6 year follow up period.

In a case report, a female patient's initial BPRS score of 62 dropped to 39 after 4 weeks of clozapine, and to 21 after four months (50). Another case report described similar results with a female patient whose mood symptoms responded well and psychotic symptoms remitted after receiving clozapine (51).

Since the 2008 update, a new report of an augmentation strategy involving the addition of methylphenidate has appeared. This adds to an old report from over 40 years ago (52, 53). In the new case, there was a good effect in a female patient with psychotic depression who had failed on venlafaxine plus olanzapine combination. The patient's family had refused ECT. Her psychosis remitted with a Clinical Global Impression score of 3 and HAM-D score of 8 after 4 days, and she had no recurrence at 2-year follow up.

NODE 7: TCA, SNRI, OR SSRI MONOTHERAPY?

Sometimes monotherapy with an antidepressant will be preferred (e.g. - due to side effect concerns with antipsychotics). If so, which one should be selected?

Node 7A: TCA Monotherapy? TCAs seem to be effective for many cases of psychotic depression. A meta-analysis found TCAs to be superior to placebo (54) and to antipsychotic monotherapy (22).

Some evidence suggests TCAs would be preferred over SSRIs. Van Den Borek and colleagues conducted an RCT in depressed patients showing that imipramine at a plasma level of imipramine + desipramine of 192-521 ng/ml was more effective than fluvoxamine at 150-1800 mg daily (55). Cochrane analysis of the psychotic depression patients in this study (56) found that 64% (16/25) of patients on imipramine had 50% reduction in HAM-D, as compared 30% (7/23) on fluvoxamine (p=0.03).

In another RCT of depressed patients by Brujin and colleagues, imipramine was shown to be more effective than mirtazapine (57). Cochrane review's analysis of the psychotic depression patients in this study (56) showed that 9/15 patients (60%) on imipramine achieved a 50% reduction in HAM-D scores, as compared to 3/15 patients (20%) in the mirtazapine group (p=0.05).

As discussed earlier, the recent RCT comparing the TCA imipramine head-to-head with venlafaxine is hard to interpret because of conflicting data on response and remission (34).

Amoxapine as mentioned earlier has strong typical antipsychotic properties from its metabolite 7-hydroxy amoxapine (24). This product is therefore not recommended due to its possible associated risks for tardive dyskinesia.

Node 7B: An SSRI/SNRI? Studies suggesting effectiveness of SSRI or SNRI monotherapy are discussed below. Fluvoxamine (58), sertraline (59), paroxetine (59), and venlafaxine (34,60) all have some evidence.

Zanardi and colleagues conducted a double-blind controlled 6-week study comparing the responses of 66 patients with psychotic depression (DSM-III-R) to sertraline (n=24) and paroxetine (n=22) (59). The HAM-D-21 and the Dimensions of Delusional Experience Rating Scale (DDERS) were utilized for response assessment. 75% of sertraline patients and 46% of paroxetine patients responded, but the difference was not statistically significant (p=0.16). Limitations to the study include lack of placebo group, high dropout rate (41%) in the paroxetine group, and enrollment of 14 bipolar patients.

Case studies and case series have described the use of fluvoxamine monotherapy (58). In a recent case study a female patient was initially treated with fluvoxamine and risperidone for 1 year followed by fluvoxamine monotherapy maintenance for 2 years (61). At this point, she was switched to sertraline but then developed delusions. Her symptoms resolved after switching back to fluvoxamine. In a case series, 5 patients treated with fluvoxamine all showed reduction in HAM-D and BPRS scores (62).

Zanardi and colleagues conducted another 6-week RCT with 28 inpatients with DSM-IV psychotic depression (60). Subjects received either 300 mg of fluvoxamine or 300 mg of venlafaxine. 79% of the fluvoxamine group (n=11) and 58% of the venlafaxine (n=7) showed response with a reduction in HAM-D-21 score to ≤ 8 and DDRS score of 0. No statistically significant difference was found between the two drugs (p=0.40). Limitations to the study included small sample size, lack of placebo control, and enrollment of 6 bipolar patients.

Kantrowitz and colleagues examined the risk for psychosis exacerbation with TCA and serotonergic antidepressant monotherapy in a systemic review on psychotic depression (63). Of the 20 studies reviewed, patients assigned to a tricyclic antidepressant were more likely to experience psychosis exacerbation (8/78) than patients on serotonergic antidepressants (1/93), p=0.01. 6/6 patients treated with MAOIs experienced psychosis exacerbation.

In conclusion, there may be some efficacy for SSRI or venlafaxine monotherapy, but the evidence appears slightly stronger for TCA monotherapy. However, TCAs have the previously noted safety issues and there may also be some increased risk of psychosis exacerbation with TCA monotherapy. The strongest evidence supports initial use of combination therapy with an antidepressant and an antipsychotic, if ECT is not used.

FINAL COMMENTS

This update to the 2008 PAPHSS algorithm further refines the previous analysis of the available evidence for pharmacological treatment of psychotic depression. However, the validity of the conclusions are limited by the quality and quantity of studies and evidence available. Head-to-head prospective trials in psychotic depression are still relatively few in number. Yet, the alternative to relying as best as possible on this evidence-base would be to make decisions solely on the individual practitioner's clinical experience. This can be an unreliable basis for decision-making (64). Andreescu and colleagues in 2007 found that only 57% of 100 patients with psychotic depression received at least one combination of an antidepressant and an antipsychotic, and only 5% received a full dose of the antipsychotic (65). Mulsant and colleagues showed similar results in 1997, when 4% of 53 patients received adequate combination therapy (66). Therefore, this algorithm update hopes to inform clinicians about the evidence available for the psychopharmacology of psychotic depression. It organizes that evidence in a systematic manner, but it is flexible enough in its recommendations to leave ample opportunity to add individual judgment based on clinical experience.

REFERENCES

1. Hamoda HM, Osser DN. The Psychopharmacology Algorithm Project at the Harvard South Shore Program: an update on psychotic depression. Harv Rev Psychiatry. 2008;16:235-47.
2. Osser DN, Patterson RD. Algorithms for the pharmacotherapy of depression: Part One Directions in Psychiatry. 1998;18:303-18.
3. Johnson J, Jowarth E, Weissman MM. The validity of major depression with psychotic features based on a community study Arch Gen Psychiatry. 1991;48:1075-81.
4. Ohayon MM, Schatzberg AF. Prevalence of depressive episodes with psychotic features in the general population. Am J Psychiatry. 2002;159:1855-61.
5. Coryell W, Lavori P, Endicott J, Keller M, VanEerdewegh M. Outcome in schizoaffective, psychotic, and nonpsychotic depression. Course during a six- to 24-month follow-up. Arch Gen Psychiatry. 1984;41:787-91.
6. Ruggero CJ, Kotov R, Carlson GA, Tanenberg-Karant M, Gonzalez DA, Bromet EJ. Diagnostic consistency of major depression with psychosis across 10 years. J Clin Psychiatry. 2011;72:1207-13.

7. Tohen M, Khalsa HM, Salvatore P, Vieta E, Ravichandran C, Baldessarini RJ. Two-year outcomes in first-episode psychotic depression the McLean-Harvard First-Episode Project. J Affect Disord. 2012;136:1-8.

8. Ansari A, Osser DN. The psychopharmacology algorithm project at the Harvard South Shore Program: an update on bipolar depression. Harv Rev Psychiatry. 2010;18:36-55.

9. Bajor LA, Ticlea AN, Osser DN. The Psychopharmacology Algorithm Project at the Harvard South Shore Program: an update on posttraumatic stress disorder. Harv Rev Psychiatry. 2011;19:240-58.

10. Osser DN, Dunlop LR. The Psychopharmacology Algorithm Project at the Harvard South Shore Program: an update on generalized social anxiety disorder. Psychopharm Review. 2010;45:91-8.

11. Osser DN, Jalali-Roudsari M, Manschreck T. The Psychopharmacology Algorithm Project at the Harvard South Shore Program: an update on schizophrenia. Harv Rev Psychiatry. 2013;21:in press.

12. Petrides G, Fink M, Husain MM, Knapp RG, Rush AJ, Mueller M, et al. ECT remission rates in psychotic versus nonpsychotic depressed patients: a report from CORE. J ECT. 2001;17:244-53.

13. Perry P, Morgan D, Smith R, Tsuang M. Treatment of unipolar depression accompanied by delusions. J Affect Disord. 1982;4:195- 200.

14. Olfson M, Marcus S, Sackeim HA, Thompson J, Pincus HA. Use of ECT for the inpatient treatment of recurrent major depression. Am J Psychiatry. 1998;155:22-9.

15. Keller J, Schatzberg AF, Maj M. Current issues in the classification of psychotic major depression. Schizophr Bull. 2007;33:877-85.

16. Navarro V, Gasto C, Torres X, Masana G, Penades R, Guarch J, et al. Continuation/maintenance treatment with nortriptyline versus combined nortriptyline and ECT in late-life psychotic depression: a two-year randomized study. Am J Geriatr Psychiatry. 2008;16:498-505.

17. Meyers BS, Klimstra SA, Gabriele M, Hamilton M, Kakuma T, Tirumalasetti F, et al. Continuation treatment of delusional depression in older adults. American Journal of Geriatric Psychiatry. 2001;9:415-22.

18. Sackeim HA, Haskett RF, Mulsant BH, Thase ME, Mann JJ, Pettinati HM, et al. Continuation pharmacotherapy in the prevention of relapse following electroconvulsive therapy: a randomized controlled trial. JAMA. 2001;285:1299-307.

19. American Psychiatric Association. Practice guideline for the treatment of patients with major depressive disorder, third edition. Am J Psychiatry. 2010;167:1-118.

20. National Collaborating Centre for Mental Health. The treatment and management of depression in adults: NICE clinical guideline 90. London; Leicester, UK: Gaskell and the British Psychological Society, 2009.

21. Farahani A, Correll CU. Are antipsychotics or antidepressants needed for psychotic depression? A systematic review and meta-analysis of trials comparing antidepressant or antipsychotic monotherapy with combination treatment. J Clin Psychiatry. 2012;73:486-96.

22. Wijkstra J, Lijmer J, Balk FJ, Geddes JR, Nolen WA. Pharmacological treatment for unipolar psychotic depression: Systematic review and meta-analysis. Br J Psychiatry. 2006;188:410-5.

23. Spiker DG, Weiss JC, Dealy RS, Griffin SJ, Hanin I, Neil JF, et al. The pharmacological treatment of delusional depression. Am J Psychiatry. 1985;142:430-6.

24. Anton R, Burch E. Amoxapine vs amitriptyline combined with perphenazine in the treatment of psychotic depression. Am J Psychiatry. 1990;147:1203-8.

25. Nelson JC, Price L, Jatlow P. Neuroleptic dose and desipramine concentration during combined treatment of unipolar delusional depression. Am J Psychiatry. 1986;143:1151-4.

26. Mulsant BH, Sweet RA, Rosen J, Pollock BG, Zubenko GS, Flynn T, et al. A double-blind randomized comparison of nortriptyline plus perphenazine versus nortriptyline plus placebo in the treatment of psychotic depression in late life. J Clin Psychiatry. 2001;62:597- 604.

27. Anderson IM. SSRIS versus tricyclic antidepressants in depressed inpatients: a meta-analysis of efficacy and tolerability. Depress Anxiety. 1998;7 Suppl 1:11-7.

28. Vermeiden M, van den Broek WW, Mulder PG, Birkenhager TK. Influence of gender and menopausal status on antidepressant treatment response in depressed inpatients. J Psychopharmacol. 2010;24:497-502.

29. Rothschild AJ, Samson JA, Bessette MP, Carter-Campbell JT. Efficacy of the combination of fluoxetine and perphenazine in the treatment of psychotic depression. J Clin Psychiatry. 1993;54:338- 42.

30. Wolfersdorf M, Barg T, Konig F, Leibfarth M, Grunewald I. Paroxetine as antidepressant in combined antidepressant-neuroleptic therapy in delusional depression: observation of clinical use. Pharmacopsychiatry. 1995;28:56-60.

31. Rothschild AJ, Williamson DJ, Tohen MF, Schatzberg A, Andersen SW, Van Campen LE, et al. A double-blind, randomized study of olanzapine and olanzapine/fluoxetine combination for major depression with psychotic features. J Clin Psychopharmacol. 2004;24:365-73.

32. Meyers BS, Flint AJ, Rothschild AJ, Mulsant BH, Whyte EM, Peasley-Miklus C, et al. A double-blind randomized controlled trial of olanzapine plus sertraline vs olanzapine plus placebo for psychotic depression: the study of pharmacotherapy of psychotic depression (STOP-PD). Arch Gen Psychiatry. 2009;66:838-47.

33. Blumberger DM, Mulsant BH, Emeremni C, Houck P, Andreescu C, Mazumdar S, et al. Impact of prior pharmacotherapy on remission of psychotic depression in a randomized controlled trial. J Psychiatr Res. 2011;45:896-901.

34. Wijkstra J, Burger H, van den Broek WW, Birkenhager TK, Janzing JG, Boks MP, et al. Treatment of unipolar psychotic depression: a randomized, double-blind study comparing imipramine, venlafaxine, and venlafaxine plus quetiapine. Acta Psychiatr Scand. 2010;121:190-200.

35. Correll CU, Leucht S, Kane JM. Lower risk for tardive dyskinesia associated with second-generation antipsychotics: a systematic review of 1-year studies. Am J Psychiatry. 2004;161:414-25.

36. Chiu CC, Chen KP, Liu HC, Lu ML. The early effect of olanzapine and risperidone on insulin secretion in atypical-naive schizophrenic patients. J Clin Psychopharmacol. 2006;26:504-7.

37. Smith E, Rothschild AJ, Heo M, Peasley-Miklus C, Caswell M, Papademetriou E, et al. Weight gain during olanzapine treatment for psychotic depression: effects of dose and age. Int Clin Psychopharmacol. 2008;23:130-7.

38. Correll CU, Manu P, Olshanskiy V, Napolitano B, Kane JM, Malhotra AK. Cardiometabolic risk of second-generation antipsychotic medications during first-time use in children and adolescents. JAMA. 2009;302:1765-73.

39. Moeller O, Evers S, Deckert J, Baune BT, Dannlowski U, Nguyen DH, et al. The impact of ziprasidone in combination with sertraline on visually-evoked event-related potentials in depressed patients with psychotic features. Prog Neuropsychopharmacol Biol Psychiatry. 2007;31:1440-3.

40. Matthews JD, Siefert C, Dording C, Denninger JW, Park L, van Nieuwenhuizen AO, et al. An open study of aripiprazole and escitalopram for psychotic major depressive disorder. J Clin Psychopharmacol. 2009;29:73-6.

41. Goto M, Yoshimura R, Kakihara S, Shinkai K, Yamada Y, Kaji K, et al. Risperidone in the treatment of psychotic depression. Prog Neuropsychopharmacol Biol Psychiatry. 2006;30:701-7.

42. Wijkstra J, Burger H, van den Broek WW, Birkenhager TK, Janzing JG, Boks MP, et al. Long-term response to successful acute pharmacological treatment of psychotic depression. J Affect Disord. 2010;123:238-42.

43. Aronson T, Shukla S, Hoff A. Continuation therapy after ECT for delusional depression: a naturalistic study of prophylactic treatments and relapse. Convulsive Therapy. 1987;3:251-9.

44. Schatzberg AF, Rothschild AF. Psychotic (delusional) major depression: should it be included as a distinct syndrome in DSM- IV? Am J Psychiatry. 1992;149:733-45.

45. Khan A, Cohen S, Stowell M, Capwell R, Avery D, Dunner DL. Treatment options in severe psychotic depression. Convulsive Therapy. 1987;3:93-9.

46. Price LH, Charney DS, Heninger GR. Variability of response to lithium augmentation in refractory depression. Am J Psychiatry. 1986;143:1387-92.

47. Price L, Conwell Y, Nelson JC. Lithium augmentation of combined neuroleptic-tricyclic treatment in delusional depression. Am J Psychiatry. 1983;140:318-22.

48. Birkenhager TK, van den Broek WW, Wijkstra J, Bruijn JA, van Os E, Boks M, et al. Treatment of unipolar psychotic depression: an open study of lithium addition in refractory psychotic depression. J Clin Psychopharmacol. 2009;29:513-5.

49. Ranjan R, Meltzer HY. Acute and long-term effectiveness of clozapine in treatment-resistant psychotic depression. Biol Psychiatry. 1996;40:253-8.

50. Jeyapaul P, Vieweg R. A case study evaluating the use of clozapine in depression with psychotic features. Ann Gen Psychiatry. 2006;5:20.

51. Dassa D, Kaladjian A, Azorin JM, Giudicelli S. Clozapine in the treatment of psychotic refractory depression. British Journal of Psychiatry. 1993;163:822-4.

52. Huang CC, Shiah IS, Chen HK, Mao WC, Yeh YW. Adjunctive use of methylphenidate in the treatment of psychotic unipolar depression. Clin Neuropharmacol. 2008;31:245-7.

53. Wharton R, Perel J, Dayton P, Malitz S. A potential clinical use for methylphenidate with tricyclic antidepressants. Am J Psychiatry. 1971;127:1619-25.

54. Khan A, Noonan C, Healey W. Is a single tricyclic antidepressant trial an active treatment for psychotic depression? Progress in Neuro-Psychopharmacology and Biological Psychiatry. 1991;15:765-70.

55. van den Broek WW, Birkenhager TK, Mulder PG, Bruijn JA, Moleman P. A double-blind randomized study comparing imipramine with fluvoxamine in depressed inpatients. Psychopharmacology (Berl). 2004;175:481-6.

56. Wijkstra J, Lijmer J, Balk F, Geddes J, Nolen WA. Pharmacological treatment for psychotic depression. The Cochrane Database of Systematic Reviews, 2004: Art. No.:CD004044.pub2. DOI:10.1002/14651858.CD004044.pub2.

57. Bruijn JA, Moleman P, Mulder PG, van den Broek WW, van Hulst AM, van der Mast RC, et al. A double-blind, fixed blood-level study comparing mirtazapine with imipramine in depressed in-patients. Psychopharmacology (Berl). 1996;127:231-7.

58. Gatti F, Bellini L, Gasperini M, Perez J, Zanardi R, Smeraldi E. Fluvoxamine alone in the treatment of delusional depression. Am J Psychiatry. 1996;153:414-6.

59. Zanardi R, Franchini L, Gasperini M, Perez J, Smeraldi E. Double- blind controlled trial of sertraline versus paroxetine in the treatment of delusional depression. Am J Psychiatry. 1996;153:1631-3.

60. Zanardi R, Franchini L, Serretti A, Perez J, Smeraldi E. Venlafaxine versus fluvoxamine in the treatment of delusional depression: a pilot double-blind controlled study. J Clin Psychiatry. 2000;61:26-9.

61. Kishimoto A, Todani A, Miura J, Kitagaki T, Hashimoto K. The opposite effects of fluvoxamine and sertraline in the treatment of psychotic major depression: a case report. Ann Gen Psychiatry. 2010;9:23.

62. Furuse T, Hashimoto K. Fluvoxamine monotherapy for psychotic depression: the potential role of sigma-1 receptors. Ann Gen Psychiatry.2009;8:26.

63. Kantrowitz JT, Tampi RR. Risk of psychosis exacerbation by tricyclic antidepressants in unipolar Major Depressive Disorder with psychotic features. J Affect Disord. 2008;106:27279-84.

64. Osser DN. Why physicians do not follow some algorithms and guidelines. Drug Benefit Trends. 2009;21:345-54.

65. Andreescu C, Mulsant BH, Peasley-Miklus C, Rothschild AJ, Flint AJ, Heo M, et al. Persisting low use of antipsychotics in the treatment of major depressive disorder with psychotic features. J Clin Psychiatry. 2007;68:194-200.

66. Mulsant BH, Haskett RF, Prudic J, Thase ME, Malone KM, Mann JJ, et al. Low use of neuroleptic drugs in the treatment of psychotic major depression. Am J Psychiatry. 1997;154:559-61.

UPDATE

PSYCHOTIC DEPRESSION ALGORITHM

In the seven years since the publication of the last version of this algorithm, the recommendations and flowchart remain the same. There have been no new studies that seem to change the overall sequences of the nodes. However, there have been some studies adding support to what was proposed in the 2012 algorithm.

The importance of correctly diagnosing and treating psychotic depression in the most evidence-supported way was reinforced by a recent meta-analysis of 20 relevant studies finding the rate of suicide attempts is more than double the rate in nonpsychotic depressed patients (1). This was true in all age groups, and was not associated with any particular features of the episodes, such as severity, presence or absence of hallucinations, cognitive dysfunction, or physical or psychiatric comorbidity. Completed suicide was also greater in the psychotic depression group, with an odds ratio of 1.7 (if an outlying large study was excluded) (2).

NODE 2B: FIRST-LINE TREATMENT WITH A COMBINATION OF AN SSRI ANTIDEPRESSANT AND AN ANTIPSYCHOTIC

At this node, the authors considered the evidence supporting the combination of a selective serotonin reuptake inhibitor (SSRI) as the antidepressant, and an antipsychotic. The evidence with different antipsychotics was reviewed. In the STOP-PD study, sertraline was the SSRI and olanzapine was the antipsychotic, and this combination was compared with olanzapine alone (3). Consistent with other studies of antidepressant/antipsychotic combinations, the remission rate on the combination was superior to antipsychotic monotherapy, with an odds ratio (OR) of 1.3. A new study called STOP-PD II was published in 2019 (4). This new trial was sponsored by the National Institute of Mental Health, whereas STOP-PD was sponsored by the manufacturer of olanzapine, which explains the selection of this particularly side-effect prone second-generation antipsychotic (SGA) and the design of the study which focused on finding how effective olanzapine could be as a monotherapy. In STOP-PD II, the purpose was to see if patients remitting on the combination of sertraline and olanzapine could be maintained on the antidepressant alone without the olanzapine versus staying on the combination, for 9 months.

In STOP-PD II, 269 subjects (mostly inpatients, aged 18–85) were recruited from 4 centers and treated open-label with sertraline (150–200 mg) plus olanzapine (15–20 mg). Those who were remitted or near-remitted for 8 weeks were randomized to stay on their combination or have their olanzapine tapered off over 4 weeks using identical-appearing placebos. The relapse rate on the combination was 20% compared with 55% on the sertraline plus placebo, which was an impressive number-needed-to-treat of 2.8. Almost all of the relapses occurred within the first 2 months. On the downside for the combination, patients gained an additional (mean of) 6 lb on olanzapine versus 3 lb on placebo. Patients had already gained a mean of 12 lb in the open-label phase involving the olanzapine. This study adds strong support for the algorithm's recommendation of using a combination of an antipsychotic and an antidepressant for psychotic depression, and further suggests it should be continued for at least 4 months before any thought of trying to taper off the antipsychotic.

An editorial advises that clinicians consider using a less hazardous SGA than olanzapine, for example aripiprazole (5), even though the quantity of evidence available from studies is greatest with olanzapine. The use of another SGA might reduce the incentive to taper and eliminate the antipsychotic beyond 4 months. This was also the suggestion in the 2012 algorithm. If the patient had suicidal ideation when depressed, one should be particularly reluctant to remove the antipsychotic. The editorial author also points out that patients with hallucinations were excluded from STOP-PD II, though they are allowed in the DSM-IV and -V criteria for psychotic depression; this slightly reduces the applicability of the results.

The study did not include bipolar depressed patients, and the treatment approach should be different. The editorial suggests that lithium can be just as effective as antipsychotics for such patients (5). See the chapter in this book on the algorithm for bipolar depression, which is in accord with that view.

REFERENCES

1. Gournellis R, Tournikioti K, Touloumi G, Thomadakis C, Michalopoulou PG, Christodoulou C, et al. Psychotic (delusional) depression and suicidal attempts: a systematic review and meta-analysis. Acta Psychiatr Scand. 2018;137:18-29.
2. Gournellis R, Tournikioti K, Touloumi G, Thomadakis C, Michalopoulou PG, Michopoulos I, et al. Psychotic (delusional) depression and completed suicide: a systematic review and meta-analysis. Ann Gen Psychiatry. 2018;17:39.
3. Meyers BS, Flint AJ, Rothschild AJ, Mulsant BH, Whyte EM, Peasley-Miklus C, et al. A double-blind randomized controlled trial of olanzapine plus sertraline vs olanzapine plus placebo for psychotic depression: the study of pharmacotherapy of psychotic depression (STOP-PD). Arch Gen Psychiatry. 2009;66:838-47.
4. Flint AJ, Meyers BS, Rothschild AJ, Whyte EM, Alexopoulos GS, Rudorfer MV, et al. Effect of continuing olanzapine vs placebo on relapse among patients with psychotic depression in remission: the STOP-PD II randomized clinical trial. JAMA. 2019;322:622-31.
5. Coryell WH. Maintenance treatment for psychotic depressive disorders: progress and remaining challenges. JAMA. 2019;322:615-7.

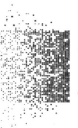

The Psychopharmacology Algorithm Project at the Harvard South Shore Program: An Update on Schizophrenia

David N. Osser, MD, Mohsen Jalali Roudsari, MD, and
Theo Manschreck, MD

This article is an update of the algorithm for schizophrenia from the Psychopharmacology Algorithm Project at the Harvard South Shore Program. A literature review was conducted focusing on new data since the last published version (1999–2001). The first-line treatment recommendation for new-onset schizophrenia is with amisulpride, aripiprazole, risperidone, or ziprasidone for four to six weeks. In some settings the trial could be shorter, considering that evidence of clear improvement with antipsychotics usually occurs within the first two weeks. If the trial of the first antipsychotic cannot be completed due to intolerance, try another until one of the four is tolerated and given an adequate trial. There should be evidence of bioavailability. If the response to this adequate trial is unsatisfactory, try a second monotherapy. If the response to this second adequate trial is also unsatisfactory, and if at least one of the first two trials was with risperidone, olanzapine, or a first-generation (typical) antipsychotic, then clozapine is recommended for the third trial. If neither trial was with any these three options, a third trial prior to clozapine should occur, using one of those three. If the response to monotherapy with clozapine (with dose adjusted by using plasma levels) is unsatisfactory, consider adding risperidone, lamotrigine, or ECT. Beyond that point, there is little solid evidence to support further psychopharmacological treatment choices, though we do review possible options.

Keywords: algorithms, antipsychotics, psychopharmacology, schizophrenia

The evolution of clinical therapeutics in schizophrenia challenges clinicians to remain current and evidence based in their psychopharmacological practices. New medicines have been added to the array of available antipsychotic drugs, and the older medications have been the subject of new studies and meta-analyses of their comparative efficacy and safety. Heightened awareness of side effects associated with long-term administration of medications suggests an increased need for advance planning for individuals at risk for a shortened life span from these complications.

From Harvard Medical School; VA Boston Healthcare System, Brockton Division, Brockton, MA (Drs. Osser and Manschreck); Laboratory for Clinical and Experimental Psychopathology, Corrigan Mental Health Center, Fall River, MA (Drs. Jalali Roudsari and Manschreck); Harvard Commonwealth Center of Excellence in Clinical Neuroscience and Psychopharmacological Research, Beth Israel Deaconess Medical Center, Boston, MA (Drs. Jalali Roudsari and Manschreck).

Original manuscript received 27 December 2011; revised manuscript received 18 August 2012, accepted for publication 24 September 2012.

Correspondence: David N. Osser, MD, VA Boston Healthcare System, Brockton Division, 940 Belmont St., Brockton, MA 02301. Email: David. Osser@va.gov

©2013 President and Fellows of Harvard College

DOI: 10.1097/HRP.0b013e31827fd915

Also, there is increasing evidence that integrative approaches, utilizing psychosocial and cognitive-behavioral techniques to augment drug treatment, hold promise to produce better outcomes. For example, psychoeducation interventions, cognitive-behavioral therapy, and, more recently, cognitive-rehabilitation[1] protocols have demonstrated significant advances in helping patients. However, success with nonpharmacological strategies relies fundamentally on the effectiveness and tolerability of medication treatment. Psychiatrists consequently need to have both broad knowledge about adjunctive and supplemental therapeutics and expertise concerning the complex issues of drug treatment.

In this article, we present a newly updated algorithm to guide clinicians in the pharmacological dimension of care for patients with schizophrenia. This version is part of our ongoing series of revisions of a schizophrenia psychopharmacology algorithm, first published in 1988.[2–7] It has also been influenced by the schizophrenia algorithm of the International Psychopharmacology Algorithm Project (2005–06, at www.ipap.org), for which one of the authors (DNO) was a co-chair. We have integrated newer, more extensive evidence with these earlier efforts, but the present algorithm differs substantially in focus, design, and complexity from its predecessors. It is intended to stand alone as an interpretation of that evidence and does not require reference to previous versions.

METHODS

This algorithm is one of several being developed by the Psychopharmacology Algorithm Project at the Harvard South Shore Program (PAPHSS). The latest methods have been described in recent PAPHSS publications.[8–11] Literature searches were conducted using PubMed and other databases, focusing on new randomized, controlled trials (RCTs) published since the last version about ten years ago. We also examined systematic reviews of pertinent clinical issues as well as other published guidelines and algorithms. This algorithm begins with an approach to newly diagnosed individuals with schizophrenia and then suggests strategies to counter unsatisfactory treatment responses. The primary target of interest for the algorithm is positive symptoms, although we discuss management of persistent negative, cognitive, and other symptoms. For each decision point or node, we specify strategies that appear to accord with the best evidence. Since schizophrenia is a chronic illness, and patients are likely to require medications indefinitely, recommendations prioritize use of medications with demonstrated effectiveness but also those with the most acceptable long-term side effects. The authors favored putting greater emphasis on choice of an antipsychotic with a milder long-term side-effect profile for the first antipsychotic trial. Thereafter, for the next trial and those beyond, we placed greater emphasis on efficacy (while still heightening awareness of the toxicities of some of those agents).

All hierarchical and other clinical recommendations are the result of full agreement by the three authors. In addition, the peer review process that followed submission of this article was an important part of the validation assessment for this algorithm (and other PAPHSS algorithms): if the reasoning, based on the evidence interpretations provided, was plausible to all reviewers, then it was retained. When there were differences of opinion on any particular issue, adjustments were made or further exploration of relevant evidence was done until consensus was achieved or the authors could present a stronger argument in support of their position.

The algorithm is built around questions that might be asked by a psychopharmacology consultant equipped with knowledge of the evidence base. The consultant responds to questions either with another question or with an appraisal of evidence pertinent to the optimal treatment of the clinical scenario at hand. Then, recommendations are made that are derived from this appraisal.

FLOWCHART OF THE ALGORITHM

The algorithm appears in Figure 1. Each numbered node reflects a decision point in treatment. The questions and rationale for recommendations at each node will be presented below.

At the threshold, accurate diagnosis is essential for the application of evidence-based psychopharmacology. Characterization of possible comorbid conditions is also critical, including both medical and psychiatric diseases.[12,13] The presence of these comorbidities may influence response to medication and may alter treatment selection in the algorithm. Table 1 summarizes common comorbid considerations in patients with schizophrenia and how they may influence the algorithm.

NODE 1: FIRST EPISODE/FIRST TRIAL

Having reviewed these preliminary considerations related to diagnosis and comorbidity, we turn to an analysis of the evidence base for selecting the initial antipsychotic for the patient with new-onset schizophrenia.

Crossley and colleagues[63] performed a meta-analysis of 15 RCTs comparing first-generation, or typical, antipsychotics (FGAs) and second-generation, or atypical, antipsychotics (SGAs) in early psychosis and found no differences in acute efficacy. In comparison to FGAs, however, SGAs appear to show greater long-term advantages, such as increased time to relapse, better treatment retention, and greater probability of staying in remission.[64-68] Four studies in first-episode patients suggest that FGAs are less effective than SGAs in preventing a second episode.[69] SGAs also have a lower incidence of drug-induced movement disorders and tardive dyskinesia.[64,65,68,70-73] FGAs are associated with higher use of adjunctive anticholinergic medications in these studies, which present an increased risk of adverse cognitive and peripheral anticholinergic effects.[74] While helping with the secondary negative symptoms due to extrapyramidal side effects, anticholinergics may also blunt the antipsychotic effect of FGAs on positive symptoms.[75] Even very low doses of haloperidol (1.7 mg) in first-episode patients were associated with a high incidence of tardive dyskinesia at one year (12%).[76] Not all studies confirm this risk difference between FGAs and SGAs,[77] however, and earlier studies, reviewed by Correll and colleagues in 2004,[71] may have been flawed by the use of high doses of haloperidol or by biases in study design associated with industry sponsorship. Nevertheless, given the direction

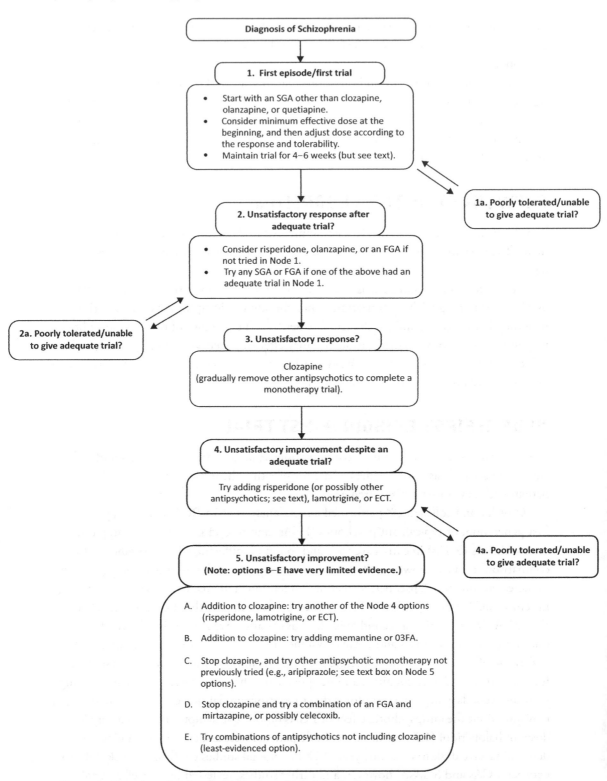

Figure 1. Flowchart for the algorithm for schizophrenia. ECT, electroconvulsive therapy; FGA, first-generation antipsychotic; O3FA, omega-3 fatty acid; SGA, second-generation antipsychotic.

Table 1 | Comorbidity and Other Features in Schizophrenia, and How They Affect the Algorithm

Comorbid conditions	Evidence considerations	Recommendations
Suicidality[14-16]	Clozapine reduced suicidal symptoms and behavior more than olanzapine in the InterSePT study. Benzodiazepine use was associated with increased mortality from suicide in schizophrenia.	For schizophrenia patients with active suicidal thoughts or behaviors, consider clozapine earlier (e.g., at Node 2) even if the patient is not treatment resistant. Avoid benzodiazepines.
Hostile, aggressive behavior[17-19]	Clozapine was more effective for improving aggressive behavior than olanzapine, risperidone, and haloperidol. Olanzapine seems to be the next best.	Consider clozapine for persistent hostility and violent behavior even if the patient is not treatment resistant. The small early-efficacy advantage for olanzapine over the others must be weighed against its long-term adverse effects.
Agitation requiring rapid management[20-25]	IM lorazepam, IM haloperidol, and IM SGAs are superior to placebo in controlling agitation in schizophrenia. Combination of lorazepam and haloperidol seemed more beneficial than either haloperidol or lorazepam alone. IM SGAs have a significantly lower risk of acute EPS compared to haloperidol when used without lorazepam or antiparkinson agents. However, this risk difference becomes insignificant when adding an anticholinergic agent or lorazepam. Note: patients prefer oral agents.	IM haloperidol plus lorazepam is still the treatment of choice for efficacy and for rapid, cost-effective treatment of severe agitation in schizophrenia. Oral PRN antipsychotics are often used but are usually unnecessary for less severe agitation.[26]
Secondary negative symptoms (i.e., due to underlying causes such as positive symptoms, EPS, or depression)[27]	FGAs and SGAs vary in their ability to cause secondary negative symptoms.[28]	Treat positive symptoms (e.g., paranoia producing asocial behavior) with standard algorithm. Treat EPS with appropriate agents, or change to antipsychotic with lower EPS risk. Manage sedation by eliminating, if possible, unnecessary sedatives.
Primary negative symptoms (i.e., "deficit" symptoms, including enduring decrease in motivation, decreased affective intensity and emotional range, and paucity of communication)[27]	Primary negative symptoms respond poorly to all antipsychotics, even clozapine.[29] The evidence base suggests some efficacy for adding antidepressants in some patients.[30,31] Possible experimental treatments for primary negative symptoms include memantine, d-serine, sarcosine, selegiline,[32] dehydroepiandrosterone,[33] ginkgo biloba, and minocycline.[35]	Might try adding SSRI, mirtazapine, trazodone, or fluvoxamine to FGAs or risperidone; efficacy even less clear for these additions to other SGAs, including clozapine. Use caution if combining clozapine with fluvoxamine, fluoxetine, or paroxetine, due to pharmacokinetic interactions. Citalopram increases clozapine levels and prolongs QTc at doses above 40 mg daily, as noted in package insert warnings.

(continued)

Table 1 | Comorbidity and Other Features in Schizophrenia, and How They Affect the Algorithm (*continued*)

Comorbid conditions	Evidence considerations	Recommendations
Major depression[36-38]	Overall, the literature is limited. Several studies found no efficacy for adding antidepressants to FGAs. Older studies did find improvement in depression in patients with "post-psychotic depression" who received a tricyclic added to ongoing treatment. Imipramine showed a positive effect versus placebo in a maintenance trial. SGAs may be more effective than classical neuroleptics in treating comorbid depression.[39] FGAs may cause more secondary depressive and negative symptoms.	First, ensure antipsychotic compliance and dose optimization. Treat post-psychotic depression with an antidepressant. Consider a tricyclic if an SSRI fails. Consider pharmacokinetic and pharmacodynamic interactions if antidepressants are added. An SSRI may be effective in mildly depressed older patients with chronic illness.[40]
Treatment of women of child-bearing potential[41-52]	Although the safety of antipsychotics in pregnancy has not been clearly established (due to many limitations in the studies), the wide use of FGAs over several decades suggests that teratogenic risks are small. Both FGAs and SGAs seem to be associated with an increased risk of perinatal complications. Some FGAs are associated with neonatal dyskinesias or neonatal jaundice. The SGAs that cause weight gain appear to increase risk of gestational metabolic complications, including diabetes and babies large for gestational age. Olanzapine may be associated with low and high birth weight and with a small risk of malformations, including hip dysplasia, meningocele, ankyloblepharon, and neural tube defects. Clozapine may be associated with increased risk of neonatal seizures but seems to show no increased risk of congenital malformations. The FDA has given it a B rating for pregnancy safety.	Prescribe as few drugs as possible. Use the lowest effective dose of the drugs with lowest risk. During the first trimester of pregnanacy, try to avoid all drugs. Adjust doses as pregnancy progresses: blood volume expands 30% in third trimester; plasma level monitoring is helpful. FGAs may still be preferred over SGAs in pregnancy; however, when pregnancy occurs during antipsychotic treatment, it is usually best to continue the existing therapy to avoid exposure to multiple agents. Consider the risk of relapse or withdrawal when switching medications or changing doses. Anticholinergic drugs should not be prescribed to pregnant women except for acute, short-term needs. Depot antipsychotics should not be routinely used in pregnancy, as infants may show extrapyramidal symptoms for several months.

Table 1	Comorbidity and Other Features in Schizophrenia, and How They Affect the Algorithm (*continued*)	
Comorbid conditions	*Evidence considerations*	*Recommendations*
Active substance abuse or dependence[53-55]	Substance abuse or dependence occurs in approximately 50%-70% of patients with schizophrenia. Active substance abuse is associated with poorer outcome with antipsychotic treatment. Tobacco-dependence rates may be as high as 90%; this addiction increases risk of cardiac death in schizophrenia patients 12-fold. The hydrocarbons in tobacco smoke (but not the nicotine) induce metabolism of clozapine (strongly) and olanzapine at the P450 1A2 enzyme.[56] Benzodiazepines are associated with higher risk for mortality in schizophrenia.[16]	Almost no studies of medication use have been done in patients actively using substances other than tobacco; hence, this algorithm may not be applicable to them. Treatment of the substance misuse, insofar as possible, is therefore a high priority. Clozapine levels must be monitored when smokers start or stop smoking. Naltrexone may be helpful for alcohol-abusing schizophrenia patients.[57] Bupropion is effective for smoking cessation,[58] as is varenicline.[59] Avoid benzodiazepines.
Cardiac disease or presence of QTc-prolonging drugs[60]	In a meta-analysis of 15 studies comparing six SGAs for their effect on QTc prolongation, only aripiprazole had significantly less effect than other antipsychotics. A seventh SGA, quetiapine, had five relevant studies, but the manufacturer refused to provide authors with QTc data. In 2011, however, the quetiapine package insert was amended with new QTc prolongation warnings and requirements for monitoring. FGAs—especially thioridazine, pimozide, and parenteral haloperidol—also prolong QTc.	Consider aripiprazole as the antipsychotic to use in these patients.
Older patients[61]	Elderly patients with schizophrenia have greater risk of EPS, metabolic syndrome, and tardive dyskinesia (from FGAs). Antipsychotics probably increase cerebrovascular events in this age group, especially if there is comorbid dementia or a history of stroke.	Use antipsychotics with great caution and close monitoring, especially if there is comorbid dementia. Behavioral symptoms and mild depression may respond to addition of an SSRI.[40,62]

EPS, extrapyramidal side effects; FGA, first-generation antipsychotic; IM, intramuscular; SGA, second-generation antipsychotic; SSRI, selective serotonin reuptake inhibitor.

of the preponderance of data cited above, we favor SGAs over FGAs for first-line, Node 1 use in this algorithm.

Some differences among SGAs influence their selection for use in first-onset patients. We focus on differences in side effects and ability to prevent future episodes. Both are important considerations in view of the long-term nature of this illness and the need to minimize both the serious medical morbidity from long-term use and the harm caused by exacerbations and relapses. Unfortunately, no SGAs are optimal in both respects. Four SGAs, on balance, appear slightly more advantageous, at least if properly dosed and monitored: amisulpride, aripiprazole, risperidone, and ziprasidone.[63,68,78,79] We will explain the reasoning supporting these choices and the problems with other options.

It is proposed, in agreement with others,[80] that *olanzapine* not be used for first-episode patients. Olanzapine, compared to other antipsychotics, is associated with much greater weight gain and other metabolic side effects in these patients.[68,78,79,81] Weight gain is almost twice as high as with quetiapine and risperidone,[78] which are considered to have intermediate risk for weight gain. The risks of glucose dysregulation and insulin resistance are also high with olanzapine—and occur early even in the absence of weight gain—placing the patient at risk for diabetes.[82] Risperidone is associated with less change in serum triglycerides and HDL cholesterol level than olanzapine and quetiapine.[78] In the open-label European First-Episode Schizophrenia Trial, Kahn and colleagues[68] reported, regarding glucose regulation, that amisulpride, haloperidol, olanzapine, quetiapine, and ziprasidone can all disturb fasting glucose status in first-episode patients. Nevertheless, there were significant differences in weight gain. After one year of treatment, ziprasidone was associated with a mean weight gain of 10 pounds, compared to 16 pounds for haloperidol, 21 for amisulpride, 23 for quetiapine, and 31 for olanzapine (p < .0001). In two other RCTs with first-episode patients, olanzapine produced significantly more metabolic problems than haloperidol.[67,83]

Quetiapine induces fewer movement disorders than other SGAs (especially compared to olanzapine, risperidone, and ziprasidone). It also induces less prolactin elevation than risperidone. It is associated, however, with higher weight gain and associated problems than risperidone and ziprasidone: in the CAFE study of early psychosis, 50% of patients on quetiapine experienced more than 7% increase in body weight at one year, second only to olanzapine with 80% of patients.[84] A recent concern is noted in a new package insert warning for quetiapine in July 2011 regarding QTc elevation; it suggests that the product should not be combined with a list of 12 specified medications. The list should also include citalopram because it has a similar QTc warning issued in September 2011. In an analysis of the evidence base on different antipsychotics time to rehospitalization or relapse after initiations, quetiapine seemed the least likely, or among the least, to maintain patients in an improved state.[85] For example, in an open-label, four-year maintenance study of 674 patients who had responded to quetiapine in several acute treatment protocols, 92% discontinued from all causes, most of them within three months.[86] Almost half of the withdrawals were due to lack of efficacy. For these reasons (side effects, poor maintenance effectiveness), quetiapine should not be among the recommended Node 1 antipsychotics.

The recommended list includes *risperidone*. As will be discussed in Node 2, it may be one of the more effective antipsychotics in patients having acute exacerbations of recurrent illness,[87,88] and it is also one that may have a relatively rapid effect in the inpatient setting.[7] In a study of patients having first exposure to an SGA in an eight-week RCT, risperidone was not different from olanzapine and was superior to quetiapine.[89] Side-effect issues include higher risk than olanzapine, quetiapine, ziprasidone, and even low-dose haloperidol of inducing prolactin elevation in first-episode psychosis.[66,78] Prolactin elevation is one of several factors associated with (but it may not be a cause of) sexual dysfunction in males,[90,91] and it causes menstrual dysfunction, gynecomastia, galactorrhea, and increases risk of osteoporosis.[90,91] Sexual dysfunction and loss of libido occurred in patients with higher levels of pathology and in association with most antipsychotics in the European First-Episode Schizophrenia Trial.[90,91] Investigation into these problems in this patient group could include evaluation for hypogonadism, which can be a consequence of hyperprolactinemia. When present, and if the risk of relapse from switching to a different antipsychotic is considered unacceptable, testosterone replacement could be helpful.[92] Extrapyramidal side effects are greater with risperidone than other SGAs, especially if excessive doses are used (e.g., over 2 mg in a first-onset patient, or over 4 mg in a patient with previous exposure to antipsychotics with strong D2 receptor-blocking properties). In summary, risperidone is highly effective but has important side effects. However, long-term risperidone side effects may be more easily managed or are generally not as serious as those of olanzapine or quetiapine.

Limited data are available concerning *aripiprazole* in first-episode patients. Komossa and colleagues,[93] in a systematic review comparing aripiprazole and other antipsychotics for schizophrenia, reported that aripiprazole may be less effective than olanzapine but more tolerable in terms of metabolic effects and sedation. Though aripiprazole is associated with little weight gain in chronic schizophrenia patients, its use in children and adolescents who have not previously been exposed to antipsychotics is associated with considerable weight gain.[94] In a study by Correll and colleagues,[94] after a median of 11 weeks, youths aged 4 to 19 with various diagnoses gained a mean of 10 pounds on aripiprazole, though that was less than the 12 pounds on risperidone, 13 pounds on quetiapine, and 19 pounds on olanzapine. No evidence indicates any difference in efficacy for aripipazole compared to risperidone, but the former has a more favorable profile in terms of dystonia, lipid and prolactin increases, and QTc prolongation. Aripiprazole is the safest SGA with respect to QTc prolongation,[60] which may be one of the long-term risk factors for sudden cardiac death with antipsychotics.[95]

In a Cochrane systematic review, Komossa and colleagues[96] reported that *ziprasidone* may be slightly less efficacious than amisulpride, olanzapine, and risperidone. It was also more likely to be discontinued than olanzapine and risperidone. In a recent double-blind study by Grootens and colleagues in patients with recent-onset schizophrenia,[97] however, it was found that ziprasidone and olanzapine have comparable therapeutic efficacy but that they differ in their side-effect profiles. Ziprasidone was associated with lower levels of triglycerides, cholesterol, and transaminases, whereas these parameters increased in the olanzapine group. Other studies support the finding that ziprasidone has probably the lowest tendency of any SGA to induce weight gain and associated metabolic problems such as triglyceride increase.[68] However, ziprasidone prolongs QTc to a greater extent than haloperidol, olanzapine, quetiapine, and risperidone,[98] although the evidence is not uniform. Ziprasidone needs to be administered at 80 mg twice daily with a 500 kcal meal to ensure optimal, reliable bioavailability.[99] Suboptimal dosing protocols in older studies and in usual clinical practice may account for some of the relatively poor effectiveness outcomes with ziprasidone.

Komossa and colleagues,[100] in another Cochrane review, compared *amisulpride* (not available in the United States) to olanzapine, risperidone, and ziprasidone in treating schizophrenia. They found that amisulpride was similar in effectiveness to olanzapine and risperidone and more effective than ziprasidone. Amisulpride induced less weight gain than risperidone and olanzapine, and less of an increase in glucose than olanzapine. No difference in cardiac effects and extrapyramidal symptoms was found with amisulpride compared to olanzapine, risperidone, and ziprasidone. In the European First-Episode Schizophrenia Trial, amisulpride was second in effectiveness only to olanzapine in the primary outcome measure of all-cause discontinuation rate at one year.[68] Olanzapine had a 33% discontinuation rate, whereas it was 40% with amisulpride, 45% with ziprasidone, 53% with quetiapine, and 63% with haloperidol. All SGAs were significantly better than haloperidol.

Some newer antipsychotics, though not included in our Node 1 recommended list, should be discussed. *Iloperidone*[101] has recently been approved for treating acute schizophrenia in adult patients. Although iloperidone has a low incidence of extrapyramidal symptoms, it is associated with more weight gain than risperidone. Additionally, there are concerns with QTc prolongation that appears to be dose-related and similar to those associated with ziprasidone. Twice-daily administration may be a disadvantage for some patients. Studies are needed with first-episode psychotic patients and to compare iloperidone to other SGAs.

Asenapine is a new antipsychotic, approved in 2009, for sublingual administration at a recommended dose of 5 mg twice daily.[102] The unusual mode of administration and the lack of data in first-episode patients render it inappropriate for Node 1 (see also the discussion in Node 2).

Lurasidone[103] is a new atypical antipsychotic that was approved in the United States for treatment of schizophrenia in October 2010. It may be as effective as aripiprazole, quetiapine, and ziprasidone in treating schizophrenia but seems less effective than olanzapine.[104,105] Lurasidone has a relatively well-tolerated side-effect profile with low liability for extrapyramidal symptoms, no significant QTc prolongation, once-daily administration (with 350 kcal of food, optimally at mealtime), and a benign metabolic profile (weight, lipids, and glucose). Lurasidone may be more beneficial than ziprasidone for treating cognitive deficits,[120] but comparison with other antipsychotics has not been reported.[106] Lurasidone may have the potential to replace ziprasidone on our preferred list for Node 1, but more research and clinical experience are needed to be more confident about where to position it in the algorithm. No studies in first-onset patients have been reported.

As for the dosing of antipsychotics in first-episode patients, the use of lower-than-usual doses is especially important to reduce the incidence and severity of adverse effects and to improve treatment acceptability.[107–110] Since antipsychotic side effects can have a lasting negative impact on attitudes toward antipsychotic treatment and adherence, efforts to minimize them are especially important.[111] For example, risperidone provided no greater antipsychotic benefits at doses of 4 mg or higher in first-onset patients but was associated with more neurocognitive side effects and motor impairment.[107,109,110] An exception to this suggestion for lower-than-usual dosing is quetiapine, which is not effective in first-onset patients when used in doses lower than those used in multiepisode schizophrenia.[78]

Summary: Node 1 Recommendations

For selection of antipsychotics as first-line treatment for first-episode schizophrenia—taking into account short- and long-term efficacy, side effects, and tolerability—amisulpride, aripiprazole, risperidone, and ziprasidone can be selected as the best first choices. However, if minimizing risk for weight gain is a strong priority, it may be reasonable to consider ziprasidone first, even though no head-to-head comparisons have been reported in this population. Because of its high long-term safety risks, olanzapine is not recommended as a Node 1 treatment. Quetiapine also presents significant problems with weight gain and metabolic side effects, and has the poorest record for maintenance treatment. For these reasons we also do not recommend quetiapine as a Node 1 treatment.

We do not encourage the use of FGAs as first-line treatment, because of the risk of movement disorders and tardive dyskinesia,[80] and because of inferior results compared to SGAs in preventing a second episode.[69]

Node 1a: Intolerance or Inadequate Trial of a Node 1 Antipsychotic?

Before considering a patient a poor responder and moving on to Node 2, it is important to determine whether the Node 1 antipsychotic has been given an adequate trial. A four- to six-week trial on an adequate antipsychotic dose represents a reasonable trial for most patients. Leucht and colleagues[112] found that for multiepisode patients, if the patient does not achieve a 25% reduction in symptoms in the first two weeks, outcome is likely to be poor at four weeks. Gallego and colleagues,[113] however, found that in first-episode patients, early symptom response was not a good predictor and that more time is often needed for an adequate trial. In this study of 112 subjects, 40% responded by week 8, and 65% by week 16.[113]

As for adequate dosing, FGAs can be in the range of 300–1000 mg chlorpromazine equivalents,[80] and suggested doses of SGAs can be 2–6 mg for risperidone,[114] 10–20 mg for olanzapine[115] (though perhaps preferably, at least 16 mg),[116] 10–15 mg of aripiprazole,[116] 300–750 mg for quetiapine,[80] and 160 mg for ziprasidone[117] (80 mg twice daily with a 500 kcal meal).[99]

When response is unsatisfactory—despite having optimized the dose (as allowed by side effects) and duration of trial, considered reports of adherence by patient and caretakers, and assessed for the presence of any known enzyme inducers or substance abuse—consider checking the antipsychotic plasma concentration. Aripiprazole, clozapine, haloperidol, olanzapine, and ziprasidone are among the antipsychotics with available assays.[52] In the absence of side effects, and if the plasma level is well below the range seen in patients on typical doses, suspect poor adherence or rapid metabolism. If the patient reports severe side effects that are not objectively apparent, a plasma level will help in assessing whether those are a somatization or nocebo effect. At times, unusual objectively observed side effects are worth evaluating with a plasma level: a low or zero level will suggest they are caused by something else.

Aripiprazole plasma level data are especially useful, with a suggested optimal range between 150 and 210 ng/ml.[118] Growing evidence suggests that the range for olanzapine is 20–40 ng/ml, with no greater benefit and significant toxicity associated with levels above 80 ng/ml.[119,120] Other possible ranges, less well delineated, include amisulpride at 200–320 ng/ml[121] and risperidone at 20–60 ng/ml.[52] Quetiapine levels are so variable that they do not seem useful at this time.[122]

If the problem is determined to be nonadherence, and it is not due to intolerance of side effects, consider using a long-acting injectable antipsychotic (LAI). In some cases, the use of an LAI may be necessary to complete an adequate trial at Node 1. The role of LAIs in managing schizophrenia has been investigated in new studies, to which we now turn.

Poorly Adherent Patients: The Role of Long-Acting Injectable Antipsychotics

Nonadherence to medication is one of the major problems in treating patients with schizophrenia, and LAIs are an intervention that has been thought to improve adherence. It has been argued, however, that the data actually suggest that LAIs may not be significantly superior to oral antipsychotics unless the patient is committed to accepting this form of treatment. Supporting this assertion is the study by Olfson and colleagues[123] of patients in the California Medicaid program. In this real-world, observational study—which may have important external validity—2695 marginally adherent patients were evaluated before, during, and after initiating treatment with fluphenazine decanoate, haloperidol decanoate, or LAI risperidone microspheres. The authors found that very few of these patients continued to take their LAI for six months (haloperidol, 9.7%; fluphenazine, 5.4%; and risperidone 2.6%; p < .0001). It was speculated that the particularly poor outcome with risperidone LAI may have reflected formulary restrictions in some outpatient settings. Rosenheck and colleagues,[124] however, also found disappointing results with LAI risperidone in another observational study of 369 U.S. veterans with unstable schizophrenia or schizoaffective disorder. Risperidone LAI was not superior to oral antipsychotics in the rate of rehospitalization in this study. It was also associated with more extrapyramidal effects and local injection-site pain.

Tiihonen and colleagues[125] examined the risk of rehospitalization and drug discontinuation in schizophrenia patients from Finland who had been hospitalized for the first time. They showed that the risk of rehospitalization for patients receiving depot medications was about one-third of that for patients receiving oral formulations of the same compounds (adjusted hazard ratio = 0.36; 95% confidence interval [CI], 0.17–0.75). Their patient sample may have been relatively unrepresentative, however, of more underresourced populations such as the U.S. public sector patients in the Olfson and colleagues study.[123] Leucht and colleagues[126] recently published a meta-analysis of controlled comparisons of LAIs and oral formulations in more chronic populations and concluded that LAIs are better in reducing relapse. Again, though, the patient samples in these mostly industry-sponsored RCTs were free of major comorbidity, able to cooperate with complex study procedures, and otherwise "clean" compared to the more difficult populations in underfunded public programs.

There are currently six LAIs of FGAs in international use, including flupenthixol, fluphenazine, haloperidol, perphenazine, pipotiazine, and zuclopenthixol. Among SGAs, olanzapine, risperidone, and paliperidone have LAI formulations. We will comment briefly on some pertinent issues regarding the use of some of these LAIs.

FGA LAIs might be expected to give rise to acute extrapyramidal symptoms, tardive dyskinesia, and symptoms related to hyperprolactinemia.[127,128] The frequency of movement disorders and tardive dyskinesia with FGA LAIs is similar to that seen with oral FGAs.[129] Fluphenazine decanoate and haloperidol decanoate may be associated with a relatively higher rate of movement disorders compared to other LAIs, but perhaps with a lower risk of causing weight gain.[128]

Risperidone LAI has some advantage over FGAs concerning risk of movement disorders. However, it is associated with increased plasma prolactin similar to, albeit somewhat lower in magnitude than, that seen with oral risperidone.[128] Risperidone LAI is affected by delayed release:[128] it takes about 3–6 weeks from the first injection of risperidone to produce a therapeutic plasma level.[52] Though often impractical, supplementation with oral risperidone during this crossover period appears essential to get optimal results.[130] A recent RCT found that patients stabilized on FGA LAIs had more treatment discontinuations when randomized to six months of risperidone LAI (31%) compared to staying on their original FGA LAI (10%).[131] Risperidone patients gained significantly more weight but had no difference in new-onset extrapyramidal side effects.

Paliperidone palmitate is the LAI associated with paliperidone, the major active metabolite of risperidone. It may be initiated with two weekly injections to achieve therapeutic concentration rapidly, and unlike risperidone LAI, it does not require supplementation with oral antipsychotics. Subsequent injections occur at four-week intervals, an advantage over the two-week interval with risperidone LAI. The tolerability and safety of paliperidone palmitate was generally similar to risperidone LAI.[132,133]

LAI olanzapine is similar to oral olanzapine both in effectiveness and in adverse effects,[128,129,134] with the exception of a new side effect: post-injection delirium/sedation syndrome (incidence = 1.4% of patients treated), which involves sedation, confusion, dizziness, dysarthria, somnolence, and possible unconsciousness.[128,134,135] This syndrome results from occasional inadvertent intravascular injection of olanzapine. Patients must be observed for three hours after each injection, and medical referral must be immediately available. All patients have recovered, but some have required up to three days of hospitalization.

In conclusion, LAIs may not have a marked benefit over oral medications, especially in chronically ill, poorly-compliant patients. We do not recommend their routine use in the algorithm, but they may have a role in evaluating acute antipsychotic efficacy if poor results are clearly due to nonadherence. Evidence does suggest that their initiation early in the course of schizophrenia *in relatively cooperative patients* may improve long-term outcome.[125] This effect may be due to their prevention of covert nonadherence.[127] When presenting treatment options for the first or second antipsychotic trial to the patient, we think it reasonable to include a discussion of the LAIs as an approach that could reduce early rehospitalization and relapse. LAIs should be discussed in a way that tries to overcome the stigma associated with the idea of receiving medication by injection. Before recommending and selecting an LAI, however, it is also important to be aware of any systems-related barriers that may impede follow-up care with LAIs.[136] Community care systems will vary in the availability of nurses to give injections and of funding and reliable monitoring processes.

If an LAI is chosen, haloperidol decanoate and paliperidone palmitate are advantageous because of their four-week periods of effectiveness.[123,125] Cost considerations strongly favor the former option at this time. The least effective appears to be risperidone LAI, perhaps because of its delayed release.

Additional Issues for the Node 1 Trial

Some clinicians might consider raising doses above the recommended ranges when patients fail to respond well to usual doses at Node 1 despite adequate time and blood levels sufficient to demonstrate bioavailability. No significant clinical evidence, however, supports this strategy.[80] Higher doses are not associated with greater improvement with aripiprazole, quetiapine, risperidone, or olanzapine, and they often result in increased side effects.[114,119,137,138] Administering a different antipsychotic is a preferable approach.

Text Box 1	Antipsychotic-Induced Akathisia in Schizophrenia	
Evidence Considerations	*Recommendations*
Akathisia is a feeling of discomfort, often a tingling sensation, especially in the legs, relieved somewhat by motor activity.[141]	Start with smaller dose, and increase the dose gradually, particularly in drug-naive patients.[139] Consider beta-adrenergic antagonists[139,148] —for example, propranolol.
At its extreme, it may precipitate aggressive, violent, and suicidal behaviors.[142,143]	
To diagnose, ask patient to cease moving and to describe subjective sensations, if any. Differentiate psychotic agitation, anxiety, drug withdrawal syndromes, some neurological disorders, or tardive dyskinesia.[144] Akathisia can be misdiagnosed as psychotic agitation, which may lead to an inappropriate increase in antipsychotic therapy.[144,145]	Consider benzodiazepines[139] —for example, clonazepam, lorazepam, or diazepam (especially if associated with anxiety).
Akathisia has been found to occur at antipsychotic doses that produce full occupancy of striatal D2 receptors.[146] However, this full occupancy has no mechanistic implications for akathisia; other neurotransmitter systems (norepinephrine, serotonin) likely contribute to its pathophysiology.[147-149]	Consider antimuscarinic agents[139,147,151,152]—for example, benztropine (particularly if akathisia is associated with parkinsonism). However, the evidence base for their use is weak.[139]
The development of akathisia may be a possible predictor of an unsatisfactory response to a neuroleptic.[140] Even if the dose is raised (after treating the akathisia), the antipsychotic response may still be unsatisfactory.[150] It is unclear if these findings apply to the akathisia-like symptoms associated with some SGAs.	There are other possible options for treatment-resistant akathisia: trazodone,[153] cyproheptadine,[148] mirtazapine,[149] zolmitriptan,[154] and vitamin B6.[155]

Intolerance of the side effects of the antipsychotic can cause poor adherence and early discontinuation.[52] If the patient discontinues a trial prematurely despite dosage adjustment or other management strategies (e.g., changing the time of dosing, or stopping or reducing other medications that may be contributing to the side effect), then Node 1 has not been completed, and another trial should occur with one of the recommended agents.

Akathisia is an antipsychotic-induced adverse effect that particularly affects adherence. The first adjustment should be to reduce the dose if possible. If that fails, it seems reasonable to try to treat the akathisia.[139] See Text Box 1 for a review of treatment options. It should be noted, however, that akathisia was found to be a predictor of, or marker for, patients who will have poor outcome from FGA therapy despite usual treatment efforts.[140] It is unclear if the same is true with akathisia from SGAs.

NODE 2: UNSATISFACTORY RESPONSE TO AN ADEQUATE TRIAL OF A NODE 1 ANTIPSYCHOTIC?

Relatively limited evidence is available to guide selection of the next antipsychotic after failure of the first adequate antipsychotic trial. We will review some of that evidence.

In 2006, Mc Cue and colleagues,[88] in an open-label randomized prospective trial (n = 327), compared five SGAs and haloperidol in newly admitted, acutely ill patients with schizophrenia, schizoaffective disorder, or schizophreniform disorder. This real-world effectiveness study employed the somewhat unorthodox and perhaps bias-prone primary outcome measure of whether the patients were able to be discharged from inpatient care within three weeks. The results were that three medications did significantly better than three others: olanzapine (mean dose = 19 mg; 92% discharged), haloperidol (16 mg; 89%), and risperidone (5.2 mg; 88%) did the best, whereas aripiprazole (22 mg; 64%), quetiapine (650 mg; 63%), and ziprasidone (150 mg; 64%) were significantly less effective on this measure. Dosing was robust for all six medications. This study suggests that there may be important differences in the effectiveness of antipsychotics in the acute inpatient setting. These findings are not inconsistent with those of an often cited meta-analysis by Leucht and colleagues[28] of primarily industry-sponsored trials comparing different antipsychotics, except for its finding that haloperidol, an FGA, was as effective as the better SGAs. However, the differences in favor of the better options were sharper in the data from McCue and colleagues[88] than in the meta-analysis.[28]

Suzuki and colleagues,[89] in a randomized, open-label study, evaluated the effectiveness of sequential switch among three SGAs. Japanese patients (n = 78) who had never had a full trial of any SGA were randomized to robust doses of olanzapine, risperidone, or quetiapine for up to eight weeks. Then, unsatisfactory responders to this trial were randomized to one of the other two antipsychotics for up to eight more weeks. Poor responders after the second trial were given the third antipsychotic. The study found that 50% (n = 39) of the patients responded to the first round of antipsychotic therapy. Olanzapine and risperidone were not different in their response rates, and both were superior to quetiapine. Among first-round nonresponders, 38% (n = 14) responded to the second randomized SGA trial. Quetiapine was the most effective second-line option, with a surprisingly good response rate of 60%. Only two patients responded in the third trial. Suzuki and colleagues concluded that after failure on an initial trial with an SGA, a second trial is a reasonable strategy, but that after two failed trials, a third trial has minimal chance of success. If patients received either olanzapine or risperidone first, the findings did not support favoring risperidone or olanzapine over quetiapine as a second choice. If patients received quetiapine first, the findings suggest a switch to either olanzapine or risperidone.

As noted earlier, ziprasidone, which was not included in the above study, has generally not fared well in comparisons to other antipsychotics: a Cochrane analysis of 11 comparative trials in established, as opposed to first-onset, patients concluded that ziprasidone was not as effective as other antipsychotics.[96] These results may be due in part to the failure to employ optimal administration parameters: 160 mg daily[117] (which is at the high end of the recommended range) in two doses, taken with 500 kcal meals.[156] Even if these conditions can be met, ziprasidone may still not be the best choice for Node 2.

In a similarly designed, randomized, open-label, eight-week study—also from Japan, and involving newly admitted, acutely ill psychotic patients—olanzapine and risperidone were again significantly superior to aripiprazole and quetiapine in the outcome as measured by time to discontinuation.[87]

Overall, these data, which are derived from studies with good external validity, support the proposition that if the Node 1 trial was not with one of the proposed more effective SGAs (olanzapine, risperidone, or an FGA), a second trial should involve one of these. The success of perphenazine in Phase 1 of the Clinical Antipsychotic Trials of Intervention Effectiveness (CATIE), compared to the SGAs olanzapine, risperidone, quetiapine, and ziprasidone, has convinced some clinicians that perphenazine is now the FGA of choice over the more traditional haloperidol.[157] In this context, it is worth noting that bioavailability of perphenazine can also be assessed with plasma levels. The proposed optimal range is 1–3 ng/ml, with levels above that producing no additional benefit and perhaps greater probability of side effects.[158,159]

Therapeutic drug monitoring with haloperidol has a long and complicated history.[160] Haloperidol was once thought, based on six early studies, to have a curvilinear plasma level/response relationship (i.e., a therapeutic window), with a proposed therapeutic range of 5–15 ng/ml. Subsequent efforts to confirm this range have had mixed results.[161] Haloperidol levels remain at least as useful as other antipsychotic levels for confirming compliance and bioavailabilty. The consensus is that levels higher than 15 ng/ml bring no additional benefit,[160] but the lower limit is probably lower than 5 ng/ml for patients experiencing first exposure to strong D2 receptor–occupying FGAs. Attention might also be paid to the presence of parkinsonian side effects (cogwheeling, akinesia), which, if present, indicate greater than 75% D2 occupancy and suggest that no matter how low (or high) the plasma level, raising the dose would be of little advantage.[6] By the same token, the absence of parkinsonism suggests lower striatal D2 occupancy and potential value to raising the dose.

Lurasidone, one of the newer SGAs, was discussed earlier as a potential Node 1 antipsychotic because of some advantages over ziprasidone. We do not favor it, however, as a Node 2 choice. In the only randomized comparison (n = 478) with any of the antipsychotics that performed better in the effectiveness studies reviewed above,[87–89] lurasidone at either dose (40 or 120 mg) appeared inferior to olanzapine 15 mg[105]—despite the study's sponsorship by the manufacturer of lurasidone.

In 2006, Stroup and colleagues,[162] in phase 2T of the CATIE study, examined patients (n = 444) who had failed their first SGA and then were randomized to a different SGA. Patients who switched to olanzapine or risperidone did better than those switched to quetiapine or ziprasidone. However, a methodological issue with CATIE is that a high proportion of the patients who did better on olanzapine in the second trial had been on olanzapine before entering the study.[163] This limitation was not present in the study by Suzuki and colleagues,[89] which did not find an advantage to olanzapine or risperidone for the second trial.

It is unclear at this time if asenapine is a reasonable option for Node 2. Placebo-controlled RCTs with haloperidol and risperidone have been published showing comparable efficacy. Since the haloperidol trial excluded patients who had a history of failing on another antipsychotic, the patients would not be comparable to Node 2 patients.[164] Three unpublished trials in over 1000 patients involved comparison with olanzapine, and in two of them asenapine was described as less effective than olanzapine.[165] Thus, the potential categorization of asenapine as one of the more effective antipsychotics awaits the publication of more of its trials and more extensive clinical experience.[102] On September 30, 2011, the U.S. Food and Drug Administration added a warning because of 52 cases of allergic reactions, 19 of which resulted in emergency room visits or hospitalization.

Summary: Node 2 Recommendations

Some evidence supports trying a carefully selected second antipsychotic. If not tried before, an FGA, olanzapine, or risperidone is recommended. If one of these was tried in Node 1, any antipsychotic except clozapine may be selected for Node 2.

If olanzapine is selected, consider taking steps to try to prevent weight gain or to prevent further gain if it begins right away—that is, within early weeks of treatment. Diet and exercise are recommended for those few patients sufficiently motivated to make these lifestyle changes. Topiramate and metformin have been tried, both initially and after weight gain develops. One RCT compared adding topiramate 100 mg or placebo to 72 patients when they were started on olanzapine.[166] Remarkably, the topiramate patients did not gain any weight, whereas those on placebo had the usual weight gain. This study needs replication but is promising, although topiramate has many potential side effects. Metformin has had beneficial effects on weight and metabolic parameters.[167,168] Although these studies were short term, positive results are likely to continue over time, and metformin may have infrequent side effects.[169]

Node 2a: Intolerance or Inadequate Trial of Node 2 Antipsychotic?

If the patient could not complete an adequate trial (as defined in Node 1a) of a Node 2 option, choose another antipsychotic from the recommended options before going to Node 3.

NODE 3: UNSATISFACTORY RESPONSE TO AN ADEQUATE SECOND ANTIPSYCHOTIC TRIAL?

Treatment-resistant schizophrenia (TRS) denotes patients with failure to respond to at least two adequate trials of different antipsychotics. Approximately 30% (range 10%–45%) of schizophrenia patients meet this criterion.[170,171] Clozapine is more effective than FGAs[172–174] and other SGAs[175–177] for TRS. Kane and colleagues,[172] in the first double-blind RCT in TRS, demonstrated that clozapine (30%) was more effective than chlorpromazine (4%) in patients who had been refractory to prior trials of FGAs, including haloperidol. Chakos and colleagues,[173] in a review and meta-analysis of subsequent randomized trials, found that clozapine continued to be superior to FGAs in controlling symptoms in patients with chronic schizophrenia. In Phase 2 of CATIE, McEvoy and colleagues[175] compared clozapine, olanzapine, risperidone, and quetiapine in a group of schizophrenia patients who had failed to improve after the initial trial with one of four SGAs or perphenazine. Patients receiving clozapine were less likely to discontinue treatment because of inadequate therapeutic response than patients receiving any of the other SGAs.

Lewis and colleagues,[176] in the large CUtLASS RCT, compared clozapine with amisulpride, olanzapine, quetiapine, and risperidone. Clozapine produced significantly greater reductions in Positive and Negative Syndrome Scale total scores than other agents (–4.93 points; CI, –8.82 to –1.05; p = .013).

Thus, the evidence appears to be substantial that clozapine is the one and only clearly effective option for TRS as defined by failure to respond to two adequate trials of antipsychotics as in this algorithm.[80] Though six studies have compared olanzapine in various doses to clozapine— some of which showed olanzapine's effectiveness to be closer than other SGAs to clozapine—these studies had methodological problems, including low clozapine doses and small sample sizes.[80] Conley and colleagues,[177] in one of those small comparison studies, used a double-blind, crossover design with 13 patients to compare the efficacy of clozapine (450 mg) versus high-dose olanzapine (50 mg) in well-defined TRS. Clozapine was much more effective than olanzapine. Thirty percent of patients responded to clozapine, the same percentage as in Kane and colleagues' study of TRS mentioned above,[172] and no patients improved on olanzapine.[177] Also, 46% of patients dropped out in the olanzapine phase, versus none while on clozapine.

Clozapine is also more effective than haloperidol, olanzapine, and risperidone for persistent aggressive and hostile behavior in treatment-resistant schizophrenia[18] and is more effective than haloperidol and olanzapine for this behavior in non-treatment-resistant schizophrenia patients.[17]

Clozapine is associated with reduced suicide rates in schizophrenia. There is a threefold reduction in the risk of suicidal behaviors compared to other antipsychotic medications.[15] In an international randomized, single-blind study of schizophrenia and schizoaffective disorder patients at high risk for suicide (n = 980), clozapine produced significantly fewer suicidal thoughts and actions than those randomized to olanzapine.[14] In this study, only 27% of subjects had TRS.

Patients with TRS are often poorly compliant with antipsychotic therapy. Adherence with clozapine, however, may be better.[178]

Clozapine blood levels are useful in efforts to improve therapeutic response. They assist with assessing unusual side effects, detecting adherence problems, and evaluating the impact of metabolic inhibitors (e.g., fluvoxamine) and inducers (e.g., cigarette smoke). The optimal therapeutic response usually occurs with clozapine levels above 350–450 ng/mL.[179–182] Plasma levels over 600 ng/mL have been associated with increased toxicity, including seizures.[183] The usual effective dosing range is 300–400 mg/day in divided doses. The total dose should not exceed 900 mg/day, and single doses generally should not exceed 450 mg. If the response is unsatisfactory at 600 mg/day, a blood level should be obtained before further increases are undertaken.[56]

Since clozapine is metabolized by cytochrome P450 isozymes, especially P450 1A2, co-prescription with inhibitors and inducers of these isozymes requires careful attention. Fluvoxamine is a strong inhibitor of the 1A2 enzyme and can increase clozapine levels by 500%, while cigarette smoke induces 1A2-mediated metabolism and can lower levels by over 50%.[56,184] Citalopram has recently been found to raise clozapine levels significantly due to an unknown mechanism and has a new package insert warning about this effect.

If possible, benzodiazepines should be discontinued or reduced because of the risk of respiratory depression in combination with clozapine, especially early in the trial.[185]

Clozapine is associated with adverse effects, some potentially serious and life threatening, including agranulocytosis, seizures, myocarditis, cardiomyopathy, constipation (which can cause obstruction and paralytic ileus), and weight gain/metabolic syndrome. Some less serious side effects—for example, sedation, hypersalivation, tachycardia, hypotension, dizziness, and obsessive-compulsive symptoms—can be disruptive and result in poor adherence. Clinicians should be familiar with the evidence for how optimally to manage these side effects.[186] Due to concerns about the adverse effects of clozapine and about the time and effort required to perform appropriate medical monitoring, manage adverse effects, and administer an adequate trial, this medication is underused despite its advantages.[56]

Many of the adverse effects of clozapine are dose dependent and associated with the speed of titration. Since adverse effects tend to be more common at the beginning of the therapy, it is important to start treatment at low doses and to increase slowly.[52] The starting dose of clozapine is 12.5 mg once or twice daily. For patients over the age of 60, 6.25 mg may be reasonable. Clozapine is gradually titrated upward. Efforts should be made to withdraw the previous antipsychotic gradually once effective clozapine levels are reached. Many believe, though it has not been demonstrated in appropriately designed studies, that optimal results occur with monotherapy.[187]

NODE 4: NO OR UNSATISFACTORY IMPROVEMENT DESPITE AN ADEQUATE CLOZAPINE TRIAL?

Up to 30% of people with refractory schizophrenia treated with clozapine exhibit residual positive symptoms.[188,189]

Clozapine augmentation is a common treatment approach for patients failing to respond to clozapine monotherapy. However, the evidence base supporting augmentation is limited. Meta-analyses suggest small effect sizes (at best) for all proposed options.[190-192]

The addition of risperidone has been studied in five placebo-controlled RCTs.[193-197] Josiassen[196] found an advantage of risperidone over placebo augmentation of clozapine. This study allowed doses up to 6 mg of risperidone and was the longest trial at 12 weeks. Three other trials found no advantage for risperidone, and one found a strong trend toward superiority of placebo, but doses were restricted.[195] A meta-analysis showed no difference in overall efficacy.[192] Thus, the evidence for this frequently employed option is weak, but a higher dose of risperidone for longer duration could be worth trying.

Augmentation with other antipsychotics has very limited support. In two RCTs, the only clear impact of aripiprazole as an augmentation was to blunt the severity of the adverse metabolic effects.[198] Recently, aripiprazole and haloperidol were compared as clozapine augmentations in an RCT.[199] No differences in efficacy were found, but aripiprazole had a more favorable side-effect profile. It is difficult to draw conclusions from this study, however; a placebo control is essential since most augmentation studies have found a large placebo effect.

A small study of sulpiride (which is not available in the United States) found it to be effective as an augmentation.[192]

Another augmentation option is lamotrigine. Tiihonen and colleagues,[200] in a meta-analysis of five placebo-controlled RCTs of lamotrigine augmentation of clozapine, found a small positive effect size of 0.32 by Cohen's d. The net benefit, however, was primarily due to one positive study, leading Sommer and colleagues in their meta-analysis to eliminate that study as an outlier.[192] In two large, placebo-controlled RCTs (n = 429) of lamotrigine augmentation in patients taking various antipsychotics, Goff and colleagues[201] found no advantage for lamotrigine. However, the 63 patients who were on clozapine did slightly better with lamotrigine. In conclusion, lamotrigine may be beneficial for some clozapine partial responders.

The evidence supporting clozapine augmentation with electroconvulsive therapy is weak. No RCTs have been published. However, Havaki-Kontaxaki and colleagues,[202] in a review of the case reports of the concurrent administration of clozapine and ECT in clozapine-resistant schizophrenia or schizoaffective patients, found that this combined therapy appeared to be effective and was reasonably safe. Since this option appears to have as much merit as the well-studied, but weakly efficacious, options of risperidone and lamotrigine, we have included it here at Node 4.

Transcranial magnetic stimulation (rTMS) has also been found to have some efficacy for chronic auditory hallucinations in schizophrenia.[80] Though financial barriers may prevent access for many patients in public sector settings, and much remains to be learned about parameters for optimal acute and maintenance treatment, this treatment holds promise as a Node 4 option with potentially fewer side effects.

Before considering these clozapine augmentations, we recommend a reevaluation of the diagnosis, potential substance abuse, and medication adherence.[203] Optimizing clozapine blood levels, attention to side effects, and elimination of confounding variables such as the presence of other antipsychotics may be important and should be considered before clozapine augmentation.[56,186]

NODE 5: NO OR UNSATISFACTORY IMPROVEMENT WITH CLOZAPINE AUGMENTATION?

If there have been three failed adequate trials of antipsychotics including clozapine, and one failed clozapine augmentation, the probability of improvement with further psychopharmacological interventions is low. However, unexpected positive results can occur. As noted in the flowchart in Figure 1, there are perhaps five approaches to consider at this point. We comment on them in Text Box 2, though not necessarily in order of preference. For any particular patient, the prescribing clinician should review all five options and determine which approach seems best. The clinician should also review the potential psychosocial interventions and decide whether any may have been underutilized up to this point.

Text Box 2	Options to Consider for Treatment-Resistant Schizophrenia at Node 5	
Treatment	*Comments*
Another of the augmentations from Node 4	Try risperidone, lamotrigine, or electroconvulsive therapy.
Other clozapine augmentations	*Memantine.* Lucena and colleagues,[204] in a small, double-blind trial of memantine or placebo (n = 21) as augmentation in clozapine-resistant patients, found memantine better than placebo on all outcomes, with large effect sizes (overall improvement: ES = –2.75, p = .01; positive symptoms: ES = –1.38). Note: no benefit has been found for augmentation with memantine for other SGAs.[204]
	O3FAs. Most of the interest has focused on recent use to prevent onset of schizophrenia in high-risk youth.[205] However, in a 2002 RCT, Peet and colleagues[206] evaluated the addition of O3FA to clozapine (n = 31), SGAs (n = 46), and FGAs (n = 36). Only patients on clozapine had significant benefit.
Stop clozapine, and try other single antipsychotics not previously tried	Perhaps the best antipsychotic to try after clozapine is aripiprazole, based on anecdotal data.[207] The theory is that the partial dopamine agonist effect of aripiprazole will have more benefit when the patient has not recently been treated with a strong dopamine-blocking antipsychotic, which would have produced upregulation of these receptors.[208] Consistent with this theory, one report described a patient who responded well to aripiprazole after clozapine despite failing to respond to it in a previous trial after risperidone.[209] Kane and colleagues,[210] in an RCT, compared the efficacy and safety of aripiprazole (high dose: 30 mg) or perphenazine (40 mg, double that used in CATIE) in well-established, treatment-resistant schizophrenia patients. An impressive 27% of aripiprazole- and 25% of perphenazine-treated patients responded, as defined by a 30% decrease in rating scores. Thus, either of these could be reasonable options at this point. Also, consider loxapine, which has some atypical pharmacodynamic properties[211] and some slight evidence of working when other antipsychotics have failed.[4,6]

(continued)

Text Box 2	Options to Consider for Treatment-Resistant Schizophrenia at Node 5 (*continued*)	
Treatment	*Comments*
Stop clozapine, and try a combination of an FGA and mirtazapine or, if early in course, of an SGA and celecoxib	The FGA/mirtazapine combination is thought to potentially duplicate the receptor impact of clozapine. If clozapine has been tried and failed, the likelihood of success is presumably reduced. However, if the patient is at Node 5 because clozapine was not tolerated, this option may be worth considering. Joffe and colleagues,[212] in a 6-week, placebo-controlled RCT (n = 41) of mirtazapine in patients with inadequate response to their current FGAs, found that 20% of patients (n = 4) on mirtazapine were responders vs. 5% (n = 1) on placebo. On rating-scale scores, the effect size was 1.0 (95% CI, 0.34–1.67). Another positive trial was by Terevnikov.[213] Note: small trials like these can generate higher effect sizes than larger ones. Another RCT (n = 41) did not support the use of this augmentation.[214]
	On the theory that inflammatory processes contribute to the pathogenesis of schizophrenia, anti-inflammatory agents have been tried. Aspirin (1000 mg daily) showed a small effect on positive symptoms in an RCT.[215] In an RCT with the COX-2 inhibitor celecoxib (400 mg daily compared to placebo, with both added to amisulpride), Muller and colleagues[216] treated 49 patients who had been ill for two years or less for six weeks. Significant improvements were seen. Previous studies involving more chronically ill patients showed no benefit from celecoxib.
Combination therapy with non-clozapine FGAs or SGAs	There is no good evidence that antipsychotic combination therapy not involving clozapine offers any efficacy advantage over the use of single antipsychotics. The evidence supporting such combinations consists almost entirely of open-label studies and case series.[217,218] In a persuasive, well-executed negative trial of combination therapy, Kane and colleagues[219] performed a 16-week, placebo-controlled RCT (n = 323) adding aripiprazole to risperidone or quetiapine (equal numbers of each). It could be hypothesized that, based on mechanistic speculations, aripiprazole might be a useful adjunct to either. However, no efficacy was demonstrated. In fact, by week 4, placebo was significantly superior, though over the next 12 weeks this difference gradually disappeared. Both groups improved, so "clinical experience" would have suggested to the observing clinicians that this augmentation was helpful. There are few other good data, which is unfortunate, considering how widely various combinations are used in international practice.

CATIE, Clinical Antipsychotic Trials of Intervention Effectiveness; CI, confidence interval; ES, effect size; FGA, first-generation antipsychotic; O3FA, omega-3 fatty acid; RCT, randomized, controlled trial; SGA, second-generation antipsychotic.

COMPARISON WITH OTHER GUIDELINE AND ALGORITHM RECOMMENDATIONS

The present algorithm for selecting psychopharmacological treatment for schizophrenia differs in some respects from earlier versions of the PAPHSS algorithm and from other recently published algorithms and guidelines. The 1999–2001 version of the PAPHSS algorithm recommended initial treatment of first-onset patients with an SGA, preferably either olanzapine or risperidone, and leaned toward risperidone because of evidence of a more rapid acute effect.[6,7] The patient would be eligible for clozapine after receiving either of the two preferred SGAs and one FGA. In the new version, olanzapine is no longer preferred for first-line use, and an FGA trial is not needed before consideration of clozapine.

Table 2	Comparison with Some Other Algorithms and Guidelines Published in the Last Three Years		
Algorithm/guideline	*Year*	*Comments/differences from PA algorithm*
Maudsley Prescribing Guidelines Algorithms[52]	2012	Has comprehensive discussion of antipsychotic side effects and their management. PA focus is more on the implications of those side effects for decisions at various points in the algorithm.
		In a change from their 2009 algorithm, Maudsley decided that one of the two antipsychotics before clozapine should be olanzapine. PA does not find the evidence compelling that olanzapine must be one of the two.
Evidence-Based Pharmacotherapy of Schizophrenia[220]	2011	Does not address first-episode treatment. PA suggests start first episode with SGA other than clozapine, quetiapine, or olanzapine; then second trial with risperidone, olanzapine, or FGA if not tried first.
		Makes no suggestions for managing resistance to clozapine. PA reviews evidence on different clozapine-augmentation strategies and on what to do next after stopping or not using clozapine.
		Discusses combining antipsychotics as option if they have different receptor profiles. PA finds that combining antipsychotics is not supported by the evidence and should be the last option.
		Favorable view of LAIs as "assuring" compliance. PA sees the evidence for this view to be less convincing and does not have LAIs in primary role.
Schizophrenia Patient Outcomes Research Team (PORT) recommendations[80]	2009	First episode to be treated with any antipsychotic except clozapine and olanzapine. PA adds FGAs and quetiapine to the list of medications not preferred.
		Adequate trials defined in general terms. PA definition of adequate trials adds bioavailability assessment, which may be assisted by a plasma level, after dose adjustment for response and side effects.
		Has no preference for second antipsychotic trial in multi-episode patients. PA prefers risperidone, olanzapine, or FGA for second trial.
		Because the evidence was so unclear, had no recommendations for negative symptoms, comorbid depression, or clozapine resistance. PA endeavored to offer possibly plausible strategies.
United Kingdom's National Institute for Clinical Excellence (NICE) Schizophrenia Guideline[221]	2009	Strong emphasis on psychosocial interventions, involving patients in medication decisions, and on cost-effectiveness of medications, but makes no specific recommendations on medications except for clozapine in treatment resistance. PA has many detailed recommendations at all phases of treatment, from initial to most treatment resistant, including many scenarios with comorbidity.
		Recommends two trials, including at least one SGA, in any order, prior to "offering" clozapine. PA recommends at least one of the following prior to clozapine: risperidone, olanzapine, or FGA.

FGA, first-generation antipsychotic; LAI, long-acting injectable antipsychotic; PA, Psychopharmacology Algorithm Project at the Harvard South Shore Program Algorithm; SGA, second-generation antipsychotic.

Table 2 lists several guidelines and algorithms published by different groups in the last three years that have addressed a similar scope of psychopharmacology problems to the present effort.[52,80,220,221] We have noted some points of contrast between their recommendations and ours.

CONCLUSIONS AND FINAL COMMENT

In the quarter-century since the first iteration of this heuristic, we have seen considerable improvement in the number and quality of treatment options for the psychopharmacology of schizophrenia. Nevertheless, many challenges persist. Better medications are needed with fewer side effects. Much more needs to be learned about the pathophysiology of this chronic, disabling condition and the comorbidities with which it often presents. Improvements in understanding genetics, the neurobiological underpinnings of schizophrenia, and mechanisms underlying its symptoms promise refinements in future treatments and in future algorithms. Eventually, targeted treatments for selected symptoms in this complex, multidimensional disorder will no doubt be developed.

Importantly, structured psychotherapies have made their mark in the world of comprehensive care. Their purposes include emphasis on symptom remission, efforts to educate both patients and families about the illness and its requirements for patient-based self-management, and prioritization of the family as the locus of care. These interventions mesh well with and complement the advances in pharmacological treatment.

All major guidelines and algorithms for treating schizophrenia published in the last few years propose, as do the present authors, that two monotherapy trials with FGAs and SGAs should occur, followed, if necessary, by a trial of clozapine, but they all also vary in how to accomplish these steps.[52,80,220,221] We have provided information to assist with choosing what we argue is the most evidence-supported approach as of this writing. Many clinicians deviate from the consensus view, however, that there should be two trials and then clozapine,[222] and non-evidence-supported polypharmacy continues to be common internationally. The recommendations provided here, if followed, offer a reasonable path to improve psychopharmacological outcomes for patients with schizophrenia and to reduce the time to achieve the maximum benefit obtainable from currently available medications. The authors welcome comments regarding readers' experience and any other aspects of this algorithm that could lead to its improvement in future revisions.

Declaration of interest: The authors report no conflicts of interest. The authors alone are responsible for the content and writing of the article.

REFERENCES

1. Eack SM, Hogarty GE, Cho RY, et al. Neuroprotective effects of cognitive enhancement therapy against gray matter loss in early schizophrenia: results from a 2-year randomized controlled trial. Arch Gen Psychiatry 2010;67:674–82.
2. Osser DN. Treatment resistant problems. In: Tupin JP, Shader RI, Harnett DS, eds. Clinical handbook of psychopharmacology. New York: Jason Aronson, 1988:269–328.
3. Osser DN. A systematic approach to pharmacotherapy in patients with neuroleptic-resistant psychoses. Hosp Community Psychiatry 1989;40:921–7.
4. Osser DN, Patterson RD. Pharmacotherapy of schizophrenia I: acute treatment. In: Soreff S, ed. Handbook for the treatment of the seriously mentally ill. Toronto: Hogrefe & Huber, 1996:91–119.
5. Osser DN, Patterson RD. Pharmacotherapy of schizophrenia II: an algorithm for neuroleptic resistant patients. In: Soreff S, ed. Handbook for the treatment of the seriously mentally ill. Toronto: Hogrefe & Huber, 1996:121–55.

6. Osser DN, Zarate CJ. Consultant for the pharmacotherapy of schizophrenia. Psychiatr Ann 1999;29:252–69.

7. Osser DN, Sigadel R. Short-term inpatient pharmacotherapy of schizophrenia. Harv Rev Psychiatry 2001;9:89–104.

8. Hamoda HM, Osser DN. The Psychopharmacology Algorithm Project at the Harvard South Shore Program: an update on psychotic depression. Harv Rev Psychiatry 2008;16: 235–47.

9. Ansari A, Osser DN. The Psychopharmacology Algorithm Project at the Harvard South Shore Program: an update on bipolar depression. Harv Rev Psychiatry 2010;18:36–55.

10. Osser DN, Dunlop LR. The Psychopharmacology Algorithm Project at the Harvard South Shore Program: an update on generalized social anxiety disorder. Psychopharm Rev 2010;45:91–8.

11. Bajor L, Ticlea A, Osser DN. The Psychopharmacology Algorithm Project at the Harvard South Shore Program: an update on posttraumatic stress disorder. Harv Rev Psychiatry 2011;19:240–58.

12. Gelenberg AJ. The catatonic syndrome. Lancet 1976;1: 1339–41.

13. Manschreck TC, Petri M. The paranoid syndrome. Lancet 1978;2:251–3.

14. Meltzer HY, Alphs L, Green AI, et al. Clozapine treatment for suicidality in schizophrenia: International Suicide Prevention Trial (InterSePT). Arch Gen Psychiatry 2003;60: 82–91.

15. Hennen J, Baldessarini RJ. Suicidal risk during treatment with clozapine: a meta-analysis. Schizophr Res 2005;73: 139–45.

16. Tiihonen J, Suokas JT, Suvisaari JM, Haukka J, Korhonen P. Polypharmacy with antipsychotics, antidepressants, or benzodiazepines and mortality in schizophrenia. Arch Gen Psychiatry 2012;69:476–83.

17. Krakowski MI, Czobor P, Citrome L, Bark N, Cooper TB. Atypical antipsychotic agents in the treatment of violent patients with schizophrenia and schizoaffective disorder. Arch Gen Psychiatry 2006;63:622–9.

18. Volavka J, Czobor P, Nolan K, et al. Overt aggression and psychotic symptoms in patients with schizophrenia treated with clozapine, olanzapine, risperidone, or haloperidol. J Clin Psychopharmacol 2004;24:225–8.

19. Volavka J, Czobor P, Derks EM, et al. Efficacy of antipsychotic drugs against hostility in the European First-Episode Schizophrenia Trial (EUFEST). J Clin Psychiatry 2011;72: 955–61.

20. Battaglia J, Moss S, Rush J, et al. Haloperidol, lorazepam, or both for psychotic agitation? A multicenter, prospective, double-blind, emergency department study. Am J Emerg Med 1997;15:335–40.

21. Garza-Trevino ES, Hollister LE, Overall JE, Alexander WF. Efficacy of combinations of intramuscular antipsychotics and sedative-hypnotics for control of psychotic agitation. Am J Psychiatry 1989;146:1598–601.

22. Breier A, Meehan K, Birkett M, et al. A double-blind, placebo-controlled dose-response comparison of intramuscular olanzapine and haloperidol in the treatment of acute agitation in schizophrenia. Arch Gen Psychiatry 2002;59: 441–8.

23. Andrezina R, Josiassen RC, Marcus RN, et al. Intramuscular aripiprazole for the treatment of acute agitation in patients with schizophrenia or schizoaffective disorder: a doubleblind, placebo-controlled comparison with intramuscular haloperidol. Psychopharmacology (Berl) 2006;188:281–92.

24. Satterthwaite TD, Wolf DH, Rosenheck RA, Gur RE, Caroff SN. A meta-analysis of the risk of acute extrapyramidal symptoms with intramuscular antipsychotics for the treatment of agitation. J Clin Psychiatry 2008;69:1869–79.

25. Zeller SL, Rhoades RW. Systematic reviews of assessment measures and pharmacologic treatments for agitation. Clin Ther 2010;32:403–25.

26. Thapa PB, Palmer SL, Owen RR, Huntley AL, Clardy JA, Miller LH. P.R.N. (as-needed) orders and exposure of psychiatric inpatients to unnecessary psychotropic medications. Psychiatr Serv 2003;54:1282–6.

27. Carpenter WT, Heinrichs DW, Wagman AMI. Deficit and nondeficit forms of schizophrenia—the concept. Am J Psychiatry 1988;145:578–83.

28. Leucht S, Corves C, Arbter D, Engel RR, Li C, Davis JM. Second-generation versus first-generation antipsychotic drugs for schizophrenia: a meta-analysis. Lancet 2009;373:31–41.

29. Buchanan RW, Breier A, Kirkpatrick B, Ball P, Carpenter WT Jr. Positive and negative symptom response to clozapine in schizophrenic patients with and without the deficit syndrome. Am J Psychiatry 1998;155:751–60.

30. Rado JT. Treatment of negative symptoms in schizophrenia. Psychopharm Rev 2011;46:33–9.

31. Singh SP, Singh V, Kar N, Chan K. Efficacy of antidepressants in treating the negative symptoms of chronic schizophrenia: meta-analysis. Br J Psychiatry 2010;197:174–9.

32. Bodkin JA, Siris SG, Bermanzohn PC, Hennen J, Cole JO. Double-blind, placebo-controlled, multicenter trial of selegiline augmentation of antipsychotic medication to treat negative symptoms in outpatients with schizprenia. Am J Psychiatry 2005;162:388–90.

33. Strous RD, Maayan R, Lapidus R, et al. Dehydroepiandrosterone augmentation in the management of negative, depressive, and anxiety symptoms in schizophrenia. Arch Gen Psychiatry 2003;60:133–41.

34. Doruk A, Uzun O, Ozsahin A. A placebo-controlled study of extract of ginkgo biloba added to clozapine in patients with treatment-resistant schizophrenia. Int Clin Psychopharmacol 2008;23:223–7.

35. Levkovitz Y, Mendlovich S, Riwkes S, et al. A double-blind, randomized study of minocycline for the treatment of negative and cognitive symptoms in early-phase schizophrenia. J Clin Psychiatry 2010;71:138–49.

36. Whitehead C, Moss S, Cardno A, Lewis G. Antidepressants for people with both schizophrenia and depression. Cochrane Database Syst Rev 2002;(2):CD002305.

37. Siris SG, Bermanzohn PC, Mason SE, Shuwall MA. Maintenance imipramine therapy for secondary depression in schizophrenia. A controlled trial. Arch Gen Psychiatry 1994; 51:109–15.

38. Kirli S, Caliskan M. A comparative study of sertraline versus imipramine in postpsychotic depressive disorder of schizophrenia. Schizophr Res 1998;33:103–11.

39. Moller HJ. Antidepressive effects of traditional and second generation antipsychotics: a review of the clinical data. Eur Arch Psychiatry Clin Neurosci 2005;255:83–93.

40. Zisook S, Kasckow JW, Golshan S, et al. Citalopram augmentation for subsyndromal symptoms of depression in middle-aged and older outpatients with schizophrenia and schizoaffective disorder: a randomized controlled trial. J Clin Psychiatry 2009;70:562–71.

41. Trixler M, Gati A, Fekete S, Tenyi T. Use of antipsychotics in the management of schizophrenia during pregnancy. Drugs 2005;65:1193–206.

42. Gentile S. Antipsychotic therapy during early and late pregnancy. A systematic review. Schizophr Bull 2010;36:518–44.

43. Collins KO, Comer JB. Maternal haloperidol therapy associated with dyskinesia in a newborn. Am J Health Syst Pharm 2003;60:2253–5.

44. Diav-Citrin O, Shechtman S, Ornoy S, et al. Safety of haloperidol and penfluridol in pregnancy: a multicenter, prospective, controlled study. J Clin Psychiatry 2005;66:317–22.

45. Reis M, Kallen B. Maternal use of antipsychotics in early pregnancy and delivery outcome. J Clin Psychopharmacol 2008;28:279–88.

46. Newham JJ, Thomas SH, MacRitchie K, McElhatton PR, McAllister-Williams RH. Birth weight of infants after maternal exposure to typical and atypical antipsychotics: prospective comparison study. Br J Psychiatry 2008;192:333–7.

47. Ernst CL, Goldberg JF. The reproductive safety profile of mood stabilizers, atypical antipsychotics, and broad-spectrum psychotropics. J Clin Psychiatry 2002;63 suppl 4:42–55.

48. McKenna K, Koren G, Tetelbaum M, et al. Pregnancy outcome of women using atypical antipsychotic drugs: a prospective comparative study. J Clin Psychiatry 2005;66:444–9.

49. Spyropoulou AC, Zervas IM, Soldatos CR. Hip dysplasia following a case of olanzapine exposed pregnancy: a questionable association. Arch Womens Ment Health 2006;9: 219–22.

50. Arora M, Praharaj SK. Meningocele and ankyloblepharon following in utero exposure to olanzapine. Eur Psychiatry 2006;21:345–6.

51. National Institute for Health and Clinical Excellence. Antenatal and postnatal mental health. Clinical management and service guideline. 2007. http://guidance.nice.org.uk/CG45/ NICEGuidance/pdf/ English

52. Taylor D, Paton C, Kapur S. The Maudsley prescribing guidelines in psychiatry. 11th ed. Padstow, UK: Wiley-Blackwell, 2012.

53. Kirchner JE, Owen RR, Nordquist C, Fischer EP. Diagnosis and management of substance use disorders among inpatients with schizophrenia. Psychiatr Serv 1998;49:82–5.

54. Kerfoot KE, Rosenheck RA, Petrakis IL, et al. Substance use and schizophrenia: adverse correlates in the CATIE study sample. Schizophr Res 2011;132:177–82.

55. Kelly DL, McMahon RP, Wehring HJ, et al. Cigarette smoking and mortality risk in people with schizophrenia. Schizophr Bull 2011;37:832–8.

56. Phansalkar S, Osser DN. Optimizing clozapine treatment, part one. Psychopharm Rev 2009;44:1–7.

57. Petrakis IL, O_Malley S, Rounsaville B, Poling J, McHugh- Strong C, Krystal JH. Naltrexone augmentation of neuroleptic treatment in alcohol abusing patients with schizophrenia. Psychopharmacology (Berl) 2004;172:291–7.

58. Tsoi DT, Porwal M, Webster AC. Efficacy and safety of bupropion for smoking cessation and reduction in schizophrenia: systematic review and meta-analysis. Br J Psychiatry 2010;196:346–53.

59. Weiner E, Buchholz A, Coffay A, et al. Varenicline for smoking cessation in people with schizophrenia: a double blind randomized pilot study. Schizophr Res 2011;129: 94–5.

60. Chung AK, Chua SE. Effects on prolongation of Bazett_s corrected QT interval of seven second-generation antipsychotics in the treatment of schizophrenia: a meta-analysis. J Psychopharmacol 2011;25:646–66.

61. Chahine LM, Acar D, Chemali Z. The elderly safety imperative and antipsychotic usage. Harv Rev Psychiatry 2010; 18:158–72.

62. Pollock BG, Mulsant BH, Rosen J, et al. A double-blind comparison of citalopram and risperidone for the treatment of behavioral and psychotic symptoms associated with dementia. Am J Geriatr Psychiatry 2007;15:942–52.

63. Crossley NA, Constante M, McGuire P, Power P. Efficacy of atypical v. typical antipsychotics in the treatment of early psychosis: meta-analysis. Br J Psychiatry 2010;196:434–9.

64. Emsley RA. Risperidone in the treatment of first-episode psychotic patients: a double-blind multicenter study. Risperidone Working Group. Schizophr Bull 1999;25:721–9.

65. Lieberman JA, Phillips M, Gu H, et al. Atypical and conventional antipsychotic drugs in treatment-naive first-episode schizophrenia: a 52-week randomized trial of clozapine vs chlorpromazine. Neuropsychopharmacology 2003;28: 995–1003.

66. Schooler N, Rabinowitz J, Davidson M, et al. Risperidone and haloperidol in first-episode psychosis: a long-term randomized trial. Am J Psychiatry 2005;162:947–53.

67. Green AI, Lieberman JA, Hamer RM, et al. Olanzapine and haloperidol in first episode psychosis: two-year data. Schizophr Res 2006;86:234–43.

68. Kahn RS, Fleischhacker WW, Boter H, et al. Effectiveness of antipsychotic drugs in first-episode schizophrenia and schizophreniform disorder: an open randomised clinical trial. Lancet 2008;371:1085–97.

69. Alvarez-Jimenez M, Parker AG, Hetrick SE, McGorry PD, Gleeson JF. Preventing the second episode: a systematic review and meta-analysis of psychosocial and pharmacological trials in first-episode psychosis. Schizophr Bull 2011;37: 619–30.

70. Lieberman JA, Tollefson G, Tohen M, et al. Comparative efficacy and safety of atypical and conventional antipsychotic drugs in first-episode psychosis: a randomized, double-blind trial of olanzapine versus haloperidol. Am J Psychiatry 2003; 160:1396–404.

71. Correll CU, Leucht S, Kane JM. Lower risk for tardive dyskinesia associated with second-generation antipsychotics: a systematic review of 1-year studies. Am J Psychiatry 2004; 161:414–25.

72. Gharabawi GM, Bossie CA, Zhu Y. New-onset tardive dyskinesia in patients with first-episode psychosis receiving risperidone or haloperidol. Am J Psychiatry 2006;163: 938–9.

73. Novick D, Haro JM, Bertsch J, Haddad PM. Incidence of extrapyramidal symptoms and tardive dyskinesia in schizophrenia: thirty-six-month results from the European schizophrenia outpatient health outcomes study. J Clin Psychopharmacol 2010;30:531–40.

74. Minzenberg MJ, Poole JH, Benton C, Vinogradov S. Association of anticholinergic load with impairment of complex attention and memory in schizophrenia. Am J Psychiatry 2004;161:116–24.

75. Tandon R, DeQuardo JR, Goodson J, Mann NA, Greden JF. Effect of anticholinergics on positive and negative symptoms in schizophrenia. Psychopharmacol Bull 1992;28:297–302.

76. Oosthuizen PP, Emsley RA, Maritz JS, Turner JA, Keyter N. Incidence of tardive dyskinesia in first-episode psychosis patients treated with low-dose haloperidol. J Clin Psychiatry 2003;64:1075–80.

77. Woods SW, Morgenstern H, Saksa JR, et al. Incidence of tardive dyskinesia with atypical versus conventional antipsychotic medications: a prospective cohort study. J Clin Psychiatry 2010;71:463–74.

78. McEvoy JP, Lieberman JA, Perkins DO, et al. Efficacy and tolerability of olanzapine, quetiapine, and risperidone in the treatment of early psychosis: a randomized, double-blind 52-week comparison. Am J Psychiatry 2007;164:1050–60.

79. Robinson DG, Woerner MG, Napolitano B, et al. Randomized comparison of olanzapine versus risperidone for the treatment of first-episode schizophrenia: 4-month outcomes. Am J Psychiatry 2006;163:2096–102.

80. Buchanan RW, Kreyenbuhl J, Kelly DL, et al. The 2009 schizophrenia PORT psychopharmacological treatment recommendations and summary statements. Schizophr Bull 2010;36:71–93.

81. Zipursky RB, Gu H, Green AI, et al. Course and predictors of weight gain in people with first-episode psychosis treated with olanzapine or haloperidol. Br J Psychiatry 2005;187: 537–43.

82. Fernandez-Egea E, Miller B, Garcia-Rizo C, Bernardo M, Kirkpatrick B. Metabolic effects of olanzapine in patients with newly diagnosed psychosis. J Clin Psychopharmacol 2011;31:154–9.

83. Sanger TM, Lieberman JA, Tohen M, Grundy S, Beasley C Jr, Tollefson GD. Olanzapine versus haloperidol treatment in first-episode psychosis. Am J Psychiatry 1999;156:79–87.

84. Patel JK, Buckley PF, Woolson S, et al. Metabolic profiles of second-generation antipsychotics in early psychosis: findings from the CAFE study. Schizophr Res 2009;111:9–16.

85. Kreyenbuhl J, Slade EP, Medoff DR, et al. Time to discontinuation of first- and second-generation antipsychotic medications in the treatment of schizophrenia. Schizophr Res 2011;131:127–32.

86. Kasper S, Brecher M, Fitton L, Jones AM. Maintenance of long-term efficacy and safety of quetiapine in the open-label treatment of schizophrenia. Int Clin Psychopharmacol 2004;19:281–9.

87. Hatta K, Sato K, Hamakawa H, et al. Effectiveness of second-generation antipsychotics with acute-phase schizophrenia. Schizophr Res 2009;113:49–55.

88. McCue RE, Waheed R, Urcuyo L, et al. Comparative effectiveness of second-generation antipsychotics and haloperidol in acute schizophrenia. Br J Psychiatry 2006;189:433–40.

89. Suzuki T, Uchida H, Watanabe K, et al. How effective is it to sequentially switch among olanzapine, quetiapine and risperidone? A randomized, open-label study of algorithm-based antipsychotic treatment to patients with symptomatic schizophrenia in the real-world clinical setting. Psychopharmacology (Berl) 2007;195:285–95.

90. Malik P, Kemmler G, Hummer M, Riecher-Roessler A, Kahn RS, Fleischhacker WW. Sexual dysfunction in first-episode schizophrenia patients: results from European First Episode Schizophrenia Trial. J Clin Psychopharmacol 2011;31: 274–80.

91. Spollen JJ 3rd, Wooten RG, Cargile C, Bartztokis G. Prolactin levels and erectile function in patients treated with risperidone. J Clin Psychopharmacol 2004;24:161–6.

92. Holt RI, Peveler RC. Antipsychotics and hyperprolactinaemia: mechanisms, consequences and management. Clin Endocrinol (Oxf) 2011;74:141–7.

93. Komossa K, Rummel-Kluge C, Schmid F, et al. Aripiprazole versus other atypical antipsychotics for schizophrenia. Cochrane Database Syst Rev 2009;(4):CD006569.

94. Correll CU, Manu P, Olshanskiy V, Napolitano B, Kane JM, Malhotra AK. Cardiometabolic risk of second-generation antipsychotic medications during first-time use in children and adolescents. JAMA 2009;302:1765–73.

95. Ray WA, Chung CP, Murray KT, Hall K, Stein CM. Atypical antipsychotic drugs and the risk of sudden cardiac death. N Engl J Med 2009;360:225–35.

96. Komossa K, Rummel-Kluge C, Hunger H, et al. Ziprasidone versus other atypical antipsychotics for schizophrenia. Cochrane Database Syst Rev 2009;(4):CD006627.

97. Grootens KP, van Veelen NM, Peuskens J, et al. Ziprasidone vs olanzapine in recent-onset schizophrenia and schizoaffective disorder: results of an 8-week double-blind randomized controlled trial. Schizophr Bull 2011;37:352–61.

98. Taylor D. Ziprasidone in the management of schizophrenia : the QT interval issue in context. CNS Drugs 2003;17: 423–30.

99. Citrome L. Using oral ziprasidone effectively: the food effect and dose-response. Adv Ther 2009;26:739–48.

100. Komossa K, Rummel-Kluge C, Hunger H, et al. Amisulpride versus other atypical antipsychotics for schizophrenia. Cochrane Database Syst Rev 2010;(1):CD006624.

101. Marino J, Caballero J. Iloperidone for the treatment of schizophrenia. Ann Pharmacother 2010;44:863–70.

102. Janicak PG, Rado JT. Asenapine: a review of the data. Psychopharm Rev 2009;44:89–96.

103. Meyer JM, Loebel AD, Schweizer E. Lurasidone: a new drug in development for schizophrenia. Expert Opin Investig Drugs 2009;18:1715–26.

104. Potkin SG, Ogasa M, Cucchiaro J, Loebel A. Double-blind comparison of the safety and efficacy of lurasidone and ziprasidone in clinically stable outpatients with schizophrenia or schizoaffective disorder. Schizophr Res 2011;132:101–7.

105. Meltzer HY, Cucchiaro J, Silva R, et al. Lurasidone in the treatment of schizophrenia: a randomized, double-blind, placebo- and olanzapine-controlled study. Am J Psychiatry 2011;168:957–67.

106. Harvey PD, Ogasa M, Cucchiaro J, Loebel A, Keefe RS. following in utero exposure to cognitive change in a randomized, double-blind comparison of lurasidone vs. ziprasidone. Schizophr Res 2011;127:188–94.

107. Kopala LC, Good KP, Honer WG. Extrapyramidal signs and clinical symptoms in first-episode schizophrenia: response to low-dose risperidone. J Clin Psychopharmacol 1997;17: 308–13.

108. McEvoy JP, Hogarty GE, Steingard S. Optimal dose of neuroleptic in acute schizophrenia. A controlled study of the neuroleptic threshold and higher haloperidol dose. Arch Gen Psychiatry 1991;48:739–45.

109. Merlo MC, Hofer H, Gekle W, et al. Risperidone, 2 mg/day vs. 4 mg/day, in first-episode, acutely psychotic patients: treatment efficacy and effects on fine motor functioning. J Clin Psychiatry 2002;63:885–91.

110. Reilly JL, Harris MS, Keshavan MS, Sweeney JA. Adverse effects of risperidone on spatial working memory in first- episode schizophrenia. Arch Gen Psychiatry 2006;63:1189–97.

111. Lambert M, Conus P, Eide P, et al. Impact of present and past antipsychotic side effects on attitude toward typical antipsychotic treatment and adherence. Eur Psychiatry 2004;19:415–22.

112. Leucht S, Busch R, Kissling W, Kane JM. Early prediction of antipsychotic nonresponse among patients with schizophrenia. J Clin Psychiatry 2007;68:352–60.

113. Gallego JA, Robinson DG, Sevy SM, et al. Time to treatment response in first-episode schizophrenia: should acute treatment trials last several months? J Clin Psychiatry 2011;72:1691–6.

114. Li C, Xia J, Wang J. Risperidone dose for schizophrenia. Cochrane Database Syst Rev 2009;(4):CD007474.

115. Kinon BJ, Volavka J, Stauffer V, et al. Standard and higher dose of olanzapine in patients with schizophrenia or schizoaffective disorder: a randomized, double-blind, fixed-dose study. J Clin Psychopharmacol 2008;28:392–400.

116. Davis JM, Chen N. Dose response and dose equivalence of antipsychotics. J Clin Psychopharmacol 2004;24: 192–208.

117. Citrome L, Yang R, Glue P, Karayal ON. Effect of ziprasidone dose on all-cause discontinuation rates in acute schizophrenia and schizoaffective disorder: a post-hoc analysis of 4 fixed-dose randomized clinical trials. Schizophr Res 2009;111:39–45.

118. Sparshatt A, Taylor D, Patel MX, Kapur S. A systematic review of aripiprazole—dose, plasma concentration, receptor occupancy, and response: implications for therapeutic drug monitoring. J Clin Psychiatry 2010;71:1447–56.

119. Citrome L, Stauffer VL, Chen L, et al. Olanzapine plasma concentrations after treatment with 10, 20, and 40 mg/d in patients with schizophrenia: an analysis of correlations with efficacy, weight gain, and prolactin concentration. J Clin Psychopharmacol 2009;29:278–83.

120. Patel MX, Bowskill S, Couchman L, et al. Plasma olanzapine in relation to prescribed dose and other factors: data from a therapeutic drug monitoring service, 1999–2009. J Clin Psychopharmacol 2011;31:411–7.

121. Sparshatt A, Taylor D, Patel MX, Kapur S. Amisulpride—dose, plasma concentration, occupancy and response: implications for therapeutic drug monitoring. Acta Psychiatr Scand 2009;120:416–28.

122. Sparshatt A, Taylor D, Patel MX, Kapur S. Relationship between daily dose, plasma concentrations, dopamine receptor occupancy, and clinical response to quetiapine: a review. J Clin Psychiatry 2011;72:1108–23.

123. Olfson M, Marcus SC, Ascher-Svanum H. Treatment of schizophrenia with long-acting fluphenazine, haloperidol, or risperidone. Schizophr Bull 2007;33:1379–87.

124. Rosenheck RA, Krystal JH, Lew R, et al. Long-acting risperidone and oral antipsychotics in unstable schizophrenia. N Engl J Med 2011;364:842–51.

125. Tiihonen J, Haukka J, Taylor M, Haddad PM, Patel MX, Korhonen P. A nationwide cohort study of oral and depot antipsychotics after first hospitalization for schizophrenia. Am J Psychiatry 2011;168:603–9.

126. Leucht C, Heres S, Kane JM, Kissling W, Davis JM, Leucht S. Oral versus depot antipsychotic drugs for schizophreniaVa critical systematic review and meta-analysis of randomised long-term trials. Schizophr Res 2011;127: 83–92.

127. Haddad PM, Taylor M, Niaz OS. First-generation antipsychotic long-acting injections v. oral antipsychotics in schizophrenia: systematic review of randomised controlled trials and observational studies. Br J Psychiatry Suppl 2009;52:S20–8.

128. Taylor D. Psychopharmacology and adverse effects of antipsychotic long-acting injections: a review. Br J Psychiatry Suppl 2009;52:S13–9.

129. Adams CE, Fenton MK, Quraishi S, David AS. Systematic meta-review of depot antipsychotic drugs for people with schizophrenia. Br J Psychiatry 2001;179:290–9.

130. Boaz TL, Constantine RJ, Robst J, Becker MA, Howe AM. Risperidone long-acting therapy prescribing patterns and their impact on early discontinuation of treatment in a large Medicaid population. J Clin Psychiatry 2011;72:1079–85.

131. Covell NH, McEvoy JP, Schooler NR, et al. Effectiveness of switching from long-acting injectable fluphenazine or haloperidol decanoate to long-acting injectable risperidone microspheres: an open-label, randomized controlled trial. J Clin Psychiatry 2012;73:669–75.

132. Citrome L. Paliperidone palmitate—review of the efficacy, safety and cost of a new second-generation depot antipsychotic medication. Int J Clin Pract 2010;64:216–39.

133. Bishara D. Once-monthly paliperidone injection for the treatment of schizophrenia. Neuropsychiatr Dis Treat 2010; 6:561–72.

134. Kane JM, Detke HC, Naber D, et al. Olanzapine long-acting injection: a 24-week, randomized, double-blind trial of maintenance treatment in patients with schizophrenia. Am J Psychiatry 2010;167:181–9.

135. Detke HC, McDonnell DP, Brunner E, Zhao F, Sorsaburu S, Stefaniak VJ, Corya SA. Post-injection delirium/sedation syndrome in patients with schizophrenia treated with olanzapine long-acting injection, I: analysis of cases. BMC Psychiatry 2010;10:43.

136. Glasgow RE, Vogt TM, Boles SM. Evaluating the public health impact of health promotion interventions: the REAIM framework. Am J Public Health 1999;89:1322–7.

137. Kane JM, Carson WH, Saha AR, et al. Efficacy and safety of aripiprazole and haloperidol versus placebo in patients with schizophrenia and schizoaffective disorder. J Clin Psychiatry 2002;63:763–71.

138. Lindenmayer JP, Citrome L, Khan A, Kaushik S. A randomized, double-blind, parallel-group, fixed-dose, clinical trial of quetiapine at 600 versus 1200 mg/d for patients with treatment-resistant schizophrenia or schizoaffective disorder. J Clin Psychopharmacol 2011;31:160– 8.

139. Miller CH, Fleischhacker WW. Managing antipsychotic-induced acute and chronic akathisia. Drug Saf 2000;22: 73–81.

140. Levinson DF, Simpson GM, Singh H, et al. Fluphenazine dose, clinical response, and extrapyramidal symptoms during acute treatment. Arch Gen Psychiatry 1990;47:761–8.

141. Sachdev P. The development of the concept of akathisia: a historical overview. Schizophr Res 1995;16:33–45.

142. Crowner ML, Douyon R, Convit A, Gaztanaga P, Volavka J, Bakall R. Akathisia and violence. Psychopharmacol Bull 1990;26:115–7.

143. Hansen L. A critical review of akathisia, and its possible association with suicidal behaviour. Hum Psychopharmacol 2001;16:495–505.

144. Kane JM, Fleischhacker WW, Hansen L, Perlis R, Pikalov A 3rd, Assuncao-Talbott S. Akathisia: an updated review focusing on second-generation antipsychotics. J Clin Psychiatry 2009;70:627–43.

145. Hirose S. The causes of underdiagnosing akathisia. Schizophr Bull 2003;29:547–58.

146. Farde L. Selective D1- and D2-dopamine receptor blockade both induce akathisia in humans: a PET study with [11C]SCH 23390 and [11C]raclopride. Psychopharmacology (Berl) 1992;107:23–9.

147. Adler LA, Peselow E, Rosenthal M, Angrist B. A controlled comparison of the effects of propranolol, benztropine, and placebo on akathisia: an interim analysis. Psychopharmacol Bull 1993;29:283–6.

148. Fischel T, Hermesh H, Aizenberg D, et al. Cyproheptadine versus propranolol for the treatment of acute neuroleptic-induced akathisia: a comparative double-blind study. J Clin Psychopharmacol 2001;21:612–5.

149. Poyurovsky M, Pashinian A, Weizman R, Fuchs C, Weizman A. Low-dose mirtazapine: a new option in the treatment of antipsychotic-induced akathisia. A randomized, doubleblind, placebo- and propranolol-controlled trial. Biol Psychiatry 2006;59:1071–7.

150. Van Putten T, Marder SR. Behavioral toxicity of antipsychotic drugs. J Clin Psychiatry 1987;48 suppl:13–9.

151. Sachdev P, Loneragan C. Intravenous benztropine and propranolol challenges in acute neuroleptic-induced akathisia. Clin Neuropharmacol 1993;16:324–31.

152. Rathbone J, Soares-Weiser K. Anticholinergics for neuroleptic-induced acute akathisia. Cochrane Database Syst Rev 2006;(4):CD003727.

153. Stryjer R, Rosenzcwaig S, Bar F, Ulman AM, Weizman A, Spivak B. Trazodone for the treatment of neuroleptic- induced acute akathisia: a placebo-controlled, double-blind, crossover study. Clin Neuropharmacol 2010;33:219–22.

154. Avital A, Gross-Isseroff R, Stryjer R, Hermesh H, Weizman A, Shiloh R. Zolmitriptan compared to propranolol in the treatment of acute neuroleptic-induced akathisia: a comparative double-blind study. Eur Neuropsychopharmacol 2009;19:476–82.

155. Miodownik C, Lerner V, Statsenko N, et al. Vitamin B6 versus mianserin and placebo in acute neuroleptic-induced akathisia: a randomized, double-blind, controlled study. Clin Neuropharmacol 2006;29:68–72.

156. Gandelman K, Alderman JA, Glue P, et al. The impact of calories and fat content of meals on oral ziprasidone absorption: a randomized, open-label, crossover trial. J Clin Psychiatry 2009;70:58–62.

157. Lieberman JA, Stroup TS, McEvoy JP, et al. Effectiveness of antipsychotic drugs in patients with chronic schizophrenia. N Engl J Med 2005;353:1209– 23.

158. Mazure CM, Nelson JC, Jatlow PI, Kincare P, Bowers MB Jr. The relationship between blood perphenazine levels, early resolution of psychotic symptoms, and side effects. J Clin Psychiatry 1990;51:330 –4.

159. Hansen LB, Larsen NE. Therapeutic advantages of monitoring plasma concentrations of perphenazine in clinical practice. Psychopharmacology (Berl) 1985;87:16–9.

160. Janicak PG, Marder SR, Pavuluri MN. Principles and practice of psychopharmacotherapy. 5th ed. New York: Lippincott Williams & Wilkins, 2011.

161. Janicak PG, Javaid JI, Sharma RP, Leach A, Dowd S, Davis JM. A two-phase, double-blind randomized study of three haloperidol plasma levels for acute psychosis with reassignment of initial non-responders. Acta Psychiatr Scand 1997; 95:343–50.

162. Stroup TS, Lieberman JA, McEvoy JP, et al. Effectiveness of olanzapine, quetiapine, risperidone, and ziprasidone in patients with chronic schizophrenia following discontinuation of a previous atypical antipsychotic. Am J Psychiatry 2006;163:611–22.

163. Essock SM, Covell NH, Davis SM, Stroup TS, Rosenheck RA, Lieberman JA. Effectiveness of switching antipsychotic medications. Am J Psychiatry 2006;163:2090–5.

164. Kane JM, Cohen M, Zhao J, Alphs L, Panagides J. Efficacy and safety of asenapine in a placebo- and haloperidol- controlled trial in patients with acute exacerbation of schizophrenia. J Clin Psychopharmacol 2010;30:106–15.

165. Ashih HW. Saphris and Fanapt: two new antipsychotics. Carlat Psychiatry Rep 2009;7:1–3.

166. Narula PK, Rehan HS, Unni KE, Gupta N. Topiramate for prevention of olanzapine associated weight gain and metabolic dysfunction in schizophrenia: a double-blind, placebo- controlled trial. Schizophr Res 2010;118:218–23.

167. Klein DJ, Cottingham EM, Sorter M, Barton BA, Morrison JA. A randomized, double-blind, placebo-controlled trial of metformin treatment of weight gain associated with initiation of atypical antipsychotic therapy in children and adolescents. Am J Psychiatry 2006;163:2072–9.

168. Wu RR, Zhao JP, Guo XF, et al. Metformin addition attenuates olanzapine-induced weight gain in drug-naive first-episode schizophrenia patients: a double-blind, placebo-controlled study. Am J Psychiatry 2008;165:352–8.

169. Smith RC. Metformin as a treatment for antipsychotic drug side effects: special focus on women with schizophrenia. Am J Psychiatry 2012;169:774 –6.

170. Conley RR, Buchanan RW. Evaluation of treatment-resistant schizophrenia. Schizophr Bull 1997;23:663–74.

171. Meltzer HY. Treatment-resistant schizophrenia—the role of clozapine. Curr Med Res Opin 1997;14:1–20.

172. Kane J, Honigfeld G, Singer J, Meltzer H. Clozapine for the treatment-resistant schizophrenic. A double-blind comparison with chlorpromazine. Arch Gen Psychiatry 1988;45: 789–96.

173. Chakos M, Lieberman J, Hoffman E, Bradford D, Sheitman B. Effectiveness of second-generation antipsychotics in patients with treatment-resistant schizophrenia: a review and meta-analysis of randomized trials. Am J Psychiatry 2001;158:518–26.

174. Essock SM, Hargreaves WA, Covell NH, Goethe J. Clozapine's effectiveness for patients in state hospitals: results from a randomized trial. Psychopharmacol Bull 1996;32:683–97.

175. McEvoy JP, Lieberman JA, Stroup TS, et al. Effectiveness of clozapine versus olanzapine, quetiapine, and risperidone in patients with chronic schizophrenia who did not respond to prior atypical antipsychotic treatment. Am J Psychiatry 2006;163:600–10.

176. Lewis SW, Barnes TR, Davies L, et al. Randomized controlled trial of effect of prescription of clozapine versus other second-generation antipsychotic drugs in resistant schizophrenia. Schizophr Bull 2006;32:715–23.

177. Conley RR, Kelly DL, Richardson CM, Tamminga CA, Carpenter WT Jr. The efficacy of high-dose olanzapine versus clozapine in treatment-resistant schizophrenia: a double-blind crossover study. J Clin Psychopharmacol 2003;23:668–71.

178. Meltzer HY. Dimensions of outcome with clozapine. Br J Psychiatry Suppl 1992;26:46–53.

179. Perry PJ, Miller DD, Arndt SV, Cadoret RJ. Clozapine and norclozapine plasma concentrations and clinical response of treatment-refractory schizophrenic patients. Am J Psychiatry 1991;148:231–5.

180. Kronig MH, Munne RA, Szymanski S, et al. Plasma clozapine levels and clinical response for treatment-refractory schizophrenic patients. Am J Psychiatry 1995;152: 179–82.

181. Hasegawa M, Gutierrez-Esteinou R, Way L, Meltzer HY. Relationship between clinical efficacy and clozapine concentrations in plasma in schizophrenia: effect of smoking. J Clin Psychopharmacol 1993;13:383–90.

182. Potkin SG, Bera R, Gulasekaram B, et al. Plasma clozapine concentrations predict clinical response in treatment-resistant schizophrenia. J Clin Psychiatry 1994;55 suppl B:133–6.

183. Freudenreich O, Weiner RD, McEvoy JP. Clozapine-induced electroencephalogram changes as a function of clozapine serum levels. Biol Psychiatry 1997;42:132–7.

184. Lu ML, Lane HY, Lin SK, Chen KP, Chang WH. Adjunctive fluvoxamine inhibits clozapine-related weight gain and metabolic disturbances. J Clin Psychiatry 2004;65:766–71.

185. Faisal I, lindenmayer JP, Taintor Z, Cancro R. Clozapinebenzodiazepine interactions. J Clin Psychiatry 1997;58: 547–8.

186. Phansalkar S, Osser DN. Optimizing clozapine treatment; part II. Psychopharm Rev 2009;44:9–16.

187. Meltzer HY. Treatment of the neuroleptic-nonresponsive schizophrenic patient. Schizophr Bull 1992;18:515–42.

188. Meltzer HY, Bastani B, Kwon KY, Ramirez LF, Burnett S, Sharpe J. A prospective study of clozapine in treatment-resistant schizophrenic patients. I. Preliminary report. Psychopharmacology (Berl) 1989;99 suppl:S68–72.

189. Buckley P, Miller A, Olsen J, Garver D, Miller DD, Csernansky J. When symptoms persist: clozapine augmentation strategies. Schizophr Bull 2001;27:615–28.

190. Barbui C, Signoretti A, Mule S, Boso M, Cipriani A. Does the addition of a second antipsychotic drug improve clozapine treatment? Schizophr Bull 2009;35:458–68.

191. Taylor DM, Smith L. Augmentation of clozapine with a second antipsychotic—a meta-analysis of randomized, placebo-controlled studies. Acta Psychiatr Scand 2009;119:419–25.

192. Sommer IE, Begemann MJ, Temmerman A, Leucht S. Pharmacological augmentation strategies for schizophrenia patients with insufficient response to clozapine: a quantitative literature review. Schizophr Bull 2012;38:1003–11.

193. Freudenreich O, Henderson DC, Walsh JP, Culhane MA, Goff DC. Risperidone augmentation for schizophrenia partially responsive to clozapine: a double-blind, placebo- controlled trial. Schizophr Res 2007;92:90–4.

194. Honer WG, Thornton AE, Chen EY, et al. Clozapine alone versus clozapine and risperidone with refractory schizophrenia. N Engl J Med 2006;354:472–82.

195. Anil Yagcioglu AE, Kivircik Akdede BB, Turgut TI, et al. A double-blind controlled study of adjunctive treatment with risperidone in schizophrenic patients partially responsive to clozapine: efficacy and safety. J Clin Psychiatry 2005;66: 63–72.

196. Josiassen RC, Joseph A, Kohegyi E, et al. Clozapine augmented with risperidone in the treatment of schizophrenia: a randomized, double-blind, placebo-controlled trial. Am J Psychiatry 2005;162:130–6.

197. Weiner E, Conley RR, Ball MP, et al. Adjunctive risperidone for partially responsive people with schizophrenia treated with clozapine. Neuropsychopharmacology 2010;35: 2274–83.

198. Henderson DC, Kunkel L, Nguyen DD, et al. An exploratory open-label trial of aripiprazole as an adjuvant to clozapine therapy in chronic schizophrenia. Acta Psychiatr Scand 2006;113:142–7.

199. Barbui C, Accordini S, Nose M, et al. Aripiprazole versus haloperidol in combination with clozapine for treatment-resistant schizophrenia in routine clinical care: a randomized, controlled trial. J Clin Psychopharmacol 2011;31: 266–73.

200. Tiihonen J, Wahlbeck K, Kiviniemi V. The efficacy of lamotrigine in clozapine-resistant schizophrenia: a systematic review and meta-analysis. Schizophr Res 2009;109: 10–4.

201. Goff DC, Keefe R, Citrome L, et al. Lamotrigine as add-on therapy in schizophrenia: results of 2 placebo-controlled trials. J Clin Psychopharmacol 2007;27:582–9.

202. Havaki-Kontaxaki BJ, Ferentinos PP, Kontaxakis VP, Paplos KG, Soldatos CR. Concurrent administration of clozapine and electroconvulsive therapy in clozapine-resistant schizophrenia. Clin Neuropharmacol 2006;29:52–6.

203. Moore TA, Buchanan RW, Buckley PF, et al. The Texas Medication Algorithm Project antipsychotic algorithm for schizophrenia: 2006 update. J Clin Psychiatry 2007;68: 1751–62.

204. De Lucena D, Fernandes BS, Berk M, et al. Improvement of negative and positive symptoms in treatment-refractory schizophrenia: a double-blind, randomized, placebo-controlled trial with memantine as add-on therapy to clozapine. J Clin Psychiatry 2009;70:1416–23.

205. Amminger GP, Schafer MR, Papageorgiou K, et al. Long- chain omega-3 fatty acids for indicated prevention of psychotic disorders: a randomized, placebo-controlled trial. Arch Gen Psychiatry 2010;67:146–54.

206. Peet M, Horrobin DF. A dose-ranging exploratory study of the effects of ethyl-eicosapentaenoate in patients with persistent schizophrenic symptoms. J Psychiatr Res 2002;36: 7–18.

207. Raja M. Improvement or worsening of psychotic symptoms after treatment with low doses of aripiprazole. Int J Neuro-psychopharmacol 2007;10:107–10.

208. Tadokoro S, Okamura N, Sekine Y, Kanahara N, Hashimoto K, Iyo M. Chronic treatment with aripiprazole prevents development of dopamine supersensitivity and potentially supersensitivity psychosis. Schizophr Bull 2012;38: 1012–20.

209. Jong-Yih L. Successful switch from clozapine to aripiprazole: a case report. J Clin Psychopharmacol 2009;29:93–5.

210. Kane JM, Meltzer HY, Carson WH Jr, McQuade RD, Marcus RN, Sanchez R. Aripiprazole for treatment-resistant schizophrenia: results of a multicenter, randomized, doubleblind, comparison study versus perphenazine. J Clin Psychiatry 2007;68:213–23.

211. Meltzer HY, Jayathilake K. Low-dose loxapine in the treatment of schizophrenia: is it more effective and more Batypical[than standard-dose loxapine? J Clin Psychiatry 1999;60 suppl 10:47–51.

212. Joffe G, Terevnikov V, Joffe M, Stenberg JH, Burkin M, Tiihonen J. Add-on mirtazapine enhances antipsychotic effect of first generation antipsychotics in schizophrenia: a double-blind, randomized, placebo-controlled trial. Schizophr Res 2009;108:245–51.

213. Terevnikov V, Stenberg JH, Joffe M, et al. More evidence on additive antipsychotic effect of adjunctive mirtazapine in schizophrenia: an extension phase of a randomized controlled trial. Hum Psychopharmacol 2010;25:431–8.

214. Berk M, Gama CS, Sundram S, et al. Mirtazapine add-on therapy in the treatment of schizophrenia with atypical antipsychotics: a double-blind, randomised, placebo-controlled clinical trial. Hum Psychopharmacol 2009;24:233–8.

215. Laan W, Grobbee DE, Selten JP, Heijnen CJ, Kahn RS, Burger H. Adjuvant aspirin therapy reduces symptoms of schizophrenia spectrum disorders: results from a randomized, double-blind, placebo-controlled trial. J Clin Psychiatry 2010;71:520–7.

216. Riedel M, Strassnig M, Schwarz MJ, Muller N. COX-2 inhibitors as adjunctive therapy in schizophrenia: rationale for use and evidence to date. CNS Drugs 2005;19:805–19.

217. Chan J, Sweeting M. Review: Combination therapy with non-clozapine atypical antipsychotic medication: a review of current evidence. J Psychopharmacol 2007;21:657–64.

218. Lerner V, Libov I, Kotler M, Strous RD. Combination of Batypical[antipsychotic medication in the management of treatment-resistant schizophrenia and schizoaffective disorder. Prog Neuropsychopharmacol Biol Psychiatry 2004;28: 89–98.

219. Kane JM, Correll CU, Goff DC, et al. A multicenter, randomized, double-blind, placebo-controlled, 16-week study of adjunctive aripiprazole for schizophrenia or schizoaffective disorder inadequately treated with quetiapine or risperidone monotherapy. J Clin Psychiatry 2009;70:1348–57.

220. Leucht S, Heres S, Kissling W, Davis JM. Evidence-based pharmacotherapy of schizophrenia. Int J Neuropsychopharmacol 2011;14:269–84.

221. National Institute for Health and Clinical Excellence. Schizophrenia: core interventions in the treatment and management of schizophrenia in adults in primary and secondary care (update). 2009. http://www.nice.org.uk/CG82

222. Osser DN. Why physicians do not follow some guidelines and algorithms. Drug Benefit Trends 2009;21:345–54.

UPDATE

SCHIZOPHRENIA ALGORITHM*

The algorithm for the pharmacotherapy of schizophrenia has been published six times since the first one by this author in 1988. There have been many changes over those years. However, in the seven years since its last publication in 2013, the recommendations and flowchart remain mostly the same. There have been no new studies that seem to change the overall sequences of the nodes. However, there have been a variety of studies usually adding support to what was proposed in the 2013 algorithm, but sometimes making adjustments to the risk/benefit analysis for certain recommendations. There are two new medications for adults approved in 2015 in the United States for the acute treatment of schizophrenia: cariprazine and brexpiprazole. They appear to have comparable efficacy to older antipsychotics and at this time are much more costly. They produce less weight gain than some and occasionally that may make them preferable to some lower-cost options, and cariprazine may have a role for persistent negative symptoms (to be discussed). Lurasidone is fairly new and was discussed in the previous algorithm, but in 2017 it received a new indication for schizophrenia in adolescents, and this changed its placement in the algorithm. Also, there have been several new products in the category of long-acting injectable antipsychotics (LAIs) that are discussed in this update.

There is another new antipsychotic that was just approved for the treatment of schizophrenia as this book was going to press: lumateperone. It was approved by the U.S. Food and Drug Administration in late December 2019, with expected launch in March 2020. Lumateperone is a butyrophenone, as is haloperidol, but the molecule has been adjusted and it seems to cause almost no extrapyramidal side effects, and like haloperidol it produces very little weight gain. Somnolence, though, was a side effect in 24% versus 10% with placebo. Efficacy seems comparable to antipsychotics such as quetiapine, aripiprazole, and ziprasidone. Some think it may "revolutionize" treatment of schizophrenia but future studies will be needed to make that determination.[1] It is too early to give it a place in the algorithm.

---

* I thank Robert D. Patterson, MD for his contributions to the text of this update and also for preparing the revised flowchart for the schizophrenia algorithm.

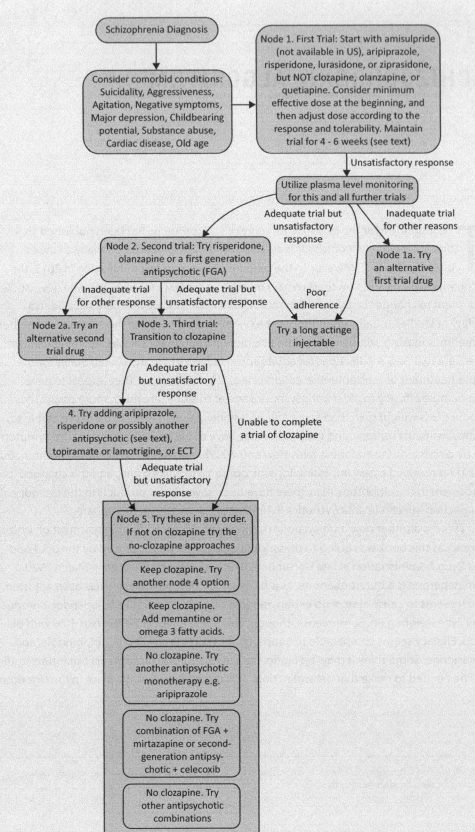

Schizophrenia Diagnosis

Consider comorbid conditions: Suicidality, Aggressiveness, Agitation, Negative symptoms, Major depression, Childbearing potential, Substance abuse, Cardiac disease, Old age

Node 1. First Trial: Start with amisulpride (not available in US), aripiprazole, risperidone, lurasidone, or ziprasidone, but NOT clozapine, olanzapine, or quetiapine. Consider minimum effective dose at the beginning, and then adjust dose according to the response and tolerability. Maintain trial for 4 - 6 weeks (see text)

Unsatisfactory response

Utilize plasma level monitoring for this and all further trials

Adequate trial but unsatisfactory response

Inadequate trial for other reasons

Node 1a. Try an alternative first trial drug

Node 2. Second trial: Try risperidone, olanzapine or a first generation antipsychotic (FGA)

Inadequate trial for other response

Adequate trial but unsatisfactory response

Poor adherence

Node 2a. Try an alternative second trial drug

Node 3. Third trial: Transition to clozapine monotherapy

Try a long acting injectable

Adequate trial but unsatisfactory response

4. Try adding aripiprazole, risperidone or possibly another antipsychotic (see text), topiramate or lamotrigine, or ECT

Unable to complete a trial of clozapine

Adequate trial but unsatisfactory response

Node 5. Try these in any order. If not on clozapine try the no-clozapine approaches

Keep clozapine. Try another node 4 option

Keep clozapine. Add memantine or omega 3 fatty acids.

No clozapine. Try another antipsychotic monotherapy e.g. aripiprazole

No clozapine. Try combination of FGA + mirtazapine or second-generation antipsychotic + celecoxib

No clozapine. Try other antipsychotic combinations

A change in the diagnostic criteria for schizophrenia occurred with the 2013 publication of the *Diagnostic and Statistical Manual of Mental Disorders Edition 5* (DSM-5). The A criteria for schizophrenia changed. In the previous version (DSM-IV), five symptoms were listed under the A criteria and at least two of five had to be present during an acute episode. The five were delusions, hallucinations, disorganized speech, grossly disorganized behavior, and negative symptoms (diminished emotional expression or avolition). In DSM-5, at least one of the first three symptoms (defined as positive symptoms) must be present. In DSM-IV, you could meet the A criteria by having both of the other two symptoms and no positive symptoms. This change actually supports the utility of this algorithm because positive symptoms were identified as the primary targets of pharmacotherapy—though management of negative and cognitive symptoms was also discussed. Thus, with DSM-5, patients diagnosed with schizophrenia are a little more likely to have the positive symptoms that the algorithm addresses. However, the quantity of patients who met the A criteria under DSM-IV by having only non-positive symptoms was very small—less than 1%.[2]

Another more important change in DSM-5 was to the D criterion for schizophrenia, which differentiates schizophrenia from schizoaffective disorder.[3] In DSM-IV, the patient had to have no mood episodes (depression or mania) during the active phase of the illness, or if they occurred, they were brief compared to the total duration of the illness (active and residual phases). In the full text of DSM-IV, an example of "brief" was given, and it was having a five-week period in a mood episode in a person who had been ill for four years. The five weeks was 2.5% of the four-year period. Note, though, that the criteria refer to a mood "episode." Depressive or manic "symptoms" (short of meeting criteria for the full syndrome of an episode) could be present even continuously and the diagnosis would still be schizophrenia if the rest of the criteria were met. In DSM-5, the D criterion changed to allowing a mood episode for a "minority" (i.e., up to 50%) of the time compared to the total length of the illness. Therefore, all the patients who were having mood episodes lasting anywhere from 2.5% to 49% of the total duration of their illness would now be reclassified as having schizophrenia and not schizoaffective disorder. The effect of this change was to significantly decrease the number of patients who will be diagnosed schizoaffective disorder.[4] The implications for the use of the schizophrenia algorithm is that these former schizoaffective patients are now candidates for schizophrenia treatment recommendations. There has, in fact, been surprisingly little study of schizoaffective disorder treatment.[5] Indeed, many experts have serious questions about whether the disorder really exists.[6] In support of this view, there is evidence the DSM-IV diagnosis of schizoaffective disorder tended to be unstable and often changed to schizophrenia over time.[7,8] Thus, patients meeting the previous as well as the present more rarefied criteria for schizoaffective are probably best classified as being either closer to the schizophrenia spectrum (and should then be treated taking into consideration this algorithm) or closer to bipolar disorder with psychosis (and those should be treated with consideration of a mania algorithm such as the one in this book).

Schizoaffective disorder is being diagnosed frequently. One study showed that up to 30% of patients admitted for psychosis received this diagnosis.[9] Many clinicians seem to think they know how to treat it, but this knowledge is not based on any substantial scientific evidence. Due to this lack of evidence, the Psychopharmacology Algorithm Project at the Harvard South Shore Program has not developed an algorithm for schizoaffective disorder.

Table 1: Comorbidity and Other Features in Schizophrenia and How They Affect the Algorithm

In Table 1, there are ten conditions that are discussed. A few deserve some additional comments.

Agitation requiring rapid management: To add to the five studies cited originally, there was a new study that came out in 2013.[10] This was a fairly large prospective randomized double-blind controlled trial evaluating four intramuscular (IM) treatments for acute agitation in an emergency room setting in Brazil. One hundred consecutive patients were randomized to either haloperidol 2.5 mg plus midazolam 7.5 mg, haloperidol 2.5 mg plus promethazine 25 mg, olanzapine 10 mg, or ziprasidone 10 mg. The majority of the patients had schizophrenia with 36% having a diagnosis of mania. One hour after the treatment, the best results were with the haloperidol plus benzodiazepine or the olanzapine. However, the odds ratio for significant side effects was 1.6 higher for olanzapine. The other two treatments were inferior in effectiveness. The odds ratio for side effects was highest (3.6) with the haloperidol plus the antiparkinsonian agent promethazine compared with the haloperidol plus midazolam. This study further supports the algorithm's recommendation that haloperidol plus a benzodiazepine (often it is lorazepam in the United States.) is still the best and safest IM treatment for acute agitation in the urgent or emergency setting.

Primary negative or "deficit" symptoms: In addition to the two citations supporting the benefit of adding an antidepressant for persisting negative symptoms in schizophrenia, there is a newer meta-analysis of several studies of mirtazapine finding it useful for this purpose.[11] Also, an evaluation of a large administrative database of Medicaid patients from 2001 to 2010 found an association with antidepressant use and reduced rehospitalization and emergency room visits.[12] The reason for the association was not at all clear and an editorial suggested that more widespread addition of antidepressants in schizophrenia to improve maintenance outcome requires more study in randomized trials before it should become routine.[13]

The new (2015) antipsychotic cariprazine had a multicenter trial in schizophrenia patients who had significant residual negative symptoms for over six months while being otherwise clinically stable with well-controlled positive symptoms.[14] About 461 patients were randomized to switch to either cariprazine (mean final dose 4.2 mg) or risperidone (mean dose 3.8 mg) for six months. In order to be sure that negative symptom improvement was not due to any difference in secondary negative symptoms from the prescribed treatment, results were controlled for depression, extrapyramidal, and positive symptoms. Negative symptoms improved significantly (>20%) in 69% of the cariprazine patients and 58% of the risperidone patients (number needed to treat = 9). This is a small difference. It seems more reasonable to try adding an antidepressant first. But cariprazine perhaps deserves a try if antidepressants fail.

Another category of medications of possible use for primary negative symptoms is dopaminergic agents. Modafinil, armodafinil, L-dopa, and pramipexole were reviewed in a recent meta-analysis.[15] Ten randomized controlled trials (six with modafinil) were assessed and the net result was that there was no significant improvement. They did not increase positive symptom scores, however.

Memantine was mentioned in 2013 as an option for negative/cognitive symptoms in Table 1. Since then, there have been more studies using it for this indication. Five controlled trials have been published, and the latest study was positive at a dose of 20 mg daily, so there are now three positive and two negative studies in the literature.[16]

Remember that primary negative symptoms are diagnosed by first excluding secondary negative symptoms. Negative symptoms can be a consequence of positive symptoms, can result from excessive sedative effects of the medication regimen, and can be produced by parkinsonian and other extrapyramidal side effects. These should all be managed first with appropriate interventions.

Major depression: The Table 1 text presented a guarded perspective on the value of adding an antidepressant for major depression or depressive symptoms occurring during the active phase of schizophrenia-related psychosis. "Postpsychotic depression," as discussed in Table 1, was (and remains) a clear target for antidepressants. A newer meta-analysis of 82 randomized controlled trials of antidepressants in schizophrenia found that antidepressants seem a little more effective for active-phase depressive symptoms than we previously thought.[17] Reduction in depressive symptoms overall had an effect size of 0.25 standardized mean difference, which translated to about one in nine patients improving. The improvement in negative symptoms in the meta-analysis was 0.30. Depressive symptoms overlap with negative symptoms and they can be difficult to distinguish clinically and in the research setting. Antidepressants were generally well tolerated, so this small rate of improvement was at a relatively small cost in terms of side effects. Therefore, the perspective on adding antidepressants for depressive symptoms has moved a bit in the direction of being more acceptable.

Women of childbearing potential: Major studies have appeared evaluating the risk of antipsychotics in pregnancy, all generally supporting the original recommendations in the table. First-generation antipsychotics (FGAs) still seem a little safer than second-generation antipsychotics (SGAs) with respect to fetal congenital malformation risk, according to a review of 1.3 million pregnancies covered by Medicaid.[18] The rate was 3.3% in those with no exposure to an antipsychotic, versus 3.8% with FGAs and 4.4% with SGAs. After adjustment for confounding variables, the rate was 0.90% for FGAs and 1.05% for SGAs. Among the SGAs, risperidone was somewhat higher (risk ratio 1.26). In another study, quetiapine had a very low rate, no different from controls.[19] However, weight gain can be very significant with SGAs, especially quetiapine and olanzapine, which were found in a study to be associated with gestational diabetes in 7% and 12%, respectively, compared with 5% with aripiprazole and 4% with ziprasidone.[20] Women on SGAs very frequently gained considerable weight prior to their pregnancy,[21] and quetiapine may raise triglycerides more than others.[22] These considerations should all be actively discussed with women of childbearing potential and collaborative decisions made taking them into account.

While on the subject of women of childbearing potential, it is worth mentioning that valproate is perhaps the most dangerous medication to use in such women. It has little proven value in schizophrenia, is associated with an increased mortality risk when used in these patients (hazard ratio 1.31),[12] and is associated with severe teratogenicity. It should be nearly a last choice compared to any other psychotropic medication.[23]

Effects of antipsychotics on QTc prolongation: Previous reviews suggested that aripiprazole was the least likely antipsychotic to prolong QTc. A new meta-analysis finds that lurasidone has the least.[24] Paliperidone and cariprazine were low, as well.

Node 1: Recommendations for the First Antipsychotic Trial in a New-Onset Patient

In addition to the medications recommended in the 2013 algorithm: amisulpride, aripiprazole, risperidone, and ziprasidone—add lurasidone. In the initial draft of the algorithm submitted for review, lurasidone was included in the first-line choices because of its reasonable effectiveness and modest side effect profile. However, reviewers pointed out that there were no studies showing effectiveness in first-onset patients. Response patterns can be different in this group, compared to patients who have had multiple past exposures to antipsychotics but who are not considered treatment resistant. In 2017, the FDA approved lurasidone for adolescents (aged 13–17) with schizophrenia based on a randomized trial of 40 or 80 mg versus placebo.[25] The subjects were not all youth who had no previous treatment for their schizophrenia, but this positive study seems to supply the missing evidence base for considering lurasidone among the first-line choices in the algorithm.

Another new study suggesting need for a slight adjustment to the first-line recommendations was by Robinson et al.[26] Both risperidone and aripiprazole were among the recommendation in 2013, but here was a head-to-head comparison of these two in 198 acutely psychotic first-onset patients who had no more than two weeks of exposure to any antipsychotic. The rate of significant response on positive symptoms was 63% with aripiprazole and 57% with risperidone. This equivalence (with slight numerical advantage to aripiprazole) could be considered somewhat unexpected because the weight of the evidence in multi episode schizophrenia patients (summarized in the algorithm paper) is that aripiprazole is somewhat inferior to risperidone. One might speculate that this difference in response to aripiprazole in antipsychotic-naïve patients has something to do with the fact that dopamine receptors can be upregulated secondary to the dopamine blockade produced by previous exposure to dopamine-blocking antipsychotics. Medications with partial dopamine agonist effect, like aripiprazole, might produce more undesirable stimulation of those upregulated receptors than they would in the antipsychotic-naïve individuals. Consistent with that, akathisia was more common with aripiprazole than with risperidone. However, metabolic side effects were greater with risperidone, and there was significantly more improvement in negative symptoms with aripiprazole ($p < .03$). The authors concluded that aripiprazole was a better initial medication with first-onset schizophrenia compared with risperidone, and this seems a reasonable conclusion. Aripiprazole also performed better than quetiapine in an open-label randomized comparison in first-episode patients, while being equally effective with ziprasidone in this three-armed trial.[27]

Among the antipsychotics not recommended for first-line use in patients having their first episode and/or getting their first treatment with an antipsychotic, olanzapine continues to stand out as undesirable for all the reasons cited in 2013, including the near-universal agreement on its undesirability with other national and international guidelines and algorithms.

An additional consideration would be a newer report that even one dose of olanzapine, 10 mg, given to healthy volunteers, produces significant insulin resistance and inflammatory abnormalities within hours after oral administration.[28] The study did not evaluate how long it took for those abnormalities to return to normal, but this "requires elucidation." Quetiapine probably has similar effects on insulin resistance,[29] and clozapine almost surely does as well.

It was also mentioned in the 2013 algorithm that quetiapine is also undesirable as a first-onset choice because it seems to be one of the antipsychotics with the least effectiveness in preventing the next episode of schizophrenia or rehospitalization. Newer studies confirm this.[30,31]

Poorly Adherent Patients: The Role of Long-Acting Injectable Antipsychotics

In the 2013 algorithm draft that was submitted for consideration for publication, the discussion of LAIs was praised by all (blinded) reviewers as particularly useful and was considered to be a reasonable statement of their appropriate place in the treatment of schizophrenia. Since then, we have many more LAIs that have been marketed but the reasoning regarding their basic roles and use seems to still be valid.

An important comment about LAI usage in the algorithm paper is that LAIs may be necessary to complete an adequate first (or second) trial of an antipsychotic on the way to seeing if clozapine is going to be indicated as the third trial. Adherence with oral trials has long been recognized as problematic. Poor adherence is often not recognized by the prescribing clinician, and it was recommended to routinely check plasma levels of oral antipsychotics as a way of evaluating possible adherence problems. Plasma levels can also suggest rapid metabolism (or slow metabolism with elevated blood levels which could explain unexpectedly severe side effects). This recommendation was, and still is, not often implemented. Hiemke et al.[32] have recently revised their comprehensive listing of psychotropic medication plasma levels and clinicians should retain their paper for reference. There was an editorial accompanying this paper, which made the following statement: "While 'individualization' or 'personalization' of treatment is a top priority on the research agenda of most psychiatric scientific societies, therapeutic drug monitoring (TDM) is indeed the only clinically proven approach for personalized treatment in psychiatry. This is in sharp contrast to the fact that—although cheap and widely available—TDM is not systematically established in routine patient care."[33]

In a recent study evaluating the value of TDM with antipsychotics, 99 patients were identified who appeared treatment-resistant and were being considered for clozapine. Plasma antipsychotic levels were measured.[34] About 35% had subtherapeutic levels, and of these 34% were unmeasurable. These patients typically were on lower-than-usual doses, and they had a higher rate of readmissions (p = .02).

TDM may also be helpful in minimizing side effects. A recent report showed that higher plasma levels of antipsychotics with strong dopamine-receptor blocking properties (such as FGAs and some SGAs like olanzapine—and probably risperidone) correlate negatively with patient subjective sense of both physical and mental well-being.[35] This is distinct from extrapyramidal side effects, and may be equivalent to what in the past has been termed "neuroleptic induced dysphoria." It is likely to be associated with higher rates of nonadherence. Higher levels of partial dopamine agonists (aripiprazole was the one studied) were correlated with impaired physical well-being, probably from akathisia. Monitoring plasma levels and keeping them at the low to medium optimal range may reduce these phenomena.

One of the best uses of an LAI, therefore, should be to correct inadequate adherence as demonstrated by a low or zero plasma level (that is not due to a genetic or drug-interaction pharmacokinetic issue) and minimize the side effect burden. This enables completion of an adequate trial so that it can be determined if the medication being used has the potential to produce a satisfactory therapeutic response and be well-tolerated over the long term. If, despite correction of a low blood level with an LAI, the response remains unsatisfactory, the patient is eligible to move on to the next node of the algorithm for another medication trial.

Patients who should continue on an LAI are those who get a satisfactory response and still need the LAI to optimize adherence. This can produce improvement in rehospitalization rates as well as reduce mortality (33% reduction compared with oral).[30,36] For this purpose, we do have more choices. For example, if the patient is started in aripiprazole and then needs an LAI, we now have several formulations of aripiprazole LAI. Injections can last four, six, or eight weeks. There is also a new formulation in which patients receive an oral dose of 30 mg at the same time that they receive a four-week injection; this results in therapeutic plasma levels developing in four days. Paliperidone now has an injection lasting 12 weeks, which can be started after the patient has been on the 4-week formulation for 4 months. Risperidone now has the first formulation of an LAI that is injected subcutaneously; it lasts four weeks.

Node 2: The Second Antipsychotic Trial

There has been no change in the recommendations here, which are to try one of the more effective antipsychotics as demonstrated in trials with patients who have had previous exposures to antipsychotics: risperidone, olanzapine, or one of the FGAs like perphenazine.[37,38] If the patient was on one of these for the first trial, then any antipsychotic may be selected for the second trial.

Node 3: The Third Antipsychotic Trial—Clozapine

In the last seven years, there have been many studies, reviews, and guidelines debating the role of clozapine, but the bottom line is that the strong recommendation for clozapine is still supported despite the considerable side effects of this medicine.[39,40] These patients have treatment-resistant schizophrenia (TRS) and nothing else has come along that is clearly effective for TRS. Despite this it remains underutilized.[41] Yet, it appears likely that real-world outcomes would be better if more clinicians utilized clozapine when indicated.[42,43] This algorithm update has provided further refinement of the parameters for adequate trials of the first two antipsychotics prior to clozapine (e.g., use of plasma levels and LAIs), and confidence in the appropriateness of turning to clozapine for the third trial should be enhanced.

Node 4: Augmentations and Alternatives to Clozapine

The 2013 algorithm offered five ideas to consider, none of which had strong support. As of this writing, some have stronger support, others weaker.

Augmentations with other antipsychotics: Previously risperidone, lamotrigine, and FGAs were considerations. There seems to have been little interest in further study of these particular options. The evidence remains as it was in the 2013 paper: The support is weak at best. Aripiprazole as an augmentation, however, has had significant new study and discussion in the literature. In a meta-analysis of four short-term (8–24 weeks) randomized placebo-controlled trials of adding aripiprazole to clozapine involving 347 patients, the improvement in positive symptoms was at a trend level (p = .12) only.[44] All-cause discontinuation rates were higher with placebo (risk ratio 1.4) but this too was nonsignificant. The patients lost a mean of three pounds but they were eight times more likely to get agitation or akathisia. These data did not seem to particularly support adding aripiprazole to the option list. However, a new meta-analysis of psychiatric rehospitalization (a measure of maintenance effectiveness) with different antipsychotics and combinations of antipsychotics involving 62,250 patients in Sweden found that aripiprazole plus clozapine was associated with the lowest rate of rehospitalization.[31] Other combinations involving clozapine, clozapine alone, and combinations involving an LAI comprised the ten best treatments associated with reduced rehospitalization. The best results on mortality and medical hospitalizations were also found with the same leading options. Editorial comment, however, urged caution and that these observational studies should be considered preliminary and more high-quality randomized controlled trials are needed to confirm the efficacy of these combinations (apart from the well-established efficacy of clozapine and the benefits of LAIs for addressing adherence issues).[13] Major newer meta-analyses of up to 62 studies of acute treatment (as opposed to relapse prevention) have found no greater efficacy for any antipsychotic combinations.[45,46]

Augmentations with anticonvulsants: Previously, lamotrigine was discussed because it has had five placebo-controlled trials as an augmentation for clozapine. New data suggest topiramate is also an option.[47] This is an addition to the previous algorithm recommendations. Zheng et al. found a significant improvement in positive symptoms (standardized mean difference: −0.37) and negative symptoms (SMD: −0.58). Patients also lost a mean of 6 pounds, and improved in other metabolic indices as well, including insulin resistance. However, there were high discontinuation rates due to paresthesias and cognitive difficulties.[48] Valproate was also studied in five trials in China and seemed comparably effective to topiramate as an augmentation of clozapine[48] but the studies were faulted for not controlling for clozapine levels, high heterogeneity of the studies, and peculiarities of ethnicity-based genetic metabolic issues with clozapine in the population treated.[49]

Augmentation with electroconvulsive therapy (ECT): The previous algorithm included ECT as an option for augmenting clozapine, based on case report data only. Since then, there was a controlled trial of ECT with clozapine continuation as the control, showing efficacy.[50] However, a small sham-controlled trial published two years later in 2017 was disappointing in showing no difference in outcome versus sham.[51] Sham produced a 28% improvement in Positive and Negative Symptom Scale scores, compared with a 19% reduction in the group getting ECT, which was a nonsignificant difference. The study diminishes enthusiasm for this strategy though it is still retained as a consideration. Sham and real ECT procedures both produced some benefit.

Switching to aripiprazole to replace clozapine after the clozapine trial must end: Though there are very little data supporting the theoretical notion that after a trial of an antipsychotic like clozapine that has weak affinity for the dopamine receptor (and which, as a consequence does not upregulate those receptors), a trial with a medicine that is both a dopamine blocker and a partial agonist at the dopamine receptor, like aripiprazole, could be timely and effective. One more case report has appeared that supports this possibility.[52]

Something really new and unexpected: A 24-year-old man with chronic TRS had a bone marrow transplantation for cancer treatment.[53] His schizophrenia remitted in a remarkable way and continued in remission at four-year follow-up. Did this have something to do with addressing immune system dysregulation? Further studies are required.

REFERENCES

1. Vyas P, Hwang BJ, Brasic JR. An evaluation of lumateperone tosylate for the treatment of schizophrenia. Expert Opin Pharmacother 2020; 21(2):139–145.
2. Tandon R, Gaebel W, Barch DM, et al. Definition and description of schizophrenia in the DSM-5. Schizophr Res 2013;150:3–10.
3. Malaspina D, Owen MJ, Heckers S, et al. Schizoaffective disorder in the DSM-5. Schizophr Res 2013;150:21–5.
4. Kotov R, Leong SH, Mojtabai R, et al. Boundaries of schizoaffective disorder: revisiting Kraepelin. JAMA Psychiatry 2013;70:1276–86.
5. Murru A, Pacchiarotti I, Nivoli AM, Grande I, Colom F, Vieta E. What we know and what we don't know about the treatment of schizoaffective disorder. Eur Neuropsychopharmacol 2011;21:680–90.
6. Cheniaux E, Landeira-Fernandez J, Lessa Telles L, et al. Does schizoaffective disorder really exist? A systematic review of the studies that compared schizoaffective disorder with schizophrenia or mood disorders. J Affect Disord 2008;106:209–17.
7. Bromet EJ, Kotov R, Fochtmann LJ, et al. Diagnostic shifts during the decade following first admission for psychosis. Am J Psychiatry 2011;168:1186–94.
8. Jager M, Haack S, Becker T, Frasch K. Schizoaffective disorder—an ongoing challenge for psychiatric nosology. Eur Psychiatry 2011;26:159–65.
9. Azorin JM, Kaladjian A, Fakra E. Current issues on schizoaffective disorder. Encephale 2005;31:359–65.
10. Mantovani C, Labate CM, Sponholz A Jr, et al. Are low doses of antipsychotics effective in the management of psychomotor agitation? A randomized, rated-blind trial of 4 intramuscular interventions. J Clin Psychopharmacol 2013;33:306–12.
11. Vidal C, Reese C, Fischer BA, Chiapelli J, Himelhoch S. Meta-analysis of efficacy of mirtazapine as an adjunctive treatment of negative symptoms in schizophrenia. Clin Schizophr Relat Psychoses 2015;9:88–95.
12. Stroup TS, Gerhard T, Crystal S, et al. Comparative effectiveness of adjunctive psychotropic medications in patients with schizophrenia. JAMA Psychiatry 2019;76:508–15.
13. Goff DC. Can adjunctive pharmacotherapy reduce hospitalization in schizophrenia?: insights from administrative databases. JAMA Psychiatry 2019;76:468–70.
14. Nemeth G, Laszlovszky I, Czobor P, et al. Cariprazine versus risperidone monotherapy for treatment of predominant negative symptoms in patients with schizophrenia: a randomised, double-blind, controlled trial. Lancet 2017;389:1103–13.

15. Sabe M, Kirschner M, Kaiser S. Prodopaminergic drugs for treating the negative symptoms of schizophrenia: systematic review and meta-analysis of randomized controlled trials. J Clin Psychopharmacol 2019;39:658–64.
16. Hassanpour F, Zarghami M, Mouodi S, et al. Adjunctive memantine treatment of schizophrenia: a double-blind, randomized placebo-controlled study. J Clin Psychopharmacol 2019;39:634–8.
17. Helfer B, Samara MT, Huhn M, et al. Efficacy and safety of antidepressants added to antipsychotics for schizophrenia: a systematic review and meta-analysis. Am J Psychiatry 2016;173:876–86.
18. Huybrechts KF, Hernandez-Diaz S, Patorno E, et al. Antipsychotic use in pregnancy and the risk for congenital malformations. JAMA Psychiatry 2016;73:938–46.
19. Cohen LS, Goez-Mogollon L, Sosinsky AZ, et al. Risk of major malformations in infants following first-trimester exposure to quetiapine. Am J Psychiatry 2018;175:1225–31.
20. Park Y, Hernandez-Diaz S, Bateman BT, et al. Continuation of atypical antipsychotic medication during early pregnancy and the risk of gestational diabetes. Am J Psychiatry 2018;175:564–74.
21. Freeman MP, Sosinsky AZ, Goez-Mogollon L, et al. Gestational weight gain and pre-pregnancy body mass index associated with second-generation antipsychotic drug use during pregnancy. Psychosomatics 2018;59:125–34.
22. Correll CU, Robinson DG, Schooler NR, et al. Cardiometabolic risk in patients with first-episode schizophrenia spectrum disorders: baseline results from the RAISE-ETP study. JAMA Psychiatry 2014;71:1350–63.
23. Balon R, Riba M. Should women of childbearing potential be prescribed valproate? A call to action. J Clin Psychiatry 2016;77:525–6.
24. Huhn M, Nikolakopoulou A, Schneider-Thoma J, et al. Comparative efficacy and tolerability of 32 oral antipsychotics for the acute treatment of adults with multi-episode schizophrenia: a systematic review and network meta-analysis. Lancet 2019;394:939–51.
25. Goldman R, Loebel A, Cucchiaro J, Deng L, Findling RL. Efficacy and safety of lurasidone in adolescents with schizophrenia: a 6-week, randomized placebo-controlled study. J Child Adolesc Psychopharmacol 2017;27:516–25.
26. Robinson DG, Gallego JA, John M, et al. A randomized comparison of aripiprazole and risperidone for the acute treatment of first-episode schizophrenia and related disorders: 3-month outcomes. Schizophr Bull 2015;41:1227–36.
27. Crespo-Facorro B, Perez-Iglesias R, Mata I, et al. Aripiprazole, ziprasidone, and quetiapine in the treatment of first-episode nonaffective psychosis: results of a 6-week, randomized, flexible-dose, open-label comparison. J Clin Psychopharmacol 2013;33:215–20.
28. Hahn MK, Wolever TM, Arenovich T, et al. Acute effects of single-dose olanzapine on metabolic, endocrine, and inflammatory markers in healthy controls. J Clin Psychopharmacol 2013;33:740–6.
29. Ngai YF, Sabatini P, Nguyen D, et al. Quetiapine treatment in youth is associated with decreased insulin secretion. J Clin Psychopharmacol 2014;34:359–64.
30. Tiihonen J, Mittendorfer-Rutz E, Majak M, et al. Real-world effectiveness of antipsychotic treatments in a nationwide cohort of 29823 patients with schizophrenia. JAMA Psychiatry 2017;74:686–93.
31. Tiihonen J, Taipale H, Mehtala J, Vattulainen P, Correll CU, Tanskanen A. Association of antipsychotic polypharmacy vs monotherapy with psychiatric rehospitalization among adults with schizophrenia. JAMA Psychiatry 2019;76:499–507.
32. Hiemke C, Bergemann N, Clement HW, et al. Consensus guidelines for therapeutic drug monitoring in neuropsychopharmacology: update 2017. Pharmacopsychiatry 2018;51:9–62.
33. Grunder G. Editorial to consensus guidelines for therapeutic drug monitoring in neuropsychopharmacology. Pharmacopsychiatry 2018;51:5–6.
34. McCutcheon R, Beck K, D'Ambrosio E, et al. Antipsychotic plasma levels in the assessment of poor treatment response in schizophrenia. Acta Psychiatr Scand 2018;137:39–46.
35. Veselinovic T, Scharpenberg M, Heinze M, et al. Dopamine D2 receptor occupancy estimated from plasma concentrations of four different antipsychotics and the subjective experience of physical and mental well-being in schizophrenia: results from the randomized NeSSy trial. J Clin Psychopharmacol 2019;39:550–60.

36. Taipale H, Mittendorfer-Rutz E, Alexanderson K, et al. Antipsychotics and mortality in a nationwide cohort of 29,823 patients with schizophrenia. Schizophr Res 2018;197:274–80.

37. Hatta K, Sato K, Hamakawa H, et al. Effectiveness of second-generation antipsychotics with acute-phase schizophrenia. Schizophr Res 2009;113:49–55.

38. McCue RE, Waheed R, Urcuyo L, et al. Comparative effectiveness of second-generation antipsychotics and haloperidol in acute schizophrenia. Br J Psychiatry 2006;189:433–40.

39. Kane JM, Agid O, Baldwin ML, et al. Clinical guidance on the identification and management of treatment-resistant schizophrenia. J Clin Psychiatry 2019;80(2).

40. Masuda T, Misawa F, Takase M, Kane JM, Correll CU. Association with hospitalization and all-cause discontinuation among patients with schizophrenia on clozapine vs other oral second-generation antipsychotics: a systematic review and meta-analysis of cohort studies. JAMA Psychiatry 2019;76:1052–62.

41. Stroup TS. Clozapine and evidence-based psychopharmacology for schizophrenia. JAMA Psychiatry 2019;76:1007–8.

42. Krivoy A, Joyce D, Tracy D, et al. Real-world outcomes in the management of refractory psychosis. J Clin Psychiatry 2019;80.

43. Wimberley T, MacCabe JH, Laursen TM, et al. Mortality and self-harm in association with clozapine in treatment-resistant schizophrenia. Am J Psychiatry 2017;174:990–8.

44. Srisurapanont M, Suttajit S, Maneeton N, Maneeton B. Efficacy and safety of aripiprazole augmentation of clozapine in schizophrenia: a systematic review and meta-analysis of randomized-controlled trials. J Psychiatr Res 2015;62:38–47.

45. Galling B, Roldan A, Rietschel L, et al. Safety and tolerability of antipsychotic co-treatment in patients with schizophrenia: results from a systematic review and meta-analysis of randomized controlled trials. Expert Opin Drug Saf 2016;15:591–612.

46. Ortiz-Orendain J, Castiello-de Obeso S, Colunga-Lozano L, Hu Y, Maayan N, Adams C. Antipsychotic combinations for schizophrenia. Schizophr Bull 2018;44:15–7.

47. Zheng W, Xiang YT, Xiang YQ, et al. Efficacy and safety of adjunctive topiramate for schizophrenia: a meta-analysis of randomized controlled trials. Acta Psychiatr Scand 2016;134:385–98.

48. Zheng W, Xiang YT, Yang XH, Xiang YQ, de Leon J. Clozapine augmentation with antiepileptic drugs for treatment-resistant schizophrenia: a meta-analysis of randomized controlled trials. J Clin Psychiatry 2017;78:e498–505.

49. Faden J. Treatment-resistant schizophrenia: a brief overview of treatment options. J Clin Psychiatry 2019;80.

50. Petrides G, Malur C, Braga RJ, et al. Electroconvulsive therapy augmentation in clozapine-resistant schizophrenia: a prospective, randomized study. Am J Psychiatry 2015;172:52–8.

51. Melzer-Ribeiro DL, Rogonatti SP, Kayo M, et al. Efficacy of electroconvulsive therapy augmentation for partial response to clozapine: a pilot randomized ECT-sham controlled trial. Arch Clin Psychiatry 2017;44:45–50.

52. Feeley RJ, Arnaout B, Yoon G. Effective switch from clozapine to aripiprazole in treatment-resistant schizophrenia and comorbid alcohol use disorder. J Clin Psychopharmacol 2017;37:729–30.

53. Miyaoka T, Wake R, Hashioka S, et al. Remission of psychosis in treatment-resistant schizophrenia following bone marrow transplantation: a case report. Front Psychiatry 2017;8:174.

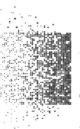

The Psychopharmacology Algorithm Project at the Harvard South Shore Program: An Algorithm for Generalized Anxiety Disorder

Harmony Raylen Abejuela, MD and David N. Osser, MD

Learning Objective: *After participating in this activity, learners should be better able to:*
• Evaluate pharmacotherapy options for patients with generalized anxiety disorder

Abstract: *This revision of previous algorithms for the pharmacotherapy of generalized anxiety disorder was developed by the Psychopharmacology Algorithm Project at the Harvard South Shore Program. Algorithms from 1999 and 2010 and associated references were reevaluated. Newer studies and reviews published from 2008–14 were obtained from PubMed and analyzed with a focus on their potential to justify changes in the recommendations. Exceptions to the main algorithm for special patient populations, such as women of childbearing potential, pregnant women, the elderly, and those with common medical and psychiatric comorbidities, were considered. Selective serotonin reuptake inhibitors (SSRIs) are still the basic first-line medication. Early alternatives include duloxetine, buspirone, hydroxyzine, pregabalin, or bupropion, in that order. If response is inadequate, then the second recommendation is to try a different SSRI. Additional alternatives now include benzodiazepines, venlafaxine, kava, and agomelatine. If the response to the second SSRI is unsatisfactory, then the recommendation is to try a serotonin-norepinephrine reuptake inhibitor (SNRI). Other alternatives to SSRIs and SNRIs for treatment-resistant or treatment-intolerant patients include tricyclic antidepressants, second-generation antipsychotics, and valproate. This revision of the GAD algorithm responds to issues raised by new treatments under development (such as pregabalin) and organizes the evidence systematically for practical clinical application.*

Keywords: algorithms, anxiety disorders, evidence-based practice, generalized anxiety disorder, psychopharmacology

G eneralized anxiety disorder (GAD) is a chronic, debilitating condition characterized by excessive and persistent worrying that interferes with many aspects of daily life.[1–7] Symptoms include both somatic (physical) symptoms, such as tremor and palpitations, and psychic (psychological) symptoms, particularly

---

From Harvard Medical School; Boston Children's Hospital, Boston, MA (Dr. Abejuela); VA Boston Healthcare System, Brockton Division, Brockton, MA (Dr. Osser).

Original manuscript received 9 October 2014; revised manuscript received 22 April 2015, accepted for publication 10 June 2015.

Correspondence: David N. Osser, MD, VA Boston Healthcare System, Brockton Division, 940 Belmont St., Brockton, MA 02301. Email: David.Osser@va.gov

Harvard Review of Psychiatry offers CME for readers who complete questions about featured articles. Questions can be accessed from the *Harvard Review of Psychiatry* website (www.harvardreviewofpsychiatry.org) by clicking the CME tab. Please read the featured article and then log into the website for this educational offering. If you are already online, click here to go directly to the CME page for further information.

DOI: 10.1097/HRP.0000000000000098

apprehensive expectations about major and minor concerns. It is the most common anxiety disorder seen in the primary care setting.[8] Nearly seven million Americans suffer from GAD.[2]

In this article, we present an algorithm for selecting medication treatments for GAD. This algorithm is an update of a 1999 version from the Psychopharmacology Algorithm Project at the Harvard South Shore Program (PAPHSS).[9] It was also influenced by a 2010 GAD algorithm from an international psychopharmacology group, to which one of the authors (DNO) contributed.[10] Although psychosocial interventions are of unquestioned importance in the armamentarium for treating GAD, this algorithm is limited to psycho-pharmacology interventions and may be applied if and when the prescribing clinician and patient determine that medication is appropriate. In some patients, combinations of medication and psychotherapy are utilized, though the effectiveness of combination treatment compared to either treatment alone is unclear.[11]

GAD is frequently comorbid with other disorders. Major depressive disorder is found in nearly 50% of patients, and over 60% have other anxiety disorders.[12] It is important to address the impact of these and other comorbidities when approaching patients with GAD.

In the United States, the selective serotonin reuptake inhibitors (SSRIs) escitalopram and paroxetine, the serotonin-norepinephrine reuptake inhibitors (SNRIs) venlafaxine XR and duloxetine, the benzodiazepine alprazolam, and buspirone are approved by the Food and Drug Administration (FDA) for GAD. Other medications such as pregabalin are approved for GAD in some other countries but available in the United States only because of approval for other indications. Other off-label options have been evaluated in GAD—including other benzodiazepines (e.g., diazepam), hydroxyzine, bupropion, tricyclic antidepressants (e.g., imipramine), kava (*Piper methysticum*), and rhodax (*Rhodiola rosea*).[1,13–17] Antipsychotics (quetiapine) have also been found to have efficacy in random-ized, controlled trials.[18] In this algorithm, the evidence for the effectiveness and safety of these and other possible options are evaluated and sequenced in accordance with their potential value in particular contexts. These contexts include the presence of various med-ical and psychiatric comorbidities, as well as other situations such as women who have the potential to become pregnant. Cost-effectiveness is occasionally a consideration when op-tions seem equivalent in overall benefit and risk.

METHODS

Prior publications have described the PAPHSS method of algorithm development.[19–24] The algorithms are structured like a hallside psychopharmacology consultation. They present a series of question about diagnoses and the history of previous treatment that the consultant might ask. The questions are designed to efficiently characterize the clinical situation. Then, recommendations are offered that are derived from an analysis of evidence pertinent to that situation. The authors reviewed their previous GAD algorithms,[9,10] con-sulted other recent algorithms and guidelines, and focused on the key randomized, con-trolled trials (RCTs), especially recent ones not considered in the previous reviews.

In constructing the decision tree, the authors considered efficacy, tolerability, and safety as the main bases for prioritizing treatments. All hierarchical and other clinical recommendations were the result of agreement by the two authors. Their conclusions were opinion-based distillations of the body of evidence reviewed that could be subject to conflicting interpretation by other experts. However, the peer-review process that follows submission of the article adds some validation to the reasoning in this algorithm and other PAPHSS algorithms. If the reasoning, based on the authors' interpretation of the pertinent evidence, is plausible to reviewers, then it is retained. When differences of opinion occur, the authors make adjustments to achieve consensus with the reviewers or have probed the relevant evidence further in order to present a stronger argument in support of their position.

At each decision point, different options are available for consideration, enabling prescribers to select what seems best and most acceptable to the patient in each particular clinical situation.

FLOW CHART FOR THE ALGORITHM

A summary and overview of the algorithm is presented in Figure 1. Each numbered "node" represents a key question or decision point that delineates patients ranging from those who are treatment naive to those who are increasingly treatment refractory. The questions and evidence-based rationales that support the recommendations at each node are presented below.

NODE 1: DOES THE PATIENT MEET DSM-5 CRITERIA FOR GENERALIZED ANXIETY DISORDER?

First, confirm a diagnosis of GAD based on the criteria present in the most recent, fifth edition of the *Diagnostic and Statistical Manual of Mental Disorders* (DSM-5),[25] and note any comorbid medical or psychiatric diagnoses that may affect decision making, as will be discussed in Node 2.

Regarding the DSM-5 diagnostic criteria, it may be that no diagnostic category changed as much as GAD between DSM-III/III-R and DSM-IV, though the changes from DSM-IV to DSM-5 were minor. The current criteria describe patients with a core problem of chronic excessive worrying, focused in a number of areas, that is difficult to control and causes impairment. If the worry is confined to the typical worries associated with other mental disorders (e.g., negative evaluation in social anxiety disorder), then GAD would not be diagnosed. In DSM-III/III-R, the condition was predominantly a disorder of autonomic, motor, or other somatic manifestations of anxiety. These symptoms turned out not to be particularly specific to GAD, and many DSM-III/III-R GAD patients would now be classified with other anxiety disorders or somatic symptom disorders.[26,27]

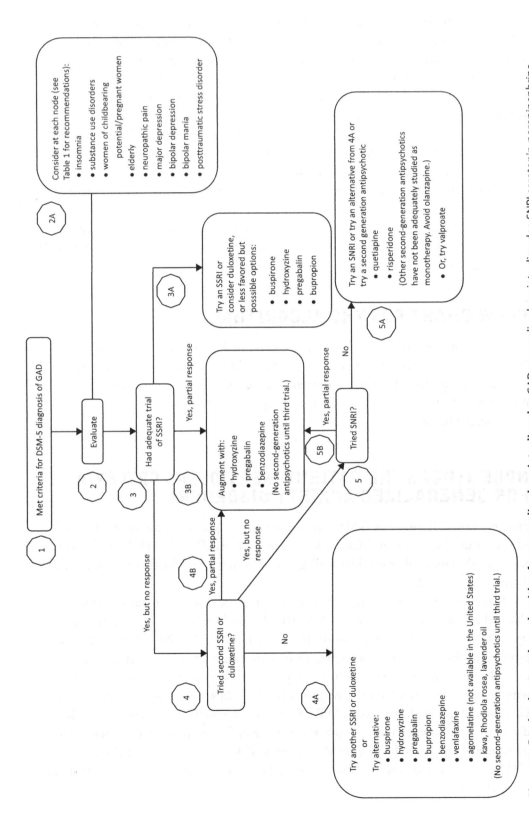

Figure 1. Psychopharmacology algorithm for generalized anxiety disorder. GAD, generalized anxiety disorder; SNRI serotonin-norepinephrine reuptake inhibitor; SSRI, selective serotonin reuptake inhibitor.

NODE 2: CONSIDER SPECIAL PATIENT POPULATIONS AND COMORBIDITIES

Table 1 summarizes common comorbid considerations in patients with GAD and how they might influence the algorithm—including insomnia, major depression, bipolar disorder, substance use disorders, and posttraumatic stress disorder. Other relevant considerations are whether patients are elderly and whether a woman has child-bearing potential. These factors should be reviewed both before beginning to consult the algorithm and subsequent to considering the next node if treatment response is unsatisfactory. A more thorough analysis of this important material is beyond the scope of this article, though the reader is encouraged to consult the cited studies and reviews.

NODE 3: HAS THE PATIENT HAD AN ADEQUATE TRIAL OF AN SSRI?

Having confirmed the diagnosis of GAD and considered the comorbidity and related issues in Node 2, the authors found that the evidence still supports SSRIs as the first-line medication for uncomplicated cases of GAD, based on their safety and tolerability, but with some reservations, as will be discussed. Two SSRIs are FDA approved for use in GAD: escitalopram and paroxetine. However, sertraline has also been used with comparable efficacy in three RCTs in comparison to placebo.[58] If a patient has not been tried on an SSRI, the recommendation is to try one, with both prescriber and patient taking into account the particular side-effect profiles of the three main options. Consider avoiding citalopram, particularly in the elderly with a history of cardiovascular disease, given concerns about its ability to prolong the QTc interval in doses >40 mg daily, as outlined in FDA guidelines announced in March 2012.[59,60] The new maximum dose in the elderly is 20 mg daily. But some controversy remains. Recently published observational data show no cardiovascular safety issues in a sample of patients who received doses over 40 mg daily,[61] and the authors of that study suggest that this finding is consistent with extensive literature. In the unpublished RCTs that the FDA relied upon to develop the new warning, however, escitalopram had much less effect on QTc than citalopram.[60]

Of the three recommended SSRIs, paroxetine produces the most side effects. Its H1 antihistaminic effects are probably the reason that it causes more weight gain, constipation, and daytime sedation than others (though unexpectedly, it can be activating and is just as likely to impair sleep as the others).[62,63] Weight gain may be as high with escitalopram, however, as with paroxetine; an observational study found both were associated with >14% of patients gaining more than 7% of body weight during extended treatment of obsessive-compulsive disorder, versus <5% with sertraline.[64] Paroxetine is associated with the most sexual side effects,[65] has more cytochrome P450 drug interactions than escitalopram or sertraline, and can produce discontinuation symptoms if a dose is missed, due to its short half-life. Additionally, paroxetine is the only SSRI with a pregnancy category D classification, because of reports of increased cardiac septal defects. Recent studies have replicated this finding.[66]

Table 1 | Comorbidity and Other Features in GAD and How They Affect the Algorithm		
Comorbid conditions and other circumstances	Evidence considerations	Recommendations
Sleep disturbance	There may be multiple contributing causes from comorbid medical and psychiatric conditions Some treatments may result in worsening or treatment-emergent insomnia (e.g., SSRIs and SNRIs)[28] More sedating agents like hydroxyzine and pregabalin may be better than SSRIs and SNRIs[29]	Evaluate and manage contributing causes to the insomnia Adjunctive trazodone added to an SSRI was helpful for improving sleep in two placebo-controlled trials[30,31] GABA agonists can work[32] but may cause rebound effects the night after discontinuation[33] Consider hydroxyzine or pregabalin[29] over SSRIs as alternative primary treatments Hydroxyzine could be an alternative hypnotic
Elderly patients	All GAD treatments have additional or increased risks or require closer monitoring in the elderly	Consider sertraline and escitalopram,[34,35] although risks could include gait impairment, GI bleeding, bone loss, and hyponatremia One small study comparing sertraline and buspirone found a trend favoring buspirone, but this result requires replication[36] The SNRI venlafaxine was also effective[37] but can be associated with a high rate of blood pressure problems when used at a mean dose of 196 mg[38] Pregabalin was effective, but caution is advised for somnolence and dizziness; falls with fracture occurred[39] Benzodiazepines can produce falls, decreased respiratory drive, substance use disorders, and additive sedation,[40] and are not recommended Quetiapine has metabolic risks, and a new warning in 2011 on QTc prolongation[41]
Neuropathic pain	Patients with neuropathic pain can respond to pregabalin[42]	Consider pregabalin rather than an SSRI
Women of childbearing potential and women who become pregnant during treatment	Benzodiazepines have a "D" rating for pregnancy due to some risk for cleft palate[43] SSRIs and SNRIs are all "C" (except paroxetine, which is "D") but are associated with some pre- and postnatal complications[44,45]	Avoid benzodiazepines and paroxetine
Active substance use disorders	15% have this comorbidity[46] Though controversial, experts concluded that benzodiazepines should be avoided in such patients[47]	Avoid benzodiazepines and related agents Avoid pregabalin, which is also a Schedule IV controlled substance
Major depression	GAD and depression can coexist and be distinguishable[27] Major depression with comorbid anxiety responds less well to antidepressants than depression without anxiety[48]	Try treating with SSRIs (second choice, SNRIs), which treat both depression and anxiety Consider adjunctive treatment focused on GAD, if necessary

Table 1 | Comorbidity and Other Features in GAD and How They Affect the Algorithm (*continued*)		
Comorbid conditions and other circumstances	*Evidence considerations*	*Recommendations*
Bipolar depression	Rates of GAD are higher in bipolar compared to unipolar depression[27] Antidepressants, including SSRIs, are usually not recommended, especially if the patient is a rapid cycler or presents with mixed features[48,49]; efficacy is doubtful, and the risk of mood switch is significant[49,50]	For the depression, consider lithium, lamotrigine, and lurasidone[21,51] For the GAD, consider pregabalin, hydroxyzine, and benzodiazepines Quetiapine was not effective in one study of patients with GAD and bipolar depression[52]
Bipolar mania	Manic patients have high rates of GAD, and response to lithium and anticonvulsants may be reduced[53] Valproate was effective compared to placebo in a small study on men with comorbid GAD[54]	Avoid antidepressants Quetiapine is effective for GAD[55] and may be preferred here Consider preferring valproate over lithium in men with mania and GAD, but not in women of childbearing potential due to teratogenicity[56]
Posttraumatic stress disorder	Prazosin is highly effective as an add-on treatment for insomnia, nightmares, disturbed awakenings, and daytime symptoms of PTSD in 4 small placebo-controlled studies[19,57]	Prazosin is recommended

GABA, gamma aminobutyric acid; GAD, generalized anxiety disorder; PTSD, posttraumatic stress disorder; SNRI, serotonin-norepinephrine reuptake inhibitor; SSRI, selective serotonin reuptake inhibitor.

The overall effect size of SSRIs in GAD in a 2007 metaanalysis was 0.36 (standardized mean difference from placebo), which is a modest effect,[67] though in some studies remission rates were as high as 50%.[68] In the elderly, in whom GAD is particularly common,[69] the evidence base with SSRIs is limited. Sertraline seemed inferior to buspirone in a small RCT without placebo control,[36] but escitalopram was effective compared to placebo in a larger study.[35]

Paroxetine was found to be effective at daily dosages of 20 mg or 40 mg, while the optimal daily dosage of escitalopram compared to placebo was 10 mg and not 20 mg.[3,4] Sertraline doses have ranged from 50–200 mg daily. A dose-response relationship has not been demonstrated for any SSRI, and no research has compared higher-dose SSRIs to longer time on the initial dose.[70]

The time required for an adequate trial of an SSRI for GAD varies with the individual. Studies with escitalopram have found that if response commences within two weeks (defined as a 20% improvement in Hamilton Anxiety Rating Scale [HAM-A] scores), the prognosis for remission is good.[71] By the same token, if there is no response in two weeks, the initial dose should be increased. If there is no response in four weeks, meta-analysis suggests that the patient is unlikely to respond.[70] Assuming that the patient has been adherent to treatment and that there is no reason to suspect the patient to be an ultra-rapid metabolizer of the medication, it is reasonable to consider such a trial to be adequate.

When prescribing SSRIs, clinicians are urged to be mindful of their typical adverse effects. Sexual side effects, in particular, are common, disturbing for many patients, and difficult to discuss, and they usually do not remit with time.[72] In addition to the other side effects noted above, upper gastrointestinal tract bleeding was nine times more common over three months in patients on an SSRI and a nonsteroidal anti-inflammatory medication than in a control group not on those medications.[73] This risk is mitigated, however, if the patient is also on an acid-controlling agent such as a proton-pump inhibitor. Even short-term use of an SSRI (7–28 days) increases the odds of a upper gastrointestinal tract bleed by 67%-84%.[74] Osteoporosis and fracture risk increase twofold with long-term SSRI use.[75] Suicidal ideation and behavior may increase in patients younger than 25 years,[76] as noted in the package-insert warning of all antidepressants.

Because of these side effects and the high placebo-response rate in GAD studies,[70] it is recommended that prescribers attempt to confirm that any apparent response of GAD to SSRI treatment was medication related and not due to nonspecific aspects of care (e.g., a placebo response). Usually, the best way to make this determination is a trial off the medication at a time when the patient is doing reasonably well and can receive suitable support and observation. Some may relapse, but many more will not and are spared the side effects. If medication-related benefit seems likely, maintenance treatment for one year or more is reasonably well established and endorsed by most evidence-based guidelines, since GAD is often a chronic condition.[3] For example, escitalopram recipients (compared to placebo) took a significantly longer time to relapse and had a markedly decreased risk of relapse than those on placebo.[77]

Node 3A: Other Options to Consider

If the risks of adverse effects from an SSRI are considered unacceptable to the prescribing clinician or patient, several reasonable options are worth considering. We will briefly discuss the rationale for each of these, their advantages and disadvantages, and when they might be considered preferable to SSRIs.

The serotonin-norepinephrine reuptake inhibitors (SNRIs) venlafaxine and duloxetine are also FDA approved for GAD and have comparable efficacy to SSRIs.[3] Of the two, the side effects of venlafaxine seem to relegate it to, at best, a second choice. While causing the same liability to sexual side effects as SSRIs, venlafaxine produces dose-related hypertension requiring clinical monitoring, and causes more problems with sweating.[78] By contrast, duloxetine was found to have significantly lower rates of sexual side effects than paroxetine, although they were higher than placebo.[79] Blood pressure effects seemed comparable to SSRIs.[79] These considerations could elevate duloxetine to a first-line option. However, risks of liver abnormalities, though small, suggest that it would be prudent to assess baseline liver function function (an inconvenience); duloxetine is contraindicated in patients with hepatic impairment.[78] Perspiration and infrequent urinary retention (0.4%) are other concerns with duloxetine.[78]

Efficacy and dosing requirements with duloxetine were demonstrated in four RCTs. The medication was effective at 60–120 mg, with no advantage to the higher dose.[4,80] The GAD symptoms earliest to respond included anxious mood and muscle tension, and the symptoms last to respond included insomnia and common gastrointestinal and autonomic symptoms (all part of the adverse-effect profile of SNRIs).[81] The most common adverse effects reported were nausea, dizziness, dry mouth, fatigue, somnolence, and constipation, but otherwise duloxetine was reported to be generally well tolerated.[80,82–84] It should be noted that despite intensive marketing to the contrary, the analgesic effects of duloxetine in depressed patients were found (in a metaanalysis of five trials) to be clinically insignificant.[85] The effect size of the analgesia was only 0.115 by Cohen's d.[85] This analysis excluded studies of patients with comorbid fibromyalgia or musculoskeletal disorders.

Buspirone is an azapirone that received FDA approval as a monotherapy agent for DSM-III GAD in 1986, with double-blind, placebo-controlled studies mostly demonstrating effectiveness comparable to benzodiazepines. A meta-analysis in 1992 of eight placebo-controlled RCTs involving buspirone in doses ranging from 15 to 60 mg daily found the typical effective dose to be 30 mg.[86] It was found very useful in a placebo-controlled trial in recently abstinent anxious alcoholics (almost half of whom met DSM-III criteria for GAD) at an average dose of 50 mg daily.[87] Advantages over benzodiazepines included no abuse potential and a good side-effect profile.[83,88] Buspirone has little overdose toxicity, no impairment of cognitive or psychomotor performance, and no sexual side effects. Only one placebo-controlled trial, however, has been undertaken to confirm buspirone's efficacy as monotherapy for DSM-IV GAD. In a comparison to venlafaxine (sponsored by the manufacturer of venlafaxine), buspirone 30 mg daily was no better than placebo on some measures, and on others it was inferior to venlafaxine.[89] Therefore, it is somewhat in doubt whether buspirone, despite its advantages in side effects, is a first-line agent in DSM-IV or DSM-5 GAD. Clinicians may nevertheless want to consider it because of its benign side effects.

Hydroxyzine is an antihistamine with mild 5-HT2 receptor blocking effects that has shown both efficacy over placebo and safety at doses around 50 mg daily in three placebo-controlled RCTs in GAD patients, one using DSM-III criteria[90] and two using DSM-IV criteria.[91,92] Given its low abuse potential, sedating properties, lack of sexual side effects, and mean effect size of 0.45 in these studies, it appears to be a viable alternative to SSRIs. Clinicians seem skeptical about this product, however, and it is not known to have any benefit for disorders like depression and other anxiety states that are common comorbidities with GAD. Nevertheless, it is commonly used as a PRN (as needed) medication on inpatient units because of its rapid onset of sedation (15–30 minutes), half-life of three hours, and duration of effect, lasting 4–6 hours with no known potential for dependence.[93] It is also prescribed this way for outpatients, with doses ranging from 37.5 mg to 75 mg.[88] In a Cochrane Review comparing hydroxyzine to other anxiolytic agents, such as benzodiazepines and buspirone, hydroxyzine was found to be equivalent in tolerability, efficacy, and acceptability among patients.[94] The third RCT[92] was particularly interesting in that, over the 12 weeks of the comparison to placebo and the benzodiazepine bromazepam, the difference between hydroxyzine and placebo gradually enlarged, suggesting an accumulating effect rather than an immediate and plateauing effect, which one might expect from a purely sedative agent. A replication trial comparing hydroxyzine to an SSRI would be of great interest.

Pregabalin is approved throughout Europe for treating GAD and is widely used there and recommended in international guidelines.[95] It has at least seven positive RCTs versus placebo and several comparators, and was at least comparably effective to other medications for both somatic and psychic symptoms of GAD.[70] Compared to SSRIs, it seemed to have a relatively rapid onset and was more beneficial for sleep.[70] Unlike antidepressants, there seemed to be a dose response relationship in GAD, where doses over 300 mg daily were more effective.[96,97] Surprisingly, the medication was not approved in the United States for GAD despite two submissions of data to the FDA. The "non-approvable letter" explaining the FDA reasoning has not been made public by the manufacturer. They are not required to disclose the letter, and the company refused to share it with the authors of this article. It has been speculated that the treatment effect size, though statistically significant, was considered too small to be clinically significant in the reviewed trials (e.g., three points or less on the HAM-A).[98]

Pregabalin was found to be effective in elderly patients in one study, though caution is required since pregabalin's most common side effects include somnolence and dizziness, and one patient fell and sustained a fracture.[39,98]

Cost considerations may result in some pharmacy-benefit managers in the United States refusing to allow use of pregabalin for GAD. It is possible that gabapentin could be used instead of pregabalin here and throughout the algorithm when pregabalin is recommended. This substitution is speculative because there are no controlled studies of gabapentin in GAD. However, gabapentin has some of the same FDA indications as pregabalin (neuropathic pain and convulsions), and it is frequently used off-label as an anxiolytic. In an RCT, Clarke and collaborators[99] found that gabapentin was effective for a variety of chronic anxiety disorders, particularly preoperative anxiety. In another RCT, gabapentin 300 mg and 900 mg were compared to placebo for anxiety symptoms in 420 breast cancer survivors.[100] Both doses were associated with significant improvements in anxiety symptoms compared to placebo, with a greater improvement reported in patients with higher baseline levels of anxiety. Notably, pregabalin is a Schedule IV controlled substance. Gabapentin is not, though some concerns have been raised about its potential for misuse by patients with tendencies in that direction.[101]

Bupropion is an antidepressant that clinicians do not tend to consider for patients with anxiety disorders.[102] However, there is an intriguing, though small, double-blind, controlled trial in 24 outpatients aged 18–64 with DSM-IV GAD.[103] They were randomized to receive either bupropion XL (extended release) 150–300 daily or escitalopram (FDA approved for GAD) 10–20 daily. The main efficacy measures used were the Clinical Global Impression of Improvement (CGI-I) and the HAM-A. Anxiety symptoms improved in both groups, but the difference in mean HAM-A scores was significant (p = .01) in favor of bupropion, which produced an endpoint score of 5.3, whereas escitalopram resulted in a mean score of 11.4. Response and remission rates as measured by the CGI-I also favored bupropion, but differences in depression ratings were nonsignificant. The study was sponsored by the manufacturer of bupropion.[103]

How seriously should one take these data? Trivedi and colleagues[104] compared the effects of bupropion and sertraline on anxiety symptoms in patients with major depression using pooled data from two eight-week, double-blind, placebo-controlled trials involving almost 700 patients. The two medications had comparable anxiolytic and antidepressant effects, and onset of improvement from both was equally rapid. There were no differences in activation side effects or insomnia. Because of these findings and other data, including bupropion's relatively low incidence of sexual side effects, Zimmerman and colleagues[102] suggested that the evidence base might actually support bupropion as the first-line antidepressant over SSRIs for most patients with major depression. Without question, sexual side effects are one of the chief concerns of patients about to try an antidepressant for depression or GAD, presuming that they are fully informed about them. Bupropion's advantage in this respect may be balanced with the modest risk of seizures associated with the longer-acting versions of bupropion,[105] though bupropion is contraindicated if the patient has a past history of seizures or a history of an eating disorder. These considerations suggest that bupropion may be a possible option to bring up with patients considering their first treatment for GAD.

Other agents with some effectiveness for GAD include benzodiazepines, mirtazapine, quetiapine, agomelatine (not available in the United States), and kava. These will be discussed as options at Node 4.

Node 3B: Did You Try an SSRI and Get a Partial Response? Consider Augmentations

Partial improvement occurs frequently in GAD—perhaps more commonly than remissions.[3] Augmentation may be considered if the partial improvement is thought to be due to the medication and not the concomitant psychotherapy or nonspecific aspects of treatment. As noted above, this determination may be difficult but is of crucial importance. As a general principle, one should avoid adding another medication when partial response to the first medication is likely a placebo response. Unnecessary polypharmacy increases the risks of adverse effects and drug interactions, reduces adherence due to complexity of the regimen, and increases costs. Clinicians should evaluate for other possible causes of incomplete response such as comorbidity, nonadherence, and pharmacokinetic/pharmacogenetic variables.

If a true partial response is nevertheless suspected, there is only weak or equivocal evidence available for guidance regarding what to choose for augmentation. Quetiapine has received the most study, with three placebo-controlled augmentation RCTs.[106–108] Though one RCT (not double-blind; n = 20) found efficacy,[106] two double-blind RCTs[107,108] did not. The larger of those two studies (n = 409) found a trend favoring quetiapine (p = .079), but the difference from placebo on the HAM-A was only one point, which seems clinically insignificant.[107] Risperidone has two augmentation studies that were positive—one of which was large.[109,110] A small, underpowered study demonstrated that olanzapine can be added to SSRIs with augmenting effects in GAD.[111] However, given the high risks of metabolic side effects, negative effects on insulin resistance in the cases of olanzapine and quetiapine,[112,113] and weight gain, among other considerations, these second-generation antipsychotics are not recommended as augmenters at this early point in the algorithm.

Buspirone was not impressive as an augmenter of citalopram in outpatients with major depression and high levels of anxiety in the STAR*D study. It produced a remission rate of only 9% over 14 weeks.[48] No studies have used buspirone as an augmenter in GAD without depression, but the STAR*D results and the general concerns raised earlier about the effectiveness of buspirone in DSM-5 GAD suggest buspirone would not be a prime option for augmentation.

It seems reasonable to consider adding one of three alternatives: hydroxyzine and pregabalin, which are well-tolerated options discussed in Node 3A above, or a benzodiazepine. Though no augmentation trials with hydroxyzine have been published, an eight-week, randomized, double-blind, placebo-controlled trial of pregabalin augmentation in GAD (150–600 mg daily) found it to be somewhat effective.[114] The changes in HAM-A scores compared to placebo were significant but not clinically impressive: -7.6 versus -6.4 (p $<$ .05). Benzodiazepines have also received no formal study of augmentation in GAD, but their use seems to be common in clinical practice. Benzodiazepines as monotherapy for GAD will be discussed in Node 4A, where it will be suggested that the usual objection to these products concerns their risks of abuse, tolerance, and dependence. However, in a recent RCT of clonazepam as an augmentation of sertraline for generalized social anxiety disorder, the clonazepam addition seemed effective and safe.[115] This study provides indirect support for the possible use of clonazepam here, but testing in GAD patients is necessary.

NODE 4: HAS THE PATIENT TRIED A SECOND SSRI OR DULOXETINE?

If the patient has had no response (or a partial response presumed to be due to placebo effect or the nonspecific effects of other aspects of care) after an adequately dosed initial trial of an SSRI, no evidence is available to help guide the second step of psychopharmacology treatment for GAD. Assuming that adherence issues and pharmacokinetic/pharmacogenetic influences on dose bioavailability have been considered, and that the diagnosis is verified, it seems reasonable to try another evidence-supported medication. Often that will be another SSRI or duloxetine because of their advantages as outlined in Node 3. Since the SSRIs are not identical in their spectra of receptor activity, it may be that a different one will have a better constellation of effects to address the patient's needs.

Node 4A: Other Options to Consider

The four alternatives suggested and discussed in Node 3A may also be considered: buspirone, hydroxyzine, pregabalin, and bupropion. To this list, some others may be added that have a sufficient evidence base for usage but that present issues or problems suggesting that they should not be alternative first-line (Node 3) agents: benzodiazepines, venlafaxine, agomelatine (not available in the United States), and kava. Some other medications, including atypical antipsychotics and tricyclic antidepressants, have evidence of efficacy but, due to their side-effect burden, are postponed for consideration later, at the next node. We will review the rationales for the four new options.

Benzodiazepines are effective for GAD and are perhaps the most widely prescribed anxiolytic agents. Alprazolam was FDA approved for GAD at the time of DSM-III. Placebo-controlled comparator trials in DSM-IV GAD with agents such as pregabalin[116] confirm their efficacy using the more recent GAD criteria. An advantage appreciated by patients is the rapid effect, appearing soon after treatment is begun. However, benzodiazepines have many disadvantages. After treatment for several months, about 40% of patients develop tolerance and dependence,[47] and they should particularly be avoided in patients with a history of substance use disorders, though with some exceptions.[9] They are also commonly associated with increased sedation, memory impairment, psychomotor incoordination resulting in increased motor vehicle accidents, and rebound anxiety.[5] Long-acting benzodiazepines such as clonazepam, however, may help decrease breakthrough anxiety during treatment with an SSRI. Both somatic and psychic symptoms may improve, although somatic symptoms may be the better targets for benzodiazepine therapy.[83,97] If benzodiazepines are to be given at this node, they are suggested primarily for patients who have no history of any substance use disorders, as noted above. They may be combined with an SSRI in the early phase of treatment (e.g., 4–8 weeks) while waiting for the SSRI to work,[88] and then tapered and discontinued if possible.

Venlafaxine XR is a reasonable alternative treatment to consider here instead of a second SSRI, though as noted earlier it seems that duloxetine would be a better choice in the SNRI class if it was not tried as initial treatment in Node 3. Overall acute efficacy of venlafaxine XR is at least as good as with the SSRIs,[67] and most studies show only minimal additional improvement at the higher doses at which side effects like hypertension are more common.[117] Notably, in a randomized, placebo-controlled trial comparing escitalopram with venlafaxine XR in patients with GAD, escitalopram was found to be better tolerated. Discontinuations due to adverse effects did not differ between escitalopram and placebo (7% vs. 5%; $p = .61$) but were significantly higher for venlafaxine XR (13%) compared to placebo ($p = .03$).[118] The study was sponsored by the makers of escitalopram.

Because relapse rates in GAD treatment after one year of follow-up are generally high, a 2010 study examined the benefits of 6 and 12 months of continued treatment with venlafaxine XR (75–225 mg/daily) or placebo in 268 patients who had achieved improvement after an initial 6 months of open-label treatment.[82] Relapse rates were over 50% for patients on placebo versus just under 10% for those who stayed on venlafaxine XR ($p < .001$). Remissions were most likely at the maximum dose of 225 mg daily. The most common adverse events in this longer trial were dry mouth, drowsiness, lightheadedness, headaches, and increased sweating.

Agomelatine is an antidepressant that works by a novel mechanism blocking serotonin 2C receptors and stimulating melatonin receptors. It has undergone 20 RCTs in depression. In the three U.S. studies, however, it did not do well, and perhaps that is why it was not granted FDA approval. In a metaanalysis, the overall effect size in depression treatment was found to be small (0.24) and inferior to SSRIs.[119] However, it was more helpful for insomnia than SSRIs or SNRIs. In GAD patients, two 12-week, placebo-controlled RCTs[17,120] and one 26-week maintenance RCT[121] have demonstrated efficacy at doses of 25–50 mg daily. It was especially useful for sleep, and side effects were minimal. In countries where it is available, agomelatine may be a reasonable alternative to an SSRI or SNRI for patients with insomnia and who want to avoid sexual side effects.

Plant-based medications, such as kava (also known as *Piper methysticum*), have shown efficacy in RCTs in GAD. Kava (120/240 mg of kavalactones per day) was compared to placebo in a recent six-week trial in 75 GAD patients without comorbid mood disorders.[14] Kava had efficacy on the HAM-A (p = .046; effect size [Cohen's d] = 0.62); 26% of participants in the kava group were classified as remitted (HAM-A < 7) versus 6% of participants in the placebo group (p = .04). Side effects that were greater in the kava group were limited to headaches. Earlier trials of kava had more mixed results, however, and a report of severe hepatotoxicity was concerning.[122]

Rhodax (also known as *Rhodiola rosea*) is another herbal medication that has been studied in GAD. In a small study from the UCLA Anxiety Disorders Program of 10 GAD subjects aged 34 to 44, Rhodax extract (340 mg) was given daily for 10 weeks. Rhodax-treated patients improved significantly on the HAM-A (p = .01), but there were some anticholinergic side effects.[15] Riluzole, a glutamate modulator, was promising as a treatment for GAD in an open-label trial in 18 patients.[123] Eighty percent responded positively, and 53% remitted, though this result needs replication. Lavender oil was reported to be effective compared to placebo and at least as good as 20 mg of paroxetine in a recent German study involving 539 patients.[124]

Node 4B: Did You Try an SSRI and Get a Partial Response? Consider Augmentations

If the second SSRI or SNRI trial resulted in a partial response that is thought to be credited to the medication, the same augmentations may be considered as in Node 3B. See Figure 1.

NODE 5: HAS THE PATIENT TRIED AN SNRI?

If the patient has had two trials (from among the recommended first- and second-line treatments in Nodes 3 and 4) and has not had a trial of an SNRI, the next trial might be with an SNRI. Their advantages and disadvantages were reviewed in earlier nodes. The growing list of alternatives that can be considered at this point includes benzodiazepines, bupropion, buspirone, hydroxyzine, pregabalin, agomelatine (not available in the United States), and herbs such as kava. Some other options will be reviewed below.

Node 5A: Other Options to Consider

The first new option at this point is a second-generation antipsychotic (SGA). Quetiapine has been the most studied, with five double-blind, placebo-controlled RCTs as monotherapy for GAD, four of which demonstrated efficacy.[58,125,126] As noted earlier, the weight gain, insulin resistance, and other metabolic side effects, as well as the 2011 package insert warning on QTc prolongation, all suggest quetiapine should not be an early choice in treating GAD. Because of the toxicity, both the FDA and the European regulatory agency did not approve quetiapine for any use in GAD. Quetiapine has good efficacy data, however, and it may be a reasonable option for a treatment-resistant patient at this node of the algorithm.

Risperidone was found effective in two augmentation trials when added to an SSRI in GAD.[109,110] It has not been studied as a monotherapy but might be a reasonable second-choice SGA here. Ziprasidone was used in a small, placebo-controlled trial as monotherapy for GAD; the trend toward efficacy[127] supported the findings of an earlier open-label trial.[128] Ziprasidone had no efficacy, however, in a cohort of patients in which it was used to augment an antidepressant; a larger study was recommended.[127] Risperidone has moderate metabolic side effects and significant issues with prolactin elevation, but ziprasidone has more tendency to elevate QTc, and many patients do not tolerate its side effects.[129]

Some tricyclic antidepressants have been found effective in GAD. Of all the TCAs, imipramine is the only one with significant data for decreasing overall anxiety, particularly for the psychic symptoms (anxious mood, muscle tension, difficulty concentrating, and insomnia). Prior studies have compared imipramine to benzodiazepines for GAD and found that while both medications significantly decreased the somatic symptoms of GAD and the HAM-A scores, imipramine was more effective at decreasing anxiety symptoms starting at two weeks. Other studies have found that imipramine at a dose of 90–135 mg has efficacy for GAD similar to that of benzodiazepines.[5] However, given the many side effects of TCAs—including anticholinergic effects (e.g., urinary retention), alpha-adrenergic blockade (e.g., postural hypotension), seizures, cardiac conduction delay, other cardiac-related problems, and fatality risk with overdose—TCAs are still not particularly favored even at this node. If other alternative options are viable and have not been tried, then the recommendation is to try those first.[5,88,100]

Among the first-generation antipsychotics, trifluoperazine was found effective for "anxiety neurosis" decades ago. The lack of studies with more modern definitions of GAD, coupled with the risk of tardive dyskinesia, precludes considering first-generation antipsychotics even at this point in the algorithm.[130]

Node 5B: Did You Try an SNRI and Get a Partial Response? Consider Augmentations

As in Nodes 3B and 4B, it is reasonable to consider augmenting what appears to be a partial but real response to the chosen Node 5 treatment. To the list of previous augmentation options, one could add SGAs at this point: the patient is quite treatment resistant now, having had three trials. Quetiapine, though side-effect prone, may be acceptable. A small study in 2011 investigated 24 GAD outpatient adults who had failed at least one eight-week treatment trial of an SSRI (citalopram) or an SNRI (venlafaxine) for their GAD.[131] These patients received quetiapine XR to augment their antidepressant for

12 weeks. Primary outcome measures were CGI-S and HAM-A scores. At 4 weeks, there was a significant and rapid decrease of their anxiety symptoms as measured by CGI-S and HAM-A scores, with improvements maintained at week 12. In this study there were no significant weight changes after 12 weeks.

A small (n = 18) augmentation trial with ziprasidone or placebo over eight weeks in treatment-resistant GAD patients on SSRIs or other medications, including benzodiazepines, found no efficacy and many more side effects than when ziprasidone was used as a monotherapy (60% vs. 28%).[127]

Risperidone was studied in an RCT with placebo control in 40 treatment-resistant patients with primarily GAD.[109] While staying on their previous medications, they were given risperidone 0.5–1.5 mg daily or placebo for five weeks. Patients in the risperidone group showed greater improvements on the HAM-A and other anxiety scales at endpoint. Risperidone was also generally well tolerated, with the most common complaint being somnolence, followed by dizziness and blurred vision. In an open-label trial, a few patients seemed to respond to risperidone at a dose of 0.25 to 3 mg daily.[132]

Aripiprazole has been used with promising results in two small, open-label 6–8 week trials as an augmenting agent at doses near 10 mg daily.[5,133,134]

Pollack and colleagues[5,111] examined olanzapine as an augmentation for fluoxetine in treatment-refractory GAD in a placebo-controlled RCT involving 46 patients. After six weeks (mean dose = 8.7 ± 7.1 mg daily), there were no statistically significant differences from placebo on the HAM-A, but remission rates (HAM-A of 7 or less) were higher on olanzapine. The mean weight gain for those on olanzapine augmentation was greater (11.0 ± 5.1 lb vs. −0.7±2.4 lb on placebo; p < .001).

Should SGA augmentation be considered, it would be important to monitor for weight gain, body mass index, fasting glucose, hemoglobin A1C, and triglycerides.[18]

A final option for a treatment-resistant male patient with GAD would be valproate, which has one small RCT demonstrating efficacy.[54] Side effects might include weight gain and elevated liver enzymes.

COMPARISON TO THE RECOMMENDATIONS IN OTHER ALGORITHMS AND GUIDELINES

The present algorithm for selecting psychopharmacology treatment for GAD summarizes and organizes the available evidence for effectiveness and safety of the available medications in a sequence of steps from first treatment to very treatment-resistant cases. It differs in some respects from other published algorithms and guidelines. Its proposal of SSRIs as first-line treatment is in agreement with a 2010 international consensus algorithm[10] but differs from another by Linden and colleagues in 2013[135] that recommends pregabalin first-line, followed by hydroxyzine and then venlafaxine. The present algorithm suggests pregabalin as an alternate agent for first-line use. The authors of this algorithm found reasons to think about bupropion as an option for first-line use, whereas others did not. This algorithm positions venlafaxine lower than on other algorithms due to side effects, but agrees with having duloxetine as a first-line option. The British National Institute for Health and Clinical Excellence guideline for GAD (2011) is more similar to this algorithm in that it recommends an SSRI first, then another SSRI or SNRI, and then pregabalin (not FDA approved for GAD); benzodiazepines are not recommended except for short-term use, and SGAs should not be offered, at least in[136] primary care.

The latest (2014) revision of guidelines for treatment of GAD from the British Association for Psychopharmacology (BAP)[95] suggests considering SSRIs for first-line and SNRIs and pregabalin, especially in higher doses, as alternatives. The present algorithm adds buspirone, hydroxyzine, and bupropion as other possible, though less favored, options because their side-effect profiles may be more acceptable for some patients even if their efficacy is much less well established. The present algorithm places venlafaxine lower in the options than the BAP guideline because of its greater risk of hypertension, gastrointestinal side effects, and discontinuation symptoms after abrupt withdrawal. Also, some treatments recommended by the BAP because of their evidence base—such as tricyclics and atypical antipsychotics—are placed low in priority in the present algorithm because of their side effects. In this algorithm, gabapentin—despite the lack of evidence for its efficacy—is mentioned as a possible option to be considered when pregabalin, due to formulary restrictions, is not allowed.[95]

FINAL COMMENT

Results in the few studies of evidence-based, algorithm-guided psychopharmacology care have modestly favored the algorithms compared to treatment-as-usual.[137] Clinicians in the control groups often selected treatments that were fairly similar to those selected by algorithm consulters. Better results with algorithms have occurred when considerable time is spent educating users in the accurate use of the algorithms and educating patients about the reasoning involved, since they may have their own opinions about what is best for them.[137] In other branches of medicine, promoting the use of evidence-supported treatment algorithms has produced impressive economic results.[138]

This heuristic may serve clinicians as an anchor to the evidence base for the psychopharmacology treatment of GAD. It should be kept in mind, however, that medication has an important, but fairly modest, role in altering the course of the lives of people with this disorder. At any point, psychosocial interventions may take precedence over, or at least add to, the options discussed here. Practitioners should be alert to new evidence and new research that may improve outcomes and alter the recommendations provided here. Clinical experience remains an important consideration in managing patients with GAD: such experience can contradict, support, or add to what is derived from the scientific evidence. Consideration of the evidence base is viewed as necessary, but by no means sufficient, for clinical decision making.

Declaration of interest: The authors report no conflicts of interest. The authors alone are responsible for the content and writing of the article.

REFERENCES

1. Lakhan SE, Vieira KF. Nutritional and herbal supplements for anxiety and anxiety-related disorders: systematic review. Nutr J 2010;9:42.

2. Reinhold JA, Mandos LA, Rickels K, Lohoff FW. Pharmacological treatment of generalized anxiety disorder. Expert Opin Pharmacother 2011;12:2457–67.

3. Baldwin DS, Waldman S, Allgulander C. Evidence-based pharmacological treatment of generalized anxiety disorder. Int J Neuropsychopharmacol 2011;14:697–710.

4. Stein DJ, Lerer B, Stahl SM. Essential evidence-based psychopharmacology. 2nd ed. Cambridge, New York: Cambridge University Press, 2012.

5. Huh J, Goebert D, Takeshita J, Lu BY, Kang M. Treatment of generalized anxiety disorder: a comprehensive review of the literature for psychopharmacologic alternatives to newer antidepressants and benzodiazepines. Prim Care Companion CNS Disord 2011;13(2).

6. Bereza BG, Machado M, Einarson TR. Systematic review and quality assessment of economic evaluations and quality-of-life studies related to generalized anxiety disorder. Clin Ther 2009;31:1279–308.

7. Pollack MH. Refractory generalized anxiety disorder. J Clin Psychiatry 2009;70 suppl 2:32–8.

8. Wittchen HU, Hoyer J. Generalized anxiety disorder: nature and course. J Clin Psychiatry 2001;62 suppl 11:15–9 discussion 20–1.

9. Osser DN, Renner JA Jr, Bayog R. Algorithms for the pharmacotherapy of anxiety disorders in patients with chemical abuse and dependence. Psychiatr Ann 1999;29:285–300.

10. Davidson JR, Zhang W, Connor KM, et al. A psychopharmacological treatment algorithm for generalised anxiety disorder (GAD). J Psychopharmacol 2010;24:3–26.

11. Bandelow B, Seidler-Brandler U, Becker A, Wedekind D, Ruther E. Meta-analysis of randomized controlled comparisons of psychopharmacological and psychological treatments for anxiety disorders. World J Biol Psychiatry 2007;8:175–87.

12. Kessler RC, Keller MB, Wittchen HU. The epidemiology of generalized anxiety disorder. Psychiatr Clin North Am 2001;24:19–39.

13. Sarris J, Kavanagh DJ. Kava and St. John's Wort: current evidence for use in mood and anxiety disorders. J Altern Complement Med 2009;15:827–36.

14. Sarris J, Stough C, Bousman CA, et al. Kava in the treatment of generalized anxiety disorder: a double-blind, randomized, placebo-controlled study. J Clin Psychopharmacol 2013;33:643–8.

15. Bystritsky A, Kerwin L, Feusner JD. A pilot study of Rhodiola rosea (Rhodax) for generalized anxiety disorder (GAD). J Altern Complement Med 2008;14:175–80.

16. Amsterdam JD, Li Y, Soeller I, Rockwell K, Mao JJ, Shults J. A randomized, double-blind, placebo-controlled trial of oral Matricaria recutita (chamomile) extract therapy for generalized anxiety disorder. J Clin Psychopharmacol 2009;29: 378–82.

17. Stein DJ, Ahokas AA, de Bodinat C. Efficacy of agomelatine in generalized anxiety disorder: a randomized, double-blind, placebo-controlled study. J Clin Psychopharmacol 2008;28:561–6.

18. Khan A, Joyce M, Atkinson S, Eggens I, Baldytcheva I, Eriksson H. A randomized, double-blind study of once-daily extended release quetiapine fumarate (quetiapine XR) monotherapy in patients with generalized anxiety disorder. J Clin Psychopharmacol 2011;31:418–28.

19. Bajor LA, Ticlea AN, Osser DN. The Psychopharmacology Algorithm Project at the Harvard South Shore Program: an update on posttraumatic stress disorder. Harv Rev Psychiatry 2011;19:240–58.

20. Hamoda HM, Osser DN. The Psychopharmacology Algorithm Project at the Harvard South Shore Program: an update on psychotic depression. Harv Rev Psychiatry 2008;16:235–47.

21. Ansari A, Osser DN. The Psychopharmacology Algorithm Project at the Harvard South Shore Program: an update on bipolar depression. Harv Rev Psychiatry 2010;18:36–55.

22. Osser DN, Roudsari MJ, Manschreck T. The Psychopharmacology Algorithm Project at the Harvard South Shore Program: an update on schizophrenia. Harv Rev Psychiatry 2013;21:18–40.

23. Mohammad OM, Osser DN. The Psychopharmacology Algorithm Project at the Harvard South Shore Program: an algorithm for acute mania. Harv Rev Psychiatry 2014;22:274–94.

24. Osser DN, Dunlop LR. The Psychopharmacology Algorithm Project at the Harvard South Shore Program. Psychopharm Rev 2010;45:91–8.

25. American Psychiatric Association. Diagnostic and statistical manual of mental disorders. 5th ed. Arlington, VA: APA, 2013.

26. Brown TA, Barlow DH, Liebowitz MR. The empirical basis of generalized anxiety disorder. Am J Psychiatry 1994;151:1272–80.

27. Goldberg D, Kindler KS, Sirovatka PJ, Regier DA, eds. Diagnostic issues in depression and generalized anxiety disorder. Arlington, VA: American Psychiatric Publishing, 2010.

28. Allgulander C, Dahl AA, Austin C, et al. Efficacy of sertraline in a 12-week trial for generalized anxiety disorder. Am J Psychiatry 2004;161:1642–9.

29. Holsboer-Trachsler E, Prieto R. Effects of pregabalin on sleep in generalized anxiety disorder. Int J Neuropsychopharmacol 2013;16:925–36.

30. Kaynak H, Kaynak D, Gozukirmizi E, Guilleminault C. The effects of trazodone on sleep in patients treated with stimulant antidepressants. Sleep Med 2004;5:15–20.

31. Nierenberg AA, Adler LA, Peselow E, Zornberg G, Rosenthal M. Trazodone for antidepressant-associated insomnia. Am J Psychiatry 1994;151:1069–72.

32. Pollack M, Kinrys G, Krystal A, et al. Eszopiclone coadministered with escitalopram in patients with insomnia and comorbid generalized anxiety disorder. Arch Gen Psychiatry 2008;65:551–62.

33. Walsh JK, Krystal AD, Amato DA, et al. Nightly treatment of primary insomnia with eszopiclone for six months: effect on sleep, quality of life, and work limitations. Sleep 2007;30:959–68.

34. Schuurmans J, Comijs H, Emmelkamp PM, et al. A randomized, controlled trial of the effectiveness of cognitive-behavioral therapy and sertraline versus a waitlist control group for anxiety disorders in older adults. Am J Geriatr Psychiatry 2006;14: 255–63.

35. Lenze EJ, Rollman BL, Shear MK, et al. Escitalopram for older adults with generalized anxiety disorder: a randomized controlled trial. JAMA 2009;301:295–303.

36. Mokhber N, Azarpazhooh MR, Khajehdaluee M, Velayati A, Hopwood M. Randomized, single-blind, trial of sertraline and buspirone for treatment of elderly patients with generalized anxiety disorder. Psychiatry Clin Neurosci 2010;64: 128–33.

37. Katz IR, Reynolds CF 3rd, Alexopoulos GS, Hackett D. Venlafaxine ER as a treatment for generalized anxiety disorder in older adults: pooled analysis of five randomized placebo-controlled clinical trials. J Am Geriatr Soc 2002;50:18–25.

38. Johnson EM, Whyte E, Mulsant BH, et al. Cardiovascular changes associated with venlafaxine in the treatment of late-life depression. Am J Geriatr Psychiatry 2006;14:796–802.

39. Montgomery S, Chatamra K, Pauer L, Whalen E, Baldinetti F. Efficacy and safety of pregabalin in elderly people with generalised anxiety disorder. Br J Psychiatry 2008;193:389–94.

40. Benitez CI, Smith K, Vasile RG, Rende R, Edelen MO, Keller MB. Use of benzodiazepines and selective serotonin reuptake inhibitors in middle-aged and older adults with anxiety disorders: a longitudinal and prospective study. Am J Geriatr Psychiatry 2008;16:5–13.

41. Hasnain M, Vieweg WV, Howland RH, et al. Quetiapine, QTc interval prolongation, and torsade de pointes: a review of case reports. Ther Adv Psychopharmacol 2014;4:130–8.

42. Wettermark B, Brandt L, Kieler H, Boden R. Pregabalin is increasingly prescribed for neuropathic pain, generalised anxiety disorder and epilepsy but many patients discontinue treatment. Int J Clin Pract 2014;68:104–10.

43. Wikner BN, Kallen B. Are hypnotic benzodiazepine receptor agonists teratogenic in humans? J Clin Psychopharmacol 2011;31:356–9.

44. Suri R, Altshuler L, Hellemann G, Burt VK, Aquino A, Mintz J. Effects of antenatal depression and antidepressant treatment on gestational age at birth and risk of preterm birth. Am J Psychiatry 2007;164:1206–13.

45. Palmsten K, Hernandez-Diaz S, Huybrechts KF, et al. Use of antidepressants near delivery and risk of postpartum hemorrhage: cohort study of low income women in the United States. BMJ 2013;347:f4877.

46. Kessler RC, Nelson CB, McGonagle KA, Edlund MJ, Frank RG, Leaf PJ. The epidemiology of co-occurring addictive and mental disorders: implications for prevention and service utilization. Am J Orthopsychiatry 1996;66:17–31.

47. Salzman C. Benzodiazepine dependence, toxicity, and abuse: a task force report of the American Psychiatric Association. Washington, DC: American Psychiatric Association, 1990.

48. Fava M, Rush AJ, Alpert JE, et al. Difference in treatment outcome in outpatients with anxious versus nonanxious depression: a STAR*D report. Am J Psychiatry 2008;165:342–51.

49. Leverich GS, Altshuler LL, Frye MA, et al. Risk of switch in mood polarity to hypomania or mania in patients with bipolar depression during acute and continuation trials of venlafaxine, sertraline, and bupropion as adjuncts to mood stabilizers. Am J Psychiatry 2006;163:232–9.

50. Pacchiarotti I, Bond DJ, Baldessarini RJ, et al. The International Society for Bipolar Disorders (ISBD) task force report on antidepressant use in bipolar disorders. Am J Psychiatry 2013;170:1249–62.

51. Ketter TA, Wang PW, Miller S. Bipolar therapeutics update 2014: a tale of 3 treatments. J Clin Psychiatry 2015;76: 69–70.

52. Gao K, Wu R, Kemp DE, et al. Efficacy and safety of quetiapine-XR as monotherapy or adjunctive therapy to a mood stabilizer in acute bipolar depression with generalized anxiety disorder and other comorbidities: a randomized, placebo-controlled trial. J Clin Psychiatry 2014;75:1062–8.

53. Keck PE Jr, Strawn JR, McElroy SL. Pharmacologic treatment considerations in co-occurring bipolar and anxiety disorders. J Clin Psychiatry 2006;67 suppl 1:8–15.

54. Aliyev NA, Aliyev ZN. Valproate (depakine-chrono) in the acute treatment of outpatients with generalized anxiety disorder without psychiatric comorbidity: randomized, doubleblind placebo-controlled study. Eur Psychiatry 2008;23: 109–14.

55. Bandelow B, Chouinard G, Bobes J, et al. Extended-release quetiapine fumarate (quetiapine XR): a once-daily monotherapy effective in generalized anxiety disorder. Data from a randomized, double-blind, placebo- and active-controlled study. Int J Neuropsychopharmacol 2010;13:305–20.

56. Jentink J, Loane MA, Dolk H, et al. Valproic acid monotherapy in pregnancy and major congenital malformations. N Engl J Med 2010;362:2185 - 93.

57. Raskind MA, Peterson K, Williams T, et al. A trial of prazosin for combat trauma PTSD with nightmares in active-duty soldiers returned from Iraq and Afghanistan. Am J Psychiatry 2013;170:1003–10.

58. Van Ameringen M, Mancini C, Patterson B, Simpson W, Truong C. Pharmacotherapy for generalized anxiety disorder. In: Stein DJ, Hollander E, Rothbaum BO, eds. Textbook of anxiety disorders. Washington, DC: American Psychiatric Publishing, 2010;193–218.

59. U.S. Food and Drug Administration. FDA drug safety communication: revised recommendations for Celexa (citalopram hydrobromide) related to a potential risk of abnormal heart rhythms with high doses. 2012. http://www.fda.gov/Drugs/DrugSafety/ucm297391.htm

60. Bird ST, Crentsil V, Temple R, Pinheiro S, Demczar D, Stone M. Cardiac safety concerns remain for citalopram at dosages above 40 mg/day. Am J Psychiatry 2014;171:17–9.

61. Zivin K, Pfeiffer PN, Bohnert AS, et al. Safety of high-dosage citalopram. Am J Psychiatry 2014;171:20–2.

62. Fava M, Judge R, Hoog SL, Nilsson ME, Koke SC. Fluoxetine versus sertraline and paroxetine in major depressive disorder: changes in weight with long-term treatment. J Clin Psychiatry 2000;61:863–7.

63. Preskorn SH. Outpatient management of depression: a guide for the practitioner. 2nd ed. Professional Communications: Caddo, OK, 1999.

64. Maina G, Albert U, Salvi V, Bogetto F. Weight gain during long-term treatment of obsessive-compulsive disorder: a prospective comparison between serotonin reuptake inhibitors. J Clin Psychiatry 2004;65:1365–71.

65. Serretti A, Chiesa A. Treatment-emergent sexual dysfunction related to antidepressants: a meta-analysis. J Clin Psychopharmacol 2009;29:259–66.

66. Reefhuis J, Devine O, Friedman JM, Louik C, Honein M. Specific SSRIs and birth defects: Bayesian analysis to interpret new data in the context of previous reports. BMJ 2015;351:h3190.

67. Hidalgo RB, Tupler LA, Davidson JR. An effect-size analysis of pharmacologic treatments for generalized anxiety disorder. J Psychopharmacol 2007;21:864–72.

68. Baldwin DS, Huusom AK, Maehlum E. Escitalopram and paroxetine in the treatment of generalised anxiety disorder: randomised, placebo-controlled, double-blind study. Br J Psychiatry 2006;189:264–72.

69. Beekman AT, Bremmer MA, Deeg DJ, et al. Anxiety disorders in later life: a report from the Longitudinal Aging Study Amsterdam. Int J Geriatr Psychiatry 1998;13:717–26.

70. Baldwin D, Woods R, Lawson R, Taylor D. Efficacy of drug treatments for generalised anxiety disorder: systematic review and meta-analysis. BMJ 2011;342:d1199.

71. Baldwin DS, Stein DJ, Dolberg OT, Bandelow B. How long should a trial of escitalopram treatment be in patients with major depressive disorder, generalised anxiety disorder or social anxiety disorder? An exploration of the randomised controlled trial database. Hum Psychopharmacol 2009; 24:269–75.

72. Cascade E, Kalali AH, Kennedy SH. Real-world data on SSRI antidepressant side effects. Psychiatry (Edgmont) 2009;6: 16–8.

73. de Abajo FJ, Garcia-Rodriguez LA. Risk of upper gastrointestinal tract bleeding associated with selective serotonin reuptake inhibitors and venlafaxine therapy: interaction with nonsteroidal anti-inflammatory drugs and effect of acid-suppressing agents. Arch Gen Psychiatry 2008;65:795–803.

74. Wang YP, Chen YT, Tsai CF, et al. Short-term use of serotonin reuptake inhibitors and risk of upper gastrointestinal bleeding. Am J Psychiatry 2014;171:54–61.

75. Richards JB, Papaioannou A, Adachi JD, et al. Effect of selective serotonin reuptake inhibitors on the risk of fracture. Arch Intern Med 2007;167:188–94.

76. Stone M, Laughren T, Jones ML, et al. Risk of suicidality in clinical trials of antidepressants in adults: analysis of proprietary data submitted to US Food and Drug Administration. BMJ 2009;339:b2880.

77. Pelissolo A. [Efficacy and tolerability of escitalopram in anxiety disorders: a review]. Encephale 2008;34:400–8.

78. Whiskey E, Taylor D. A review of the adverse effects and safety of noradrenergic antidepressants. J Psychopharmacol 2013; 27:732–9.

79. Delgado PL, Brannan SK, Mallinckrodt CH, et al. Sexual functioning assessed in 4 double-blind placebo- and paroxetine-controlled trials of duloxetine for major depressive disorder. J Clin Psychiatry 2005;66:686–92.

80. De Berardis D, Serroni N, Carano A, et al. The role of duloxetine in the treatment of anxiety disorders. Neuropsychiatr Dis Treat 2008;4:929–35.

81. Stahl SM, Ahmed S, Haudiquet V. Analysis of the rate of improvement of specific psychic and somatic symptoms of general anxiety disorder during long-term treatment with venlafaxine ER. CNS Spectr 2007;12:703–11.

82. Rickels K, Etemad B, Khalid-Khan S, Lohoff FW, Rynn MA, Gallop RJ. Time to relapse after 6 and 12 months' treatment of generalized anxiety disorder with venlafaxine extended release. Arch Gen Psychiatry 2010;67:1274–81.

83. Hoffman EJ, Mathew SJ. Anxiety disorders: a comprehensive review of pharmacotherapies. Mt Sinai J Med 2008;75: 248–62.

84. Carter NJ, McCormack PL. Duloxetine: a review of its use in the treatment of generalized anxiety disorder. CNS Drugs 2009;23:523–41.

85. Spielmans GI. Duloxetine does not relieve painful physical symptoms in depression: a meta-analysis. Psychother Psychosom 2008;77:12–6.

86. Gammans RE, Stringfellow JC, Hvizdos AJ, et al. Use of buspirone in patients with generalized anxiety disorder and coexisting depressive symptoms. A meta-analysis of eight randomized, controlled studies. Neuropsychobiology 1992;25: 193–201.

87. Kranzler HR, Burleson JA, Del Boca FK, et al. Buspirone treatment of anxious alcoholics. A placebo-controlled trial. Arch Gen Psychiatry 1994;51:720–31.

88. Bandelow B, Boerner JR, Kasper S, Linden M, Wittchen HU, Moller HJ. The diagnosis and treatment of generalized anxiety disorder. Dtsch Arztebl Int 2013;110:300–9.

89. Davidson JR, DuPont RL, Hedges D, Haskins JT. Efficacy, safety, and tolerability of venlafaxine extended release and buspirone in outpatients with generalized anxiety disorder. J Clin Psychiatry 1999;60:528–35.

90. Darcis T, Ferreri M, Natens J. A multicenter, double-blind placebo-controlled study investigating the anxiolytic efficacy of hydroxyzine in patients with generalized anxiety. Hum Psychopharmacol 1995;10:181–7.

91. Lader M, Scotto JC. A multicentre double-blind comparison of hydroxyzine, buspirone and placebo in patients with generalized anxiety disorder. Psychopharmacology (Berl) 1998;139: 402–6.

92. Llorca PM, Spadone C, Sol O, et al. Efficacy and safety of hydroxyzine in the treatment of generalized anxiety disorder: a 3-month double-blind study. J Clin Psychiatry 2002; 63:1020–7.

93. Dowben JS, Grant JS, Froelich KD, Keltner NL. Biological perspectives: hydroxyzine for anxiety: another look at an old drug. Perspect Psychiatr Care 2013;49:75–7.

94. Guaiana G, Barbui C, Cipriani A. Hydroxyzine for generalised anxiety disorder. Cochrane Database Syst Rev 2010;12: CD006815.

95. Baldwin DS, Anderson IM, Nutt DJ, et al. Evidence-based pharmacological treatment of anxiety disorders, post-traumatic stress disorder and obsessive-compulsive disorder: a revision of the 2005 guidelines from the British Association for Psychopharmacology. J Psychopharmacol 2014;28:403–39.

96. Bech P. Dose-response relationship of pregabalin in patients with generalized anxiety disorder. A pooled analysis of four placebo-controlled trials. Pharmacopsychiatry 2007; 40:163–8.

97. Lydiard RB, Rickels K, Herman B, Feltner DE. Comparative efficacy of pregabalin and benzodiazepines in treating the psychic and somatic symptoms of generalized anxiety disorder. Int J Neuropsychopharmacol 2010;13:229–41.

98. Wensel TM, Powe KW, Cates ME. Pregabalin for the treatment of generalized anxiety disorder. Ann Pharmacother 2012;46: 424–9.

99. Clarke H, Kirkham KR, Orser BA, et al. Gabapentin reduces preoperative anxiety and pain catastrophizing in highly anxious patients prior to major surgery: a blinded randomized placebo-controlled trial. Can J Anaesth 2013;60:432–43.

100. Ravindran LN, Stein MB. The pharmacologic treatment of anxiety disorders: a review of progress. J Clin Psychiatry 2010;71:839–54.

101. Schifano F, D'Offizi S, Piccione M, et al. Is there a recreational misuse potential for pregabalin? Analysis of anecdotal online reports in comparison with related gabapentin and clonazepam data. Psychother Psychosom 2011;80:118–22.

102. Zimmerman M, Posternak MA, Attiullah N, et al. Why isn't bupropion the most frequently prescribed antidepressant? J Clin Psychiatry 2005;66:603–10.

103. Bystritsky A, Kerwin L, Feusner JD, Vapnik T. A pilot controlled trial of bupropion XL versus escitalopram in generalized anxiety disorder. Psychopharmacol Bull 2008;41:46–51.

104. Trivedi MH, Rush AJ, Carmody TJ, et al. Do bupropion SR and sertraline differ in their effects on anxiety in depressed patients? J Clin Psychiatry 2001;62:776–81.

105. Dunner DL, Zisook S, Billow AA, Batey SR, Johnston JA, Ascher JA. A prospective safety surveillance study for bupropion sustained-release in the treatment of depression. J Clin Psychiatry 1998;59:366–73.

106. Altamura AC, Serati M, Buoli M, Dell'Osso B. Augmentative quetiapine in partial/nonresponders with generalized anxiety disorder: a randomized, placebo-controlled study. Int Clin Psychopharmacol 2011;26:201–5.

107. Khan A, Atkinson S, Mezhebovsky I, She F, Leathers T, Pathak S. Extended-release quetiapine fumarate (quetiapine XR) as adjunctive therapy in patients with generalized anxiety disorder and a history of inadequate treatment response: a randomized, double-blind study. Ann Clin Psychiatry 2013;25: E7–22.

108. Simon NM, Connor KM, LeBeau RT, et al. Quetiapine augmentation of paroxetine CR for the treatment of refractory generalized anxiety disorder: preliminary findings. Psychopharmacology (Berl) 2008;197:675–81.

109. Brawman-Mintzer O, Knapp RG, Nietert PJ. Adjunctive risperidone in generalized anxiety disorder: a double-blind, placebo-controlled study. J Clin Psychiatry 2005;66:1321–5.

110. Pandina GJ, Canuso CM, Turkoz I, Kujawa M, Mahmoud RA. Adjunctive risperidone in the treatment of generalized anxiety disorder: a double-blind, prospective, placebo-controlled, randomized trial. Psychopharmacol Bull 2007;40:41–57.

111. Pollack MH, Simon NM, Zalta AK, et al. Olanzapine augmentation of fluoxetine for refractory generalized anxiety disorder: a placebo controlled study. Biol Psychiatry 2006;59:211–5.

112. Hahn MK, Wolever TM, Arenovich T, et al. Acute effects of single-dose olanzapine on metabolic, endocrine, and inflammatory markers in healthy controls. J Clin Psychopharmacol 2013;33:740–6.

113. Ngai YF, Sabatini P, Nguyen D, et al. Quetiapine treatment in youth is associated with decreased insulin secretion. J Clin Psychopharmacol 2014;34:359–64.

114. Rickels K, Shiovitz TM, Ramey TS, Weaver JJ, Knapp LE, Miceli JJ. Adjunctive therapy with pregabalin in generalized anxiety disorder patients with partial response to SSRI or SNRI treatment. Int Clin Psychopharmacol 2012;27:142–50.

115. Pollack MH, Van Ameringen M, Simon NM, et al. A doubleblind randomized controlled trial of augmentation and switch strategies for refractory social anxiety disorder. Am J Psychiatry 2014;171:44–53.

116. Rickels K, Pollack MH, Feltner DE, et al. Pregabalin for treatment of generalized anxiety disorder: a 4-week, multicenter, double-blind, placebo-controlled trial of pregabalin and alprazolam. Arch Gen Psychiatry 2005;62:1022–30.

117. Rickels K, Pollack MH, Sheehan DV, Haskins JT. Efficacy of extended-release venlafaxine in nondepressed outpatients with generalized anxiety disorder. Am J Psychiatry 2000;157:968–74.

118. Bose A, Korotzer A, Gommoll C, Li D. Randomized placebo-controlled trial of escitalopram and venlafaxine XR in the treatment of generalized anxiety disorder. Depress Anxiety 2008;25:854–61.

119. Taylor D, Sparshatt A, Varma S, Olofinjana O. Antidepressant efficacy of agomelatine: meta-analysis of published and unpublished studies. BMJ 2014;348:g1888.

120. Stein DJ, Ahokas A, Marquez MS, et al. Agomelatine in generalized anxiety disorder: an active comparator and placebo-controlled study. J Clin Psychiatry 2014;75:362–8.

121. Stein DJ, Ahokas A, Albarran C, Olivier V, Allgulander C. Agomelatine prevents relapse in generalized anxiety disorder: a 6-month randomized, double-blind, placebo-controlled discontinuation study. J Clin Psychiatry 2012;73:1002–8.

122. Russmann S, Lauterburg BH, Helbling A. Kava hepatotoxicity. Ann Intern Med 2001;135:68–9.

123. Mathew SJ, Amiel JM, Coplan JD, Fitterling HA, Sackeim HA, Gorman JM. Open-label trial of riluzole in generalized anxiety disorder. Am J Psychiatry 2005;162:2379–81.

124. Kasper S, Gastpar M, Muller WE, et al. Lavender oil preparation Silexan is effective in generalized anxiety disorder—a randomized, double-blind comparison to placebo and paroxetine. Int J Neuropsychopharmacol 2014;17:859–69.

125. Katzman MA, Brawman-Mintzer O, Reyes EB, Olausson B, Liu S, Eriksson H. Extended release quetiapine fumarate (quetiapine XR) monotherapy as maintenance treatment for generalized anxiety disorder: a long-term, randomized, placebo-controlled trial. Int Clin Psychopharmacol 2011;26:11–24.

126. Merideth C, Cutler AJ, She F, Eriksson H. Efficacy and tolerability of extended release quetiapine fumarate monotherapy in the acute treatment of generalized anxiety disorder: a randomized, placebo controlled and active-controlled study. Int Clin Psychopharmacol 2012;27:40–54.

127. Lohoff FW, Etemad B, Mandos LA, Gallop R, Rickels K. Ziprasidone treatment of refractory generalized anxiety disorder: a placebo-controlled, double-blind study. J Clin Psychopharmacol 2010;30:185–9.

128. Snyderman SH, Rynn MA, Rickels K. Open-label pilot study of ziprasidone for refractory generalized anxiety disorder. J Clin Psychopharmacol 2005;25:497–9.

129. Suppes T, McElroy SL, Sheehan DV, et al. A randomized, double-blind, placebo-controlled study of ziprasidone monotherapy in bipolar disorder with co-occurring lifetime panic or generalized anxiety disorder. J Clin Psychiatry 2014;75:77–84.

130. Gao K, Muzina D, Gajwani P, Calabrese JR. Efficacy of typical and atypical antipsychotics for primary and comorbid anxiety symptoms or disorders: a review. J Clin Psychiatry 2006;67:1327–40.

131. Gabriel A. The extended-release formulation of quetiapine fumarate (quetiapine XR) adjunctive treatment in partially responsive generalized anxiety disorder (GAD): an open label naturalistic study. Clin Ter 2011;162:113–8.

132. Simon NM, Hoge EA, Fischmann D, et al. An open-label trial of risperidone augmentation for refractory anxiety disorders. J Clin Psychiatry 2006;67:381–5.

133. Menza MA, Dobkin RD, Marin H. An open-label trial of aripiprazole augmentation for treatment-resistant generalized anxiety disorder. J Clin Psychopharmacol 2007;27:207–10.

134. Hoge EA, Worthington JJ 3rd, Kaufman RE, Delong HR, Pollack MH, Simon NM. Aripiprazole as augmentation treatment of refractory generalized anxiety disorder and panic disorder. CNS Spectr 2008;13:522–7.

135. Linden M, Bandelow B, Boerner RJ, et al. The best next drug in the course of generalized anxiety disorders: the "PN-GAD-algorithm." Int J Psychiatry Clin Pract 2013;17:78–89.

136. National Institute for Health and Clinical Excellence. Generalized anxiety disorder and panic disorder (with or without agoraphobia) in adults: management in primary, secondary and community care. NICE clinical guideline 113. London: Gaskell and British Psychological Society, 2011.

137. Osser DN, Patterson RD. On the value of evidence-based psychopharmacology algorithms. Bull Clin Psychopharmacol 2013;23:1–5.

138. Mullaney TJ. Doctors wielding data. Bus Week 2005;94:98.

UPDATE

GENERALIZED ANXIETY DISORDER ALGORITHM

I n the last four years since the publication of this algorithm, the recommendations and flowchart for the psychopharmacology of generalized anxiety disorder (GAD) remain almost the same. There have been no new studies that change the overall sequences of the nodes. However, there have been important studies adding support to what was proposed in the 2016 algorithm. One new treatment that has received study is repetitive transcranial magnetic stimulation (rTMS).

Node 2: Comorbidity and Special Patient Populations That Might Alter the Core Algorithm

In the discussion of medications to avoid in women of childbearing potential in Table 1, paroxetine is noted to have a D rating because of atrial septal defects. A newer large observational study confirmed that paroxetine does indeed have a high incidence of this fetal abnormality.[1] Contrary to previous data, though, the incidence with fluoxetine was almost as high as with paroxetine. Also, in this table, comorbidity with bipolar is considered and antidepressants are to be avoided in favor of some of the nonantidepressant options in the algorithm. A new meta-analysis of six studies in which an antidepressant was added to a mood stabilizer in bipolar patients confirmed that there is increased risk of mood stabilization to (hypo)mania if the antidepressant is continued over the long term (e.g., one year).[2] Finally, in the same table, there is discussion of management of comorbid posttraumatic stress disorder (PTSD) with GAD. Prazosin was recommended on the basis of four small placebo-controlled studies with large effect sizes in favor of prazosin. Since then, a large important multicenter trial published in 2018 found no efficacy for prazosin.[3] The evidence on prazosin is discussed in detail in the chapter on the PTSD algorithm. It is concluded that this (and perhaps similar products like doxazosin) is still first-line for PTSD patients with significant sleep problems including nightmares and disturbed awakenings, even though it is clear that it does not work for everyone. More research is needed to help define which patients are the best candidates for prazosin.[4]

Node 3a: Alternatives to an SSRI as the First-Line Choice for GAD

The first alternative discussed was duloxetine, which is FDA-approved for GAD and has comparable efficacy though somewhat different side effects. The advantages and disadvantages were discussed. It was mentioned that duloxetine is FDA-approved for a number of painful conditions which could be seen as an advantage, though a meta-analysis by Spielmans in 2008 of the effect on pain concluded that the effect size was too small to be clinically significant.[5] The author concluded that the effect on pain was not evidence-supported and that duloxetine was not likely to be useful for pain in the context of treating depression (and presumably, for treating GAD with comorbid pain as well). There is a new, much more comprehensive meta-analysis of the effect of various antidepressants on pain as an outcome measure, confirming the previous review.[6] All antidepressants had only small independent effects on pain and the effect size of duloxetine was right in the middle of the group of antidepressants studied.

Another alternative discussed was hydroxyzine, which has several controlled studies finding efficacy in GAD. In the discussion of advantages and disadvantages, there is a new concern about QT prolongation with this product. The Pharmacovigilance Risk Assessment Committee of the European Medicines Agency (comparable to the US Food and Drug Administration) of the European Union performed a detailed review and concluded that there are small but significant risks of QT prolongation and torsade de pointes with hydroxyzine.[7] They recommended that the total dose be limited to 100 mg daily (50 mg in the elderly when use cannot be avoided in this population). Risk factors for torsades include bradycardia, low potassium, and taking other medications that prolong QTc.

Node 4a: Alternatives to the First-Choice Option for the *Second* Medication Trial for GAD

After failure on the first medication trial, the recommendation is to try a different SSRI or duloxetine. But as with the first trial, there are several alternatives that may be considered, and some new ones are added for this second trial, including benzodiazepines. They were not considered appropriate for first-line use (despite their efficacy and FDA approval in the case of alprazolam) because of their many side effects including memory impairment, excessive sedation, auto accidents, falls (especially in the elderly), dependence and use disorders, discontinuation syndromes on withdrawal, respiratory depression (e.g., in patients with sleep apnea), and because they should be avoided in patients with use disorders with other substances. Also, in 2017, the FDA issued a new black box warning for benzodiazepines (e.g., clonazepam and diazepam) indicating that serious risks could occur in combination with opiates including profound sedation, respiratory depression, coma, and death. To this list of problems may be added renewed concerns about long-term memory problems that may not remit on discontinuation of the medication. Studies have been contradictory on this matter, but the latest meta-analysis of 50 different studies concluded that the odds risk over suitable controls of the development of dementia was about 1.4.[8] This was considered not likely to be an artifact of other confounding variables, and it seemed to be a reasonable concern. Reduction of inappropriate benzodiazepine use should be a goal.

Another option for the second trial could be agomelatine, though this is still not available in the United States. It was initially proposed for U.S. approval as an antidepressant, but as was noted, it did not do well in the registration studies and was not approved. However, in addition to the three studies cited for treatment of GAD, there are now two more. One found efficacy at doses as low as 10 mg (previous studies were with 25 or 50 mg),[9] and the other compared 25–50 mg of agomelatine with escitalopram 10–20 mg in a randomized (but not placebo-controlled) trial.[10] The latter found "noninferior" response (61% with agomelatine and 65% with escitalopram). Side effects were fewer with agomelatine. For prescribers in countries where agomelatine is available, it appears to compete favorably with SSRIs for GAD, and if it was not for cost considerations compared with generic SSRIs, it could be among the first-line choices.

The last option mentioned previously at this node was lavender oil, which is marketed in Germany as a treatment for GAD. There are now two placebo-controlled 10-week trials showing efficacy, and an analysis of pooled data on 925 subjects examined, for the first time, the dose–response relationship.[11] The therapeutic range seemed to be 80–160 mg daily. The extract was well tolerated.

Finally, there is a new option to add at this node—rTMS. There have been two small sham-controlled trials in patients who have failed one or more pharmacotherapies. In the first, 25 sessions of high-frequency (20 Hz) rTMS was applied to the right dorsolateral prefrontal cortex in 15 subjects and the results compared with 25 sham-treated individuals.[12] Active treatment was superior, and the results were sustained at two- and four-week follow-up. In the second trial, 10 sessions of low-frequency (1 Hz) rTMS was applied to the right parietal lobe in 18 patients and compared with 18 sham-treated controls.[13] It was effective both for the GAD and for comorbid insomnia. The optimal parameters for this investigational use of rTMS have obviously not been established as yet, these studies are small and the results difficult to generalize to other GAD patients, the procedure is very costly, and the maintenance requirements are unknown.

We did not include vilazodone as an option. There was an initial positive study in GAD patients followed by two others which barely found any difference from placebo.[14] As a result, the manufacturer did not pursue further efforts to get FDA approval for the product.

REFERENCES

1. Reefhuis J, Devine O, Friedman JM, Louik C, Honein MA. Specific SSRIs and birth defects: Bayesian analysis to interpret new data in the context of previous reports. BMJ (Clinical research ed) 2015;351:h3190.
2. McGirr A, Vohringer PA, Ghaemi SN, Lam RW, Yatham LN. Safety and efficacy of adjunctive second-generation antidepressant therapy with a mood stabiliser or an atypical antipsychotic in acute bipolar depression: a systematic review and meta-analysis of randomised placebo-controlled trials. Lancet Psychiatry 2016;3:1138–46.
3. Raskind MA, Peskind ER, Chow B, et al. Trial of prazosin for post-traumatic stress disorder in military veterans. N Engl J Med 2018;378:507–17.

4. Raskind MA, Peskind ER. Prazosin for post-traumatic stress disorder. N Engl J Med 2018;378:1649–50.

5. Spielmans GI. Duloxetine does not relieve painful physical symptoms in depression: a meta-analysis. Psychother Psychosom 2008;77:12–6.

6. Gebhardt S, Heinzel-Gutenbrunner M, Konig U. Pain relief in depressive disorders: a meta-analysis of the effects of antidepressants. J Clin Psychopharmacol 2016;36:658–68.

7. Vigne J, Alexandre J, Fobe F, et al. QT prolongation induced by hydroxyzine: a pharmacovigilance case report. Eur J Clin Pharmacol 2015;71:379–81.

8. Penninkilampi R, Eslick GD. A systematic review and meta-analysis of the risk of dementia associated with benzodiazepine use, after controlling for protopathic bias. CNS Drugs 2018;32:485–97.

9. Stein DJ, Khoo JP, Ahokas A, et al. 12-week double-blind randomized multicenter study of efficacy and safety of agomelatine (25-50mg/day) versus escitalopram (10-20mg/day) in out-patients with severe generalized anxiety disorder. Eur Neuropsychopharmacol 2018;28:970–9.

10. Stein DJ, Ahokas A, Jarema M, et al. Efficacy and safety of agomelatine (10 or 25 mg/day) in non-depressed out-patients with generalized anxiety disorder: a 12-week, double-blind, placebo-controlled study. Eur Neuropsychopharmacol 2017;27:526–37.

11. Kasper S, Moller HJ, Volz HP, Schlafke S, Dienel A. Silexan in generalized anxiety disorder: investigation of the therapeutic dosage range in a pooled data set. Int Clin Psychopharmacol 2017;32:195–204.

12. Dilkov D, Hawken ER, Kaludiev E, Milev R. Repetitive transcranial magnetic stimulation of the right dorsal lateral prefrontal cortex in the treatment of generalized anxiety disorder: a randomized, double-blind sham controlled clinical trial. Prog Neuropsychopharmacol Biol Psychiatry 2017;78:61–5.

13. Huang Z, Li Y, Bianchi MT, et al. Repetitive transcranial magnetic stimulation of the right parietal cortex for comorbid generalized anxiety disorder and insomnia: a randomized, double-blind, sham-controlled pilot study. Brain Stimul 2018;11:1103–9.

14. Zareifopoulos N, Dylja I. Efficacy and tolerability of vilazodone for the acute treatment of generalized anxiety disorder: a meta-analysis. Asian J Psychiatr 2017;26:115–22.

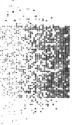

The Psychopharmacology Algorithm Project at the Harvard South Shore Program: An Update on Generalized Social Anxiety Disorder

David N. Osser, MD and Lance R. Dunlop, MD

LEARNING OBJECTIVES

After participating in this activity, the psychiatrist should be better able to:

- Evaluate the evidence base for the advantages and disadvantages of the various pharmacotherapies for generalized social anxiety disorder.
- Select first-line, second-line, and third-line medication options.
- Assess additional choices with less supporting evidence.

There is considerable interest in psychopharmacologic treatment of generalized social anxiety disorder (SAD). Some claim that the concept of SAD as a mental disorder is championed, if not invented, by the pharmaceutical industry and the proposed medication treatments are over-sold.[1] However, these assertions are adequately rebutted.[2] New evidence of impairment in neuropharmacologic and neuroanatomical systems suggests that biologic treatments may play an important role in SAD.[3,4]

In this article, we present an algorithm for the selection of medication treatments of SAD. This is an update of a previous algorithm from the Psychopharmacology Algorithm Project at the Harvard South Shore Program (PAPHSS).[5] It is also influenced by an algorithm for treating SAD in primary care to which one of the authors (D.N.O.) contributed.[6] Although psychosocial interventions are of unquestioned importance in the treatment of SAD, this algorithm is limited to pharmaceutical interventions and may be applied if and when the prescribing clinician and patient determine that medication is appropriate. In many patients, the role of medication is to facilitate psychosocial approaches such as cognitive-behavioral or psychodynamic therapies.[7,8]

Dr. Osser is Associate Professor of Psychiatry, Harvard Medical School, 150 Winding River Road, Needham, MA 02492, E-mail: dno@theworld.com; and Dr. Dunlop is Acting Medical Director, Cambria County Mental Health/Mental Retardation Clinic, Johnstown, PA 15901.

All faculty and staff in a position to control the content of this CME activity and their spouses/life partners (if any) have disclosed that they have no financial relationships with, or financial interests in, any commercial organizations pertaining to this educational activity.

The authors have disclosed that the use of citalopram, escitalopram, fluoxetine, phenelzine, clonazepam, alprazolam, buspirone, nefazodone, gabapentin, quetiapine, risperidone, pregabalin, and tiagabine for treatment of social anxiety disorder has not been approved by the U.S. Food and Drug Administration.

The algorithms developed by the PAPHSS should not be understood as discounting the importance of clinical experience. Individual experience can contradict, support, or add to what is derived from the scientific evidence. Consideration of the evidence base for practice is viewed as necessary but by no means sufficient for clinical decision making.

The roles of selective serotonin reuptake inhibitors (SSRIs) and serotonin norepinephrine reuptake inhibitors (SNRIs) in the treatment of SAD deserve special attention. Recent reviews of the treatment of major depression and posttraumatic stress disorder with these agents propose that their efficacy compared with placebo seems less robust than previously assumed.[9,10] Further, the adverse effects of SSRIs and SNRIs affect the risk-benefit analysis of their usefulness.[11] In the treatment of SAD, SSRIs are prominent in the recommendations of previous practice guidelines and algorithms. Given the concerns about these antidepressants for other disorders, is there any basis for hesitation regarding their role in SAD treatment? This will be a focus of our review.

METHODS

The method of algorithm development employed by the PAPHSS is described in previous publications.[12,13] These algorithms model the cognitive process of a psychopharmacology consultation. Each algorithm is structured with a series of questions that a consultant would ask, in the order they would be asked, to provide an evidence-supported recommendation. The evidence is provided and then appraised. In situations where the available data are contradictory, equivocal, or inadequate, this ambiguity is acknowledged.

We reviewed previous algorithms and conducted a literature search in PubMed to find all relevant studies published since the last version of the PAPHSS SAD algorithm. All proposed psychopharmacologic agents for SAD were entered in Boolean (AND) searches with the key words "social anxiety disorder." All resultant studies in English were selected. Other relevant studies or reviews referenced in those articles were also examined. A total of 1932 studies were located, entered into an Endnote library, and reviewed. The algorithm was then updated on the basis of this material.

For comparing the effectiveness of various medication treatments of SAD, this review focuses on results with the Clinical Global Impression of Improvement Scale (CGI-I), one of the primary outcome measures in almost all major psychopharmacology studies of SAD. "Improvement" on the CGI-I is generally defined as a score of 1 or 2 (very much or much improved). Meta-analysis demonstrates that CGI-I outcomes (eg, effect sizes compared with placebo) are highly comparable with the outcomes of other frequently used scales, such as the Liebowitz Social Anxiety Scale (LSAS).[14]

We reference the CGI-I improvement percentages from most of the randomized controlled trials (RCTs) reviewed here and calculated the number needed to treat (NNT) for improvement in each study. This is the number of patients who must be treated before one of them improves (ie, CGI of 1 or 2) because of the active medication rather than from a placebo effect. The NNT is easily calculated by subtracting the percentage improvement on placebo from the percentage improvement on active medication, and then taking the reciprocal of this difference. Because placebo effects are rather large in most SAD studies,[15] comparing NNTs assists with appreciating the relative ability of the various medications to produce more improvement than placebo.

It should be noted that even when patients with SAD are rated as very much improved in these studies, the patients are usually not remitted. Thus, strategies for approaching partial response will also be considered in the algorithm.

COMORBIDITY

Psychopharmacologic studies of SAD treatment typically exclude patients with common comorbidities such as unipolar and bipolar depression, alcohol and substance dependence, and other anxiety disorders. If any of these conditions are present, confidence in the basic algorithm sequence may be reduced.

Regarding *comorbid unipolar depression*, it is usually assumed that because SAD and unipolar depression are 2 disorders that respond to antidepressants, one could expect a good response when they occur together. Recent evidence from the Sequenced Treatment Alternatives to Relieve Depression (STAR*D) Study and other data, however, suggest that major depression comorbid with anxiety responds poorly to antidepressants.[16] Hence, the expectations for antidepressant effectiveness with SAD comorbid with depression may be lowered. With *comorbid bipolar I depression*, most experts conclude that antidepressants are ineffective and, in some circumstances, may destabilize the patient.[13] Although *comorbid bipolar II depression* may respond to antidepressants in the short term, long-term outcome studies are required to see whether this improvement is stable.[17] Thus, when SAD is comorbid with bipolar depression, clinicians may wish to consider the evidence for the non-antidepressant options in the algorithm or emphasize psychotherapeutic treatments.

Comorbid alcohol and substance misuse **is common in patients with SAD.** In these patients, use of benzodiazepines (BZs) is discouraged, although in general, this class of medication was not determined to be a first-line option for treatment of SAD because of adverse effects. If the patient is currently abusing or dependent on alcohol or drugs, these substances should be withdrawn, if possible, before the algorithm is applied. It seems reasonable to help the patient achieve abstinence for at least 1 week before initiating psychopharmacologic treatment of SAD. This may be the minimal time required to demonstrate drug-placebo differences in the treatment of anxiety and depressive disorders that persist after withdrawal.[5]

Finally, some evidence suggests that *comorbid anxiety disorders* (eg, panic disorder, generalized anxiety disorder) will not diminish the responsiveness of SAD to SSRIs.[18]

FLOWCHART FOR THE ALGORITHM

A flowchart of our updated psychopharmacologic treatment algorithm for SAD is presented in Figure 1. Each numbered "node" represents a key question or decision point that delineates populations of patients ranging from treatment-naive to treatment-resistant. In the following sections, the rationales for the questions and recommendations at each node are presented.

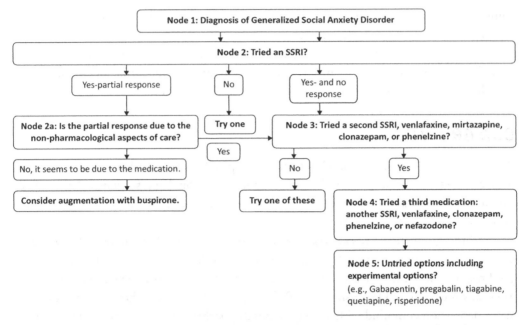

Figure 1. Flowchart showing treatment algorithm for generalized social anxiety disorder.

Node 1: Diagnosis of SAD and Comorbidities

The algorithm begins after the confirmation of a *DSM-IV-TR* criteria-based SAD diagnosis, including relevant comorbidities that affect decision making.

Node 2: SSRI Trial?

Our review concludes that the first-line medication for SAD is usually an SSRI. Three SSRIs are FDA approved for use in patients with SAD: paroxetine, sertraline, and fluvoxamine controlled release (CR). Other SSRIs (eg, citalopram, escitalopram, fluoxetine) have varying strengths of evidence but are likely effective. To assist with selection of a particular SSRI (or other antidepressant) for an individual patient, we will review the details of the antidepressant data on the treatment of SAD.

Paroxetine was the first SSRI to achieve FDA approval and has among the best effect sizes of the antidepressants, with an excellent NNT of 3 (ie, to achieve a score of 1 or 2 on the CGI-I at 8 weeks). Another 28% of patients responded by 12 weeks, compared with only 8% on placebo.[19] Doses were usually 50 to 60 mg daily after titration at clinicians' discretion during the study. Another large RCT (N = 384), using 3 fixed doses (ie, 20, 40, and 60 mg daily) versus placebo, is one of the few dose-finding studies in the SAD literature.[20] All 3 doses had similar effect sizes compared with placebo on the CGI-I (ie, an NNT of just over 3). The 40-mg dose was slightly more effective than 20 mg but produced more early dropouts, probably from adverse effects due to the protocol's rapid escalation of dose. The investigators recommend that if an initial dose of 20 mg is unsatisfactory after an adequate trial (eg, 8 weeks), an increase to 40 mg or more might be beneficial and better tolerated than in the study.

The disadvantage of paroxetine is more adverse effects compared with other SSRIs. It is associated with the most weight gain, constipation, and sedation due to its H1 antihistamine effects, and among the most sexual side effects[21] (although ejaculation delay can be an advantage for male patients with SAD who frequently have premature ejaculation).[22] Paroxetine's short half-life can result in discontinuation symptoms if the patient misses a dose, and it is the only SSRI in pregnancy category D due to reports of cardiac septal malformations in fetuses. Although more recent studies did not replicate this finding,[23] the D rating remains in place. Because a substantial number of patients with SAD are women of childbearing potential, it is important to be aware of possible pregnancy-related risks.

Sertraline demonstrated good efficacy at a mean dose of about 150 mg daily. The NNT was 4 in the best short-term study (20 weeks, 204 randomized patients).[24] In a 24-week extension of this study, responders were randomized to stay on sertraline or switch to placebo. Thirty-six percent relapsed on placebo and only 4% on sertraline.[25] It is important to note, however, that almost two-thirds of patients did well despite switching to placebo. Perhaps other aspects of their care or coincidental stress reduction resulted in a situation where they no longer needed active drug. **Thus, this study suggests that many patients with SAD who respond to SSRIs can eventually discontinue them, avoiding exposure to long-term adverse effects.**

Fluvoxamine CR is usually employed at a mean dose of 200 mg daily by the endpoint of titration. The NNT was 5 in the best study.[26] In 2 recent RCTs, one demonstrated a difference from placebo on the CGI-I and one did not.[27,28]

Regarding non-FDA-approved SSRIs, *escitalopram* was tested in 2 major acute SAD studies. One RCT (N = 358) produced a less impressive NNT of 7 for improvement on the CGI-I with a mean dose of 18 mg daily.[29] There was only a 6.6-point difference in the outcome with the LSAS versus placebo. Given that the starting scores on the LSAS were 95 to 96, this does not seem like a clinically significant difference. The second RCT was a large, dose-finding study comparing escitalopram (5, 10, or 20 mg), paroxetine (20 mg), and placebo (N = 839).[30] The 20-mg dose of escitalopram produced a better short-term result than the lower doses, suggesting that the dose-response curve for escitalopram between 5 and 20 mg was not flat. This was a surprise because, as noted earlier, the dose-response curve for paroxetine in SAD was almost flat between 20 and 60 mg.[20] Further, in the treatment of major depression with escitalopram, 10 mg is equivalent to 20 mg according to the package insert's interpretation of the available data, suggesting a flat dose-response curve in the treatment of depression.

Lader et al's study also demonstrated that the 20-mg dose of escitalopram was more effective than the 20-mg dose of paroxetine.[30] For a more objective comparison of escitalopram and paroxetine, however, they should have included 2 or more doses of each medication to evaluate the dose-response relationships in the same patient population.

Citalopram is not the subject of any placebo-controlled RCTs. In 2 open-label trials, however, the improvement rate was comparable to outcomes in RCTs with the other SSRIs.

Fluoxetine effects are less clear than for the FDA-approved SSRIs. In the largest (N = 295) study, the NNT of 5 was comparable with the others.[31] Although some patients were randomized to cognitive behavioral therapy in this study, it provided no additional benefit. In 2 smaller RCTs (both with N = 60), however, fluoxetine did not differ from placebo.

The Cochrane collaboration found a number of unpublished studies of SSRIs in SAD. Because these studies probably failed to demonstrate efficacy, "significant publication bias" in the data set for SAD is likely.[32] Thus, some caution should be added to the generally favorable impression conveyed by the published studies discussed above.

Conclusion: In Node 2, an SSRI is recommended. In this context, clinicians should be mindful of the general adverse effect profile of SSRIs. Sexual effects (eg, impotence, delayed ejaculation, loss of libido) are common, disturbing for many patients, and usually do not remit with time.[11] Cytochrome P450 drug interactions are common with paroxetine and fluoxetine, but less so with citalopram and escitalopram. Insomnia and nightmares are troublesome for many patients on SSRIs and a concomitant sedative-hypnotic is often necessary. **Upper gastrointestinal track bleeding is 9 times more common in patients on an SSRI and a nonsteroidal anti-inflammatory medication compared with a control group not on these medications.**[33] The risk is mitigated, however, by adding an acid-controlling agent such as a proton-pump inhibitor. Osteoporosis and fracture risk increase 2-fold with long-term SSRI use.[34] SSRIs may increase progression of cataracts in the elderly.[35] Suicidal ideation may increase in patients younger than 25 years, according to the new package-insert warning. For all these reasons, it is recommended that careful assessment of improvement on SSRIs is made to confirm whether response was medication-related and not due to nonspecific aspects of care. Usually, the best way to make this determination is a trial off the medication at a time when the patient is doing reasonably well and can receive suitable support and observation from the clinician and significant others.

Other options to consider at Node 2 (and later): If the risks of adverse effects from an SSRI are considered unacceptable to the prescribing clinician or patient, there are several reasonable options for first-line use, but they are not necessarily preferred in this algorithm.

Venlafaxine (an SNRI), has comparable effect sizes to SSRIs in large studies (ie, NNT of 4-7), using doses ranging from 75 to 225 mg daily.[36,37] There was no dose-response relationship, which suggests that the norepinephrine effect seen at higher doses with this medication did not affect efficacy. Short-term adverse effects are generally a little greater with venlafaxine compared with SSRIs, including nausea, other gastrointestinal symptoms, and elevated blood pressure. Therefore, it seems reasonable to use this agent second line.

Phenelzine, **a monoamine oxidase inhibitor (MAOI), has excellent efficacy with the largest effect size of any antidepressant (ie, NNT of 2.3 in one study at a dose of 65 mg daily).**[38] Three other placebo-controlled trials found comparable efficacy. The dietary requirements and risk of hypertensive crisis, however, limit this option to patients who respond poorly to the safer medications.

Mirtazapine (a tetracyclic), at a dose of 30 mg was effective compared with placebo on the LSAS in a study of 66 women with SAD, but the CGI-I was not recorded.[39] Weight gain was a significant problem with this agent.

Clonazepam (a BZ), was effective in one RCT involving 75 patients, producing the best effect size in any study on record (ie, an NNT of 1.7 on the CGI-I).[40] Seventy-eight percent responded to a dose averaging 2.4 mg daily, versus 20% on placebo. This outstanding result, however, has not been replicated. A study with *alprazolam* (dose: 4.2 mg daily) reported only a 38% response using an atypical rating instrument.[41] The problem with BZs is that they produce significant cognitive impairment and performance/coordination deficits not seen with antidepressants.[42] Further, BZs should be avoided in most patients with a history of substance or alcohol abuse or dependence. Finally, they probably do not benefit comorbid depression associated with SAD.

Node 2a: Partial response to the antidepressant trial

As noted earlier, partial improvement with antidepressant therapy occurs frequently in SAD. Augmentation may be considered if the partial improvement is thought to be due to medication and not psychotherapy and/or nonspecific aspects of treatment. This can be difficult to determine but of crucial importance. As a general principle, one should avoid adding another medication when partial response to the first medication is likely a placebo response. This is because augmentation increases the risks of adverse effects and drug interactions, reduces adherence due to complexity of the regimen, and increases cost. We recommend careful evaluation for other possible contributing factors to the unsatisfactory response such as comorbidity, nonadherence, and pharmacokinetic/ pharmacogenetic variables. Because of the earlier-mentioned issues, the algorithm indicates a preference for switching rather than augmentation, especially in the first node of psychopharmacology treatment (see Figure 1).

One possible medication augmentation strategy that is reasonably safe and inexpensive involves buspirone **added to an SSRI.** This agent, however, has not demonstrated efficacy as a monotherapy and the evidence base for it as an augmentation is quite limited. There is only one small study involving 10 patients given adjunctive buspirone (up to 60 mg daily; mean dose 45 mg) for 8 weeks with 70% responding in this uncontrolled, prospective trial.[43] Buspirone also surprised investigators by doing quite well in the STAR*D study as an augmentation to citalopram for major depression.[44] Since then, there are more frequent recommendations for this unlabeled indication.

Psychotherapy augmentation is always a viable option, but the timing of this important intervention is not addressed in this algorithm.

Node 3: Tried a Second SSRI or Venlafaxine? Considered Clonazepam or an MAOI?

If a patient fails to respond adequately to the first antidepressant, anecdotal reports support trying a different antidepressant or other medication.[45] There is, however, no systematic study of this logical approach. The lack of data is most unfortunate, and the algorithm from Node 3 onward must rely on application of general principles of conservative, safety-conscious, and cost-effective practice rather than on specific evidence pertaining to each node. It is suggested that the clinician review the efficacy and safety considerations presented in node 2 for the various options and choose the one that seems most reasonable for a specific patient. If a second SSRI is chosen, escitalopram (20 mg) may deserve consideration given the slight, and, in our view, somewhat unconvincing evidence of better results (compared with paroxetine) reported in the Lader et al study.[30] Unfortunately, 20 mg of escitalopram is very costly, because it is the only remaining branded SSRI in the US market.

See the discussion of partial response at node 2a.

Node 4: Tried a Third Medication: Another SSRI, Venlafaxine, Nefazodone, Clonazepam, or MAOI?

A third monotherapy trial is recommended. *Nefazodone* is included as one of the options here for the first time. Because of the risks of liver toxicity, this agent should not be used unless at least 2 other antidepressants were tried. Further, evidence for benefit in SAD is limited to a number of encouraging open-label trials and one placebo-controlled RCT with a negative outcome, in which 105 patients received a mean dose just under 500 mg daily[46] with no significant improvement compared with placebo. The NNT was 14 on the CGI-I.

Node 5: Have You Considered Some of the Experimental Options in Addition to Trying Another of the Options Already Discussed but Not Yet Tried?

Under the heading of experimental options, some promising choices include the following (not listed in order of preference).

Gabapentin was the subject of one placebo-controlled RCT.[47] Sixty-nine patients participated but 49% on placebo and 38% on gabapentin dropped out. The mean dose of gabapentin ranged from 600 to 3600 mg daily. On the basis of the LSAS, 32% improved on active drug and 14% on placebo (ie, NNT of 5.5).

Quetiapine monotherapy in doses up to 400 mg daily was used in a small (N = 15), placebo-controlled, 8-week RCT.[48] Although there was no difference in improvement on the primary outcome measure (the Brief Social Phobia Scale), 40% of quetiapine patients improved (score of 1 or 2) on the CGI-I versus none of the placebo patients (ie, NNT of 2.5). Because the CGI-I is the measure we used to compare the various studies, this result suggests that quetiapine may be effective, though probably rarely producing remission, as is the case with most of the other psychopharmacologic treatments. Quetiapine has significant metabolic side effects and, like other antipsychotics, may double the risk of sudden cardiac death at these doses.[49]

Risperidone at a mean dose of 1 mg was used to augment an SSRI in an 8-week, open-label trial in 7 patients.[50] LSAS scores improved from a mean of 81 to 38, which seems encouraging.

Pregabalin at a dose of 600 mg daily had slight benefits for SAD in a RCT.[51] *Tiagabine* in an open-label trial was somewhat promising.[52]

CONCLUSIONS

This algorithm summarizes and organizes the available evidence pertaining to the choice of pharmacotherapy for patients with SAD, a disabling condition that significantly affects quality of life. A structure for consideration of sequential medication options is proposed. Although SSRIs are still first-line treatments, it is evident that they have significant limitations. In general, medication seems to have an important but fairly modest role in altering the course of the lives of people with this disorder. Some patients decide that the adverse effects are not worth the benefits over the long term, whereas others are grateful for the help they receive from this approach. The prescribing clinician should be prepared to discuss the quality of the evidence base in detail and collaborate with the patient to find the treatments most acceptable and helpful to him or her.

REFERENCES

1. Lane C. Shyness: How Normal Behavior Became a Sickness. New Haven, CT: Yale University Press; 2007.
2. Campbell-Sills L, Stein MB. Justifying the diagnostic status of social phobia: a reply to Wakefield, Horwitz, and Schmitz. Can J Psychiatry. 2005;50(6):320–323; discussion 324–326.
3. Akimova E, Lanzenberger R, Kasper S. The serotonin-1A receptor in anxiety disorders. Biol Psychiatry. 2009;66(7):627–635.
4. Irle E, Ruhleder M, Lange C, et al. Reduced amygdalar and hippocampal size in adults with generalized social phobia. J Psychiatry Neurosci. 2010;35(2):126–131.
5. Osser DN, Renner JA, Bayog R. Algorithms for the pharmacotherapy of anxiety disorders in patients with chemical abuse and dependence. Psychiatric Ann. 1999;29:285–301.
6. Stein DJ, Kasper S, Matsunaga H, et al. Pharmacotherapy of social anxiety disorder: an algorithm for primary care. Prim Care Psychiatry. 2001;7(3):107–110.
7. Knijnik DZ, Blanco C, Salum GA, et al. A pilot study of clonazepam versus psychodynamic group therapy plus clonazepam in the treatment of generalized social anxiety disorder. Eur Psychiatry. 2008;23(8):567–574.
8. Blanco C, Heimberg RG, Schneier FR, et al. A placebo-controlled trial of phenelzine, cognitive behavioral group therapy, and their combination for social anxiety disorder. Arch Gen Psychiatry. 2010;67(3):286–295.
9. Fournier JC, DeRubeis RJ, Hollon SD, et al. Antidepressant drug effects and depression severity: a patient-level meta-analysis. JAMA. 2010;303(1):47–53.
10. Baker DG, Nievergelt CM, Risbrough VB. Post-traumatic stress disorder: emerging concepts of pharmacotherapy. Expert Opin Emerg Drugs. 2009;14(2):251–272.
11. Cascade E, Kalali AH, Kennedy SH. Real-world data on SSRI antidepressant side effects. Psychiatry (Edgmont). 2009;6(2):16–18.
12. Hamoda HM, Osser DN. The Psychopharmacology Algorithm Project at the Harvard South Shore Program: an update on psychotic depression. Harv Rev Psychiatry. 2008;16(4):235–247.
13. Ansari A, Osser DN. The psychopharmacology algorithm project at the Harvard South Shore Program: an update on bipolar depression. Harv Rev Psychiatry. 2010;18(1):36–55.

14. Hedges DW, Brown BL, Shwalb DA. A direct comparison of effect sizes from the Clinical Global Impression-Improvement Scale to effect sizes from other rating scales in controlled trials of adult social anxiety disorder. Hum Psychopharmacol. 2009;24(1):35–40.

15. Oosterbaan DB, van Balkom AJ, Spinhoven P, et al. The placebo response in social phobia. J Psychopharmacol. 2001;15(3):199–203.

16. Fava M, Rush AJ, Alpert JE, et al. Difference in treatment outcome in outpatients with anxious versus nonanxious depression: a STAR*D report. Am J Psychiatry. 2008;165(3):342–351.

17. Suppes T. Is there a role for antidepressants in the treatment of bipolar II depression? Am J Psychiatry. 2010;167(7):738–740.

18. Brady KT, Clary CM. Affective and anxiety comorbidity in post-traumatic stress disorder treatment trials of sertraline. Compr Psychiatry. 2003;44(5):360–369.

19. Stein DJ, Versiani M, Hair T, et al. Efficacy of paroxetine for relapse prevention in social anxiety disorder: a 24-week study. Arch Gen Psychiatry. 2002;59(12):1111–1118.

20. Liebowitz MR, Stein MB, Tancer M, et al. A randomized, double-blind, fixed-dose comparison of paroxetine and placebo in the treatment of generalized social anxiety disorder. J Clin Psychiatry. 2002;63(1):66–74.

21. Serretti A, Chiesa A. Treatment-emergent sexual dysfunction related to antidepressants: a meta-analysis. J Clin Psychopharmacol. 2009;29(3):259–266.

22. Munoz V, Stravynski A. Social phobia and sexual problems: a comparison of social phobic, sexually dysfunctional and normal individuals. Br J Clin Psychol. 2010;49(Pt 1):53–66.

23. Einarson A, Pistelli A, DeSantis M, et al. Evaluation of the risk of congenital cardiovascular defects associated with use of paroxetine during pregnancy. Am J Psychiatry. 2008;165(6): 749–752.

24. Van Ameringen MA, Lane RM, Walker JR, et al. Sertraline treatment of generalized social phobia: a 20-week, double-blind, placebo-controlled study. Am J Psychiatry. 2001;158(2):275–281.

25. Walker JR, Van Ameringen MA, Swinson R, et al. Prevention of relapse in generalized social phobia: results of a 24-week study in responders to 20 weeks of sertraline treatment. J Clin Psychopharmacol. 2000;20(6):636–644.

26. Stein MB, Fyer AJ, Davidson JR, et al. Fluvoxamine treatment of social phobia (social anxiety disorder): a double-blind, placebo-controlled study. Am J Psychiatry. 1999;156(5):756–760.

27. Davidson J, Yaryura-Tobias J, DuPont R, et al. Fluvoxamine-controlled release formulation for the treatment of generalized social anxiety disorder. J Clin Psychopharmacol. 2004;24:118–125.

28. Westenberg HG, Stein DJ, Yang H, et al. A double-blind placebo-controlled study of controlled release fluvoxamine for the treatment of generalized social anxiety disorder. J Clin Psychopharmacol. 2004;24:49–55.

29. Kasper S, Stein DJ, Loft H, et al. Escitalopram in the treatment of social anxiety disorder: randomised, placebo-controlled, flexible-dosage study. Br J Psychiatry. 2005;186(3):222–226.

30. Lader M, Stender K, Burger V, et al. Efficacy and tolerability of escitalopram in 12- and 24-week treatment of social anxiety disorder: randomised, double-blind, placebo-controlled, fixed-dose study. Depress Anxiety. 2004;19(4):241–248.

31. Davidson JR, Foa EB, Huppert JD, et al. Fluoxetine, comprehensive cognitive behavioral therapy, and placebo in generalized social phobia. Arch Gen Psychiatry. 2004;61(10):1005–1013.

32. Stein DJ, Ipser JC, Balkom AJ. Pharmacotherapy for social phobia. Cochrane Database Syst Rev. 2004;(4):CD001206.

33. de Abajo FJ, Garcia-Rodriguez LA. Risk of upper gastrointestinal tract bleeding associated with selective serotonin reuptake inhibitors and venlafaxine therapy: interaction with nonsteroidal anti-inflammatory drugs and effect of acid-suppressing agents. Arch Gen Psychiatry. 2008;65(7):795–803.

34. Richards JB, Papaioannou A, Adachi JD, et al. Effect of selective serotonin reuptake inhibitors on the risk of fracture. Arch Intern Med. 2007;167(2):188–194.

35. Etminan M, Mikelberg FS, Brophy JM. Selective serotonin reuptake inhibitors and the risk of cataracts: a nested case-control study. Ophthalmology. 2010;117(6):1251–1255.
36. Liebowitz MR, Gelenberg AJ, Munjack D. Venlafaxine extended release vs placebo and paroxetine in social anxiety disorder. Arch Gen Psychiatry. 2005;62(2):190–198.
37. Stein MB, Pollack MH, Bystritsky A, et al. Efficacy of low and higher dose extended-release venlafaxine in generalized social anxiety disorder: a 6-month randomized controlled trial. Psychopharmacology (Berl). 2005;177(3):280–288.
38. Liebowitz MR, Schneier F, Campeas R, et al. Phenelzine vs atenolol in social phobia. A placebo-controlled comparison. Arch Gen Psychiatry. 1992;49(4):290–300.
39. Muehlbacher M, Nickel MK, Nickel C, et al. Mirtazapine treatment of social phobia in women: a randomized, double-blind, placebo-controlled study. J Clin Psychopharmacol. 2005;25(6):580–583.
40. Davidson JR, Potts N, Richichi E, et al. Treatment of social phobia with clonazepam and placebo. J Clin Psychopharmacol. 1993;13(6):423–428.
41. Gelernter CS, Uhde TW, Cimbolic P, et al. Cognitive-behavioral and pharmacological treatments of social phobia. A controlled study. Arch Gen Psychiatry. 1991;48(10):938–945.
42. Hindmarch I. Cognitive toxicity of pharmacotherapeutic agents used in social anxiety disorder. Int J Clin Pract. 2009;63(7):1085–1094.
43. Van Ameringen M, Mancini C, Wilson C. Buspirone augmentation of selective serotonin reuptake inhibitors (SSRIs) in social phobia. J Affect Disord. 1996;39(2):115–121.
44. Trivedi MH, Fava M, Wisniewski SR, et al. Medication augmentation after the failure of SSRIs for depression. N Engl J Med. 2006;354(12):1243–1252.
45. Altamura AC, Pioli R, Vitto M, et al. Venlafaxine in social phobia: a study in selective serotonin reuptake inhibitor non-responders. Int Clin Psychopharmacol. 1999;14(4):239–245.
46. Van Ameringen M, Mancini C, Oakman J, et al. Nefazodone in the treatment of generalized social phobia: a randomized, placebo-controlled trial. J Clin Psychiatry. 2007;68(2):288–295.
47. Pande AC, Davidson JR, Jefferson JW, et al. Treatment of social phobia with gabapentin: a placebo-controlled study. J Clin Psychopharmacol. 1999;19(4):341–348.
48. Vaishnavi S, Alamy S, Zhang W, et al. Quetiapine as monotherapy for social anxiety disorder: a placebo-controlled study. Prog Neuro-Psychopharmacol Biol Psychiatry. 2007;31(7):1464–1469.
49. Ray WA, Chung CP, Murray KT, et al. Atypical antipsychotic drugs and the risk of sudden cardiac death. N Engl J Med. 2009;360(3):225–235.
50. Simon NM, Hoge EA, Fischmann D, et al. An open-label trial of risperidone augmentation for refractory anxiety disorders. J Clin Psychiatry. 2006;67(3):381–385.
51. Pande AC, Feltner DE, Jefferson JW, et al. Efficacy of the novel anxiolytic pregabalin in social anxiety disorder: a placebo-controlled, multicenter study. J Clin Psychopharmacol. 2004; 24(2):141–149.
52. Dunlop BW, Papp L, Garlow SJ, et al. Tiagabine for social anxiety disorder. Hum Psychopharmacol. 2007;22(4):241–244.

UPDATE

SOCIAL ANXIETY DISORDER ALGORITHM

There have been few new psychopharmacology studies of generalized social anxiety disorder (SAD) in the decade since the last publication of this algorithm. Of the relevant studies, nothing changes the basic recommendations until Node 2b, which is when you have had a partial response to the first selective serotonin reuptake inhibitor (SSRI) trial, a response that appears to be due to the effect of the SSRI rather than a placebo effect (which is often the cause of partial responses in this and many other disorders). In the previous algorithm version, buspirone was suggested as a possible augmentation on the basis of an uncontrolled case series. However, a new study came out in 2014 that resulted in an additional option at this point: clonazepam.[1]

Node 2b: Augmentation of a Partial Response to the Initial SSRI

In this large trial sponsored by the National Institute of Mental Health, 397 patients with SAD were treated with open-label sertraline at a mean dose of 180 mg for 10 weeks. Subjects were excluded if they had more than two previous medication trials—but only 25% to 30% had received any previous trials; 32% responded (50% drop in the Liebowitz Social Anxiety Scale [LSAS]) and 13% remitted. These results are notably lower than the rates of response in the initial citalopram trial for depression in the STAR*D study (47% and 28%, respectively), suggesting that SAD is a more difficult disorder to treat.[2] A total of 181 patients failed to achieve better than a partial response and agreed to be randomized to one of three treatment options for 12 weeks[2]: a *switch* to venlafaxine (mean dose eventually was 186 mg daily), *addition* of clonazepam (mean dose initially 1.5 mg and at endpoint 2.3 mg), or *addition* of placebo.

Clonazepam jumped ahead of the other two arms of the study in the first 2 weeks and stayed there for the remainder of the trial. At endpoint, there were >56% responses on clonazepam versus >36% responses on placebo (p = .027). The number needed to treat was 5. Additional patients achieving remission were 27% on clonazepam and 17% on placebo, although this was statistically nonsignificant. Number needed to treat for remission was 10. Switching to venlafaxine was not different from adding placebo (19% vs. 17% remissions). Improvement was gradual over the 12 weeks in all three arms of the study, which highlighted the importance of giving the treatments adequate time. Indeed, except for placebo, the active treatments seemed to still be on a trend toward further improvement: results had not plateaued at 12 weeks.

Side-effect differences were nonsignificant but somnolence was numerically higher with clonazepam (32%) compared with venlafaxine (23%) and placebo (15%). Discontinuations were lowest with clonazepam (10%) compared with venlafaxine (15%) and placebo (20%). Consistent with many other studies in other disorders, subjects like to stay on benzodiazepines.

There were quite a few additional exclusion criteria for this study that render the results less generalizable to "real-world" SAD patients than would be ideal. The following were excluded: women of childbearing potential not on good birth control; patients with psychosis, bipolar disorder, comorbid obsessive-compulsive disorder, suicidality, substance abuse within the last 3 months, and substance dependence within the last 6 months (8%-16% had lifetime history); and people in psychotherapy.

As a result of this study, the algorithm is changed at Node 2b and the first recommendation for an augmentation is clonazepam if the patient would have met these rather stringent criteria for inclusion in the study. If not, then there must be questions about benefits versus the risks of adding clonazepam and the prescriber should consider those before prescribing clonazepam here and consider the alternative of the next augmentation option, which is buspirone. Though uncontrolled, the response rate to adding buspirone (mean dose 45 mg) in the one study cited earlier was 70%.[3]

This study also indirectly enhances the status of clonazepam monotherapy in other places where it was mentioned as an option in the algorithm, especially Node 3.

Node 5: The Fourth Medication Trial—Some New Studies But No New Recommendations

For treatment-resistant cases of SAD, several options including gabapentin and pregabalin were suggested. There was a new, large placebo-controlled trial of pregabalin published in 2011.[4] Three doses were compared but only the top dose of 600 mg daily was significantly effective (p = .01) on the LSAS. There was also a maintenance trial with pregabalin.[5] After collecting 153 responders to open-label treatment with 450 mg daily, patients were randomized to continue on it or be switched to placebo. Various outcome measures favored pregabalin, and significant side effects were limited to dizziness (number needed to harm [NNH] = 14) and infections (NNH = 20). Currently, pregabalin is a brand product and much more expensive than gabapentin, yet their pharmacodynamic properties and approved indications are very similar.[6]

REFERENCES

1. Pollack MH, Van Ameringen M, Simon NM, et al. A double-blind randomized controlled trial of augmentation and switch strategies for refractory social anxiety disorder. Am J Psychiatry. 2014;171:44–53.
2. Trivedi MH, Rush AJ, Wisniewski SR, et al. Evaluation of outcomes with citalopram for depression using measurement-based care in STAR*D: implications for clinical practice. Am J Psychiatry. 2006;163:28–40.

3. Van Ameringen M, Mancini C, Wilson C. Buspirone augmentation of selective serotonin reuptake inhibitors (SSRIs) in social phobia. J Affect Disord. 1996;39:115–121.

4. Feltner DE, Liu-Dumaw M, Schweizer E, et al. Efficacy of pregabalin in generalized social anxiety disorder: results of a double-blind, placebo-controlled, fixed-dose study. Int Clin Psychopharmacol. 2011;26:213–220.

5. Greist JH, Liu-Dumaw M, Schweizer E, et al. Efficacy of pregabalin in preventing relapse in patients with generalized social anxiety disorder: results of a double-blind, placebo-controlled 26-week study. Int Clin Psychopharmacol. 2011;26:243–251.

6. Bockbrader HN, Wesche D, Miller R, et al. A comparison of the pharmacokinetics and pharmacodynamics of pregabalin and gabapentin. Clin Pharmacokinet. 2010;49:661–669.

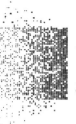

The Psychopharmacology Algorithm Project at the Harvard South Shore Program: An Update on Posttraumatic Stress Disorder

Laura A. Bajor, DO, Ana Nectara Ticlea, MD, and David N. Osser, MD

Background: *This project aimed to provide an organized, sequential, and evidence-supported approach to the pharmacotherapy of posttraumatic stress disorder (PTSD), following the format of previous efforts of the Psychopharmacology Algorithm Project at the Harvard South Shore Program.*

Method: *A comprehensive literature review was conducted to determine the best pharmacological choices for PTSD patients and to update the last published version (1999) of the algorithm. We focused on optimal pharmacological interventions to address the prominent symptoms of PTSD, with additional attention to the impact that common comorbidities have on treatment choices.*

Results: *We found that SSRIs and SNRIs are not as effective as previously thought, and that awareness of their long-term side effects has increased. New evidence suggests that addressing fragmented sleep and nightmares can improve symptoms (in addition to insomnia) that are frequently seen with PTSD (e.g., hyperarousal, reexperiencing). Prazosin and trazodone are emphasized at this initial step; if significant PTSD symptoms remain, an antidepressant may be tried. For PTSD-related psychosis, an antipsychotic may be added. In resistant cases, two or three antidepressants may be used in sequence. Following that, or with partial improvement and residual symptomatology, augmentation may be tried; the best options are antipsychotics, clonidine, topiramate, and lamotrigine.*

Conclusion: *This heuristic may be helpful in producing faster symptom resolution, fewer side effects, and increased compliance. (Harv Rev Psychiatry 2011;19:240–258.)*

Keywords: algorithms, posttraumatic stress disorder, psychopharmacology, stress disorders

INTRODUCTION

There has been considerable interest in finding effective psychopharmacological strategies for treating posttraumatic stress disorder (PTSD). It is assumed that biological treatment may have an important role, given the abnormalities in neurotransmitter, neuroendocrine, and neuroanatomical systems that have been identified in patients with PTSD.[1–3]

From Harvard Medical School; Harvard South Shore Psychiatry Residency Training Program, Brockton, MA (Drs. Bajor and Ticlea); VA Boston Healthcare System, Brockton Division, Brockton, MA (Dr. Osser)

Original manuscript received 29 November 2010, accepted for publication subject to revision 28 April 2011; revised manuscript received 16 May 2011.

Correspondence: David N. Osser, MD, VA Boston Healthcare System, Brockton Division, 940 Belmont St., Brockton, MA 02301. Email: David.Osser@va.gov

DOI: 10.3109/10673229.2011.614483

In this article the authors present a heuristic for selecting medication treatments for PTSD. This version updates a previous PTSD algorithm from the Psychopharmacology Algorithm Project at the Harvard South Shore Program (PAPHSS).[4] It was also influenced by the International Psychopharmacology Algorithm Project PTSD algorithm, to which one of the authors (DNO) contributed as a consultant.[5]

Although psychosocial interventions are effective for many patients with PTSD,[6] this algorithm focuses on medication usage and is meant to be applied if and when the prescribing clinician and patient determine that medication may be appropriate. We did not evaluate the efficacy of psychotherapy and when it should be offered, though we acknowledge that some guidelines consider psychosocial interventions as a first-line treatment for PTSD.[7-9]

At present, the only medications that the Food and Drug Administration (FDA) has approved for PTSD are the selective serotonin reuptake inhibitors (SSRIs) sertraline and paroxetine. These medications are widely recommended and used in clinical practice. In this review, we focus on the quality of the evidence for the efficacy of SSRIs and other medications used to treat PTSD. Recent systematic reviews have questioned whether standard medication treatments (e.g., SSRIs) produce results that are clinically robust and whether it is time to revisit the usual sequence of medication choices. A novel approach may be justifiable, at least for certain subpopulations of PTSD patients.[7,10,11]

Method

The PAPHSS method of algorithm development has been described in previous publications.[12-14] These algorithms model the cognitive process involved in a psychopharmacology consultation, with focus on the evidence base. Each is structured as a series of questions about the patient's diagnosis and past treatment history. If the patient has not been tried on one of the medications that is best supported by the evidence pertaining to the clinical circumstances, the algorithm suggests trying that medication. The evidence is cited and appraised, and other options that might be considered are also discussed. When the evidence for treatment at a "node" is inadequate or contradictory, this situation is acknowledged, and any recommendations offered are more tentative and flexible. For more treatment-resistant patients (higher-numbered nodes), there is greater uncertainty, more focus on treatment of residual symptoms, and more deference to the prescriber's clinical experience. The PAPHSS proposes that, as a core value, consideration of the scientific evidence is necessary, but not sufficient, for clinical decision making. The prescriber's clinical experience can support or contradict the research data and should contribute to treatment decisions.

Since PTSD is a chronic illness, and the treatment selected is likely to be continued over an extended period, factors such as short- and long-term side-effect profiles and the risks for drug/drug interactions are weighed strongly in deciding whether and at what point in treatment to include a medication.

After reviewing the previous (1999) PAPHSS algorithm, as well as other algorithms and guidelines, the authors conducted literature searches in PubMed to identify studies and reviews published since 1999. Proposed psychopharmacological agents for PTSD were entered in Boolean (AND) searches with the keywords "posttraumatic stress disorder." Resultant studies in English were selected. Other studies or reviews referenced in the selected articles were also examined. The algorithm was updated based on 103 studies and reviews published since 1999 identified in this manner.

Demographics, Symptom Clusters, and Tailoring of Treatment Approaches

The criteria for PTSD in the *Diagnostic and Statistical Manual of Mental Disorders* (4th ed.) (DSM-IV) include the symptom clusters of reexperiencing, avoidance, and hyperarousal.[15] These symptom clusters may differ in their responses to psychopharmacological treatment. It is less clear whether these differences depend on the nature of the trauma—for example, combat veterans versus survivors of rape or domestic abuse. Recently traumatized individuals may respond better than those with distant trauma, such as Vietnam veterans.[16,17] The evidence also suggests that SSRIs may be more effective with female civilian survivors of sexual or domestic violence.[16,17] It is not clear, however, whether these differences are due to gender, age at initial traumatization, possible influence of compensation for combat veterans with PTSD, or other characteristics. Unfortunately, the available evidence is insufficient to support targeting treatments based on these variables. The evidence base on psychopharmacological treatment of child and adolescent PTSD is also scant and devoid of positive controlled studies.[18]

Flowchart for the Algorithm

A summary and overview of the algorithm appears in Figure 1. Each numbered "node" represents a decision point delineating patient populations ranging from treatment naive to highly resistant. The questions, evidence analysis, and reasoning that support the recommendations at each node will be presented below.

NODE 1: DOES THE PATIENT MEET DSM-IV CRITERIA FOR POSTTRAUMATIC STRESS DISORDER?

First, confirm a diagnosis based on DSM-IV criteria, and note any co-occurring psychiatric and medical symptoms and diagnoses that may be important, including substance abuse, depression, bipolar disorder, dissociative symptoms, anger, impulsivity, and psychosis. In treating female patients of childbearing age, the potential impact of medication on pregnancy should also be considered. Table 1 provides a brief overview of treatment considerations for these situations. A more thorough description of this important material is beyond the scope of this review, but the reader is encouraged to consult the associated references.

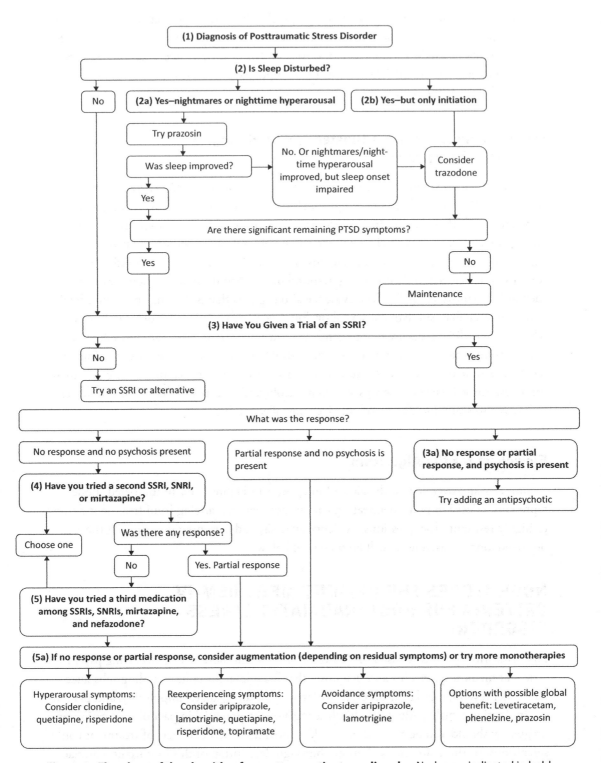

Figure 1. Flowchart of the algorithm for posttraumatic stress disorder. Nodes are indicated in bold.

Table 1	Comorbidity and Other Features in PTSD and How They Affect the Algorithm		
Comorbidity	**Considerations**	**Recommendations**
Substance abuse	Comorbidity of substance abuse is very high in PTSD patients[4] PTSD patients are at increased risk of abusing prescription medications[19] Algorithm recommendations do not apply to patients who are actively abusing substances[4]	Screen for substance abuse in PTSD patients Avoid benzodiazepines Ideally, a patient should be clean & sober at least a week before attempting to apply this algorithm[20]
Bipolar disorder	Lifetime risk for PTSD approximately double in patients with bipolar disorder, who may be exposed to more trauma & have fewer resources & social supports[21] SSRIs & other antidepressants may pose risks of destabilizing the bipolar disorder[13]	Treat nightmares & disturbed awakenings with prazosin Be more reluctant to use antidepressants for patient dually diagnosed with bipolar disorder & PTSD than in the standard algorithm
Psychosis	Psychotic symptoms in PTSD patients could indicate a comorbid psychotic disorder or could be part of the PTSD[22]	Consider skipping node 2 (sleep management) If primary psychosis, treat first with an antipsychotic
Major depressive disorder	History of major depression increases risk of developing PTSD, & PTSD diagnosis increases risk of depression[23] Dysregulation of HPA axis may cause above associations[2,24,25] Responsiveness to antidepressants is diminished in PTSD patients with comorbid depression in some studies[26–28] Children/adolescents with PTSD show more variability in response to antidepressants than those with only depression[29]	Screen for depression in PTSD patients Use antidepressants earlier in the algorithm but know that prognosis is guarded Know that patients with both diagnoses may not respond to antidepressants as well as those with only PTSD respond If psychotic depression, treat with antidepressant & antipsychotic[12]
Dissociation	Associated with more traumatic events & more serious PTSD pathology[30] Paroxetine found slightly better than placebo in one study with small *n* & high dropout rates[31] Some recommend psychotherapy as first-line treatment for the dissociative symptoms of PTSD[32]	Screen for dissociative symptoms Know that dissociation indicates more serious pathology & less predictable response to pharmacotherapy Consider psychotherapy to address these specific symptoms
Pregnancy	Physiological changes of pregnancy (e.g., decreased drug-protein binding, enhanced hepatic metabolism & renal clearance, & delayed gastric emptying) may affect drug levels in ways that are difficult to predict[33] Medications with teratogenic risks should be avoided during the first trimester, particularly weeks 3 through 9[33] Paroxetine is only SSRI categorized by FDA as "Category D" due to reports of cardiac septal malformations[33] Valproate has severe teratogenic effects[33]	Expect altered drug effects in pregnant patients, & monitor them more closely Avoid paroxetine & valproic acid

(continued)

Table 1	Comorbidity and Other Features in PTSD and How They Affect the Algorithm (*continued*)		
Comorbidity	*Considerations*	*Recommendations*
Smoking	Rates of smoking were increased in veterans with PTSD returning from Iraq & Afghanistan[34,35]	Bupropion was found to be effective for smoking-cessation efforts in one study of patients with chronic PTSD[36] One study found smoking-cessation efforts to be more successful in PTSD patients if smoking was addressed by the patients' psychiatric team rather than by referral to separate clinic[34]

FDA, Food and Drug Administration; SSRI, selective serotonin reuptake inhibitor; VA, Department of Veterans Affairs.

NODE 2: IS SLEEP DISTURBED?

Mounting evidence has implicated sleep impairment as a core symptom in PTSD and a primary source of distress and dysfunction for patients with this disorder.[37,38] It is therefore proposed that sleep problems be assessed initially and reassessed after each algorithm step if they persist and overall response remains unsatisfactory.[38] For many patients, sleep deprivation may exacerbate core daytime PTSD symptoms (hypervigilance, avoidance, reexperiencing), and these symptoms may improve when sleep improves.[39] Another justification for treating sleep difficulties first is the availability of prazosin, a psychopharmacology option that targets impaired sleep in PTSD patients and that has demonstrated substantially larger effect sizes than medications commonly thought to be effective for the general symptom profile in PTSD (SSRIs and serotonin-norepinephrine reuptake inhibitors [SNRIs]). To our knowledge, none of the previous guidelines or algorithms has placed sleep evaluation and treatment first, before the use of an SSRI.

Sleep disturbances common in PTSD include the following: hyperarousal linked to difficulties initiating or maintaining sleep; trauma-related nightmares; awakenings without nightmare recollection; and prolonged sleep latency.[40,41] Increased noradrenergic activity during sleep and while trying to fall asleep is thought to be an important mechanism.[41–43] Notably, SSRIs can sometimes exacerbate these symptoms.[39,44,45]

Other causes of insomnia may contribute to the sleep difficulties of patients with PTSD. These include sleep apnea, restless leg syndrome, periodic limb movements of sleep, sleep hygiene issues, nicotine withdrawal, and medical problems associated with sleep fragmentation (e.g., pain and nocturia). Caffeine, though frequently employed as a method of coping with daytime symptoms of sleep deprivation secondary to PTSD and other causes of insomnia, can at times become a major independent contributor. Assessment of these factors is essential in the sleep evaluation before applying the algorithm recommendations.

Node 2a

If the patient has PTSD-related nightmares or disturbed arousals, we recommend consideration of a trial of prazosin as the first-line medication treatment. Prazosin is a generic alpha-1 adrenergic antagonist previously used to treat hypertension and symptoms of benign prostatic hyperplasia. Murray Raskind and colleagues at the University of Washington reasoned that alpha antagonists might be effective for the hyperarousal symptoms of PTSD. They selected prazosin for study as it is the only commercially available alpha-1 agent that crosses the blood-brain barrier, with the consequence that it would be the most likely to have activity in the brain. To date, they have conducted three randomized, placebo-controlled studies.[42,43,46] Efficacy was demonstrated for trauma-related nightmares, overall quality of sleep, and, to some extent, general PTSD symptoms in patients with either military and civilian trauma. All studies found large effect sizes (Cohen's $d > 1.0$) on the various measures of sleep impairment. These results are summarized in Table 2.

Prazosin was well tolerated in these studies. Hypotension risks were minimized by slowly titrating the dose upward over several weeks, allowing tolerance to the blood pressure effects to develop. Details of the dosing protocols are provided in Table 2 and may be used as guidelines for clinical use. In the largest study, 2 of 20 (10%) dropped out due to subjective dizziness possibly related to blood pressure. Both studies by Raskind and colleagues[42,43] involved male veterans, whereas the study by Taylor and colleagues[46] involved civilian females. Though the reason is unclear, the dosage requirements for men and women differed, with the male veterans often requiring 10 mg or more, compared to the mean of 3 mg needed by women.

In a more recent observational study with mostly male veterans in a Department of Veterans Affairs (VA) setting ($n = 62$), the mean dose of prazosin after initial titration was 3 mg, which increased to 6 mg after up to six years of follow-up.[47] This dose is much lower than in the two controlled studies and may reflect clinicians' unawareness of the doses used in those studies. The rate of dropout due to hypotension at these doses was less than 2%.

Infrequent side effects include dizziness, drowsiness, headache, constipation, loss of appetite, fatigue, nasal congestion, dry eyes, and priapism. Noncardiac chest pain has occurred, but cardiac ischemia must be ruled out.[48] If the patient is hypertensive, coordination with the primary care clinician is advised.

Thompson and colleagues[39] showed in a small chart review study of 22 combat veterans that disturbed awakenings without nightmare recollection were also significantly reduced ($p < 0.01$) following treatment with prazosin. Although this finding needs to be confirmed in randomized, controlled trials (RCTs), the study suggests that it would be reasonable to employ prazosin in patients with these awakenings.

The study data currently available for prazosin are limited. It should be emphasized that the studies were mostly small, that they were done mostly by one group, and that the RCTs did not use monotherapy in previously untreated patients. Furthermore, dosing with prazosin is somewhat complex. Though the effect sizes with prazosin were large, it has been observed that small studies can generate higher effect sizes; such results should be interpreted with caution.[49] Nevertheless, we are proposing the consideration of prazosin for first-line use for patients with prominent nightmares and related sleep disturbances.

In support of this recommendation, we would first cite again the exceptional effect size relative to placebo of around 1.0 for significant improvement in sleep. As we will be showing later, all other medications, whether used as first-line (e.g., SSRIs) or as add-on interventions for treatment-resistant patients, fail to achieve even close to this effect size for PTSD symptoms. Next, we have emphasized the importance of sleep impairment in PTSD and the central role that it may have in the pathology of this disorder—and to that may be added the medical risks of leaving sleep problems untreated.[50] Finally, the acceptable side-effect profile of prazosin and low dropout rate that has been found in the studies to date have a favorable appearance compared to the SSRIs, with their common unacceptable sexual side effects and the high dropout rates that meta-analyses have noted.

Table 2 | Effect of Prazosin on Sleep and PTSD Symptoms in Three Placebo-Controlled, Randomized Trials					
Study	*n*	*Dropouts*	*Outcome variables*	*Effect size (Cohen's d)*	*Dosing protocol*
Raskind et al. (2003)[42]	10	0	CAPS subscales:		Start at 1 mg at bedtime x 3 days
			Recurrent distressing nightmares	1.9	Increase as follows, as tolerated:
			Difficulty falling/staying asleep	1.6	2 mg for 4 nights
			Reexperiencing /intrusion	0.7	4 mg for 7 nights
			Avoidance/numbing	0.6	6 mg for 7 nights
			Hyperarousal	0.9	4 mg at 3 pm & 6 mg at bedtime
			Total CAPS score	0.7	Mean final daily dose = 9.3 mg
			Clinical Global Impression	1.4	
Raskind et al. (2007)[43]	40	6	CAPS recurrent distressing nightmares subscale	0.94	Same as above, except:
			Pittsburg Sleep Quality Index	1.00	Day 21: one 10 mg dose at bedtime
			Clinical Global Impression	1.08	Day 28: one 15 mg given at bedtime
					Mean final dose = 13 mg
Taylor et al. (2008)[46]	13	0	Recurrent distressing nightmares	0.96	Begin with 1 mg at bedtime
			Difficulty falling/staying asleep	0.50	Increase 1 mg weekly, as tolerated
			Non-nightmare distressed awakenings	1.20	Maximum recommended dose = 4 mg
			Clinical Global Impression	1.50	Mean final dose = 3.1 mg
			PTSD Dream Rating Scale	1.40	

CAPS, Clinician-Administered PTSD Scale.

Clearly, we need larger studies with prazosin, and we need to know if alpha-1 adrenergic agents can be effective for the full spectrum of PTSD symptoms. Some studies are under way: one involving 320 veterans across 13 VA medical centers, and another studying 120 active-duty soldiers at Fort Lewis, Washington. These studies are expected to be completed in late 2012. In the interim, our view is that the current evidence is sufficiently strong to consider employing this agent as a first-line intervention.

Other alpha-1 blocking agents such as doxazosin (4–8 mg/day) and terazosin (3–7 mg/day) may have similar effects on PTSD symptoms, according to brief reports of 12 and 20 patients, respectively.[51,52] Although these products apparently do not cross the blood-brain barrier, the investigators propose that reduction of peripheral adrenergic activity, including tachycardia, may secondarily attenuate central nervous system manifestations of hyperarousal. This hypothesis requires further investigation.

If sleep has improved to an acceptable level, the patient may be maintained on prazosin. The long-term observational follow-up study of prazosin use in 62 patients for up to six years mentioned above found that almost 50% of patients took prazosin until the end of the study period, usually without adding other medications for PTSD.[47]

Node 2a, Continued: The Use of Trazodone

If prazosin fails to improve insomnia, or if it improves nightmares but without eliminating problems with sleep onset—and if other causes unrelated to PTSD have been addressed—then it may be worth considering a trial of low-dose trazodone (see Figure 1). It can be added or substituted, depending on whether prazosin is perceived to offer benefit.

Trazodone, a sedating antidepressant, has shown some effectiveness for sleep difficulties in PTSD patients in open-label studies.[53] It was the most widely prescribed medication used for hypnotic purposes in the United States in 2005.[54] Excess sedation, dizziness, and orthostasis occur frequently, and syncope occasionally. In males, priapism is a concern.[55] Milder erectile stimulation is apparently much more common; before the advent of medications such as sildenafil, trazodone was recommended for patients with erectile dysfunction.[56]

Trazodone has recently been described as an "ideal hypnotic agent." It has triple sleep-promoting actions (at the 5-HT2A, alpha-1, and H1 receptors), a short half-life, and a low risk of dependence.[57] Although it has not received FDA approval for primary insomnia, in a placebo-controlled RCT of trazodone 50 mg and zolpidem 10 mg in 278 patients with primary insomnia, the two medications had similar efficacy at two weeks, and both had a low incidence of adverse effects. The study was sponsored by the manufacturer of zolpidem.[58]

If trazodone is used, side effects should be actively reviewed and monitored. Since other medications can cause priapism, including prazosin and phosphodiesterase inhibitors (e.g., sildenafil), combining trazodone with these agents demands extra caution regarding this side effect. The combination of trazodone and prazosin may also produce additive problems with blood pressure. Trazodone is usually started at 50 mg at bedtime, with instructions to reduce to 25 mg if too sedating. The dosage of trazodone for sleep has ranged from 12.5 to 300 mg.

Node 2b

If the patient presents with difficulty falling asleep but not with nightmares or nocturnal hyperarousal, trazodone may again be considered after identifying and managing other contributing factors. Since prazosin is generally nonsedating, it may be less useful in this situation. At this early point in the algorithm, trazodone might work well enough to eliminate the need for further pharmacotherapy for a patient with sleep-onset difficulties, but the evidence for its use in these circumstances is much less compelling than for the use of prazosin in patients with nightmares.

Trazodone may also be a good choice for patients who request a sleep aid for the short term while waiting for medications (e.g., SSRIs) targeting general symptoms of PTSD to take effect. Trazodone does appear to have efficacy for SSRI-induced insomnia and nightmares, as demonstrated in two small, placebo-controlled RCTs and some open-label studies.[53,55,59,60] If, during any subsequent steps of the algorithm when SSRIs and SNRIs are employed, insomnia/nightmares either fail to improve or emerge de novo, the addition of trazodone should be considered.

Other Medications for Insomnia?

If prazosin and trazodone are not effective or not tolerated in nodes 2, 2a, and 2b, other medications with hypnotic properties may be considered—and are often used in clinical practice. The authors did not find sufficient evidence to support their use at this early point in the algorithm. We will comment briefly on several.

The tricyclic antidepressants (TCAs) imipramine and amitriptyline have some evidence of usefulness in PTSD.[61,62] However, their side effects, especially at full doses, include anticholinergic, cardiac, and seizure risks. TCAs are also undesirable in suicidal patients, who might overdose on them.

Doxepin is a TCA that has recently been studied in large, placebo-controlled RCTs as a treatment for primary insomnia in very low doses of 1–6 mg; one study included geriatric patients.[63] It was found to be safe and effective for transient or chronic insomnia and received FDA approval as a hypnotic in March 2010. It has been marketed at these doses under the new brand name Silenor, but it will still be available as a generic capsule in doses as low as 10 mg. Its mechanism of action at these doses appears to be histamine H1 blockade.[63] It may not provide any advantage over sedating antihistamines such as diphenhydramine or hydroxyzine. Tolerance to the sedative effects of antihistamines has been shown to occur quickly, making them impractical for the long-term use usually required in PTSD.[64]

Benzodiazepines (BZs) are frequently used by clinicians for sleep problems in PTSD. However, in the only placebo-controlled RCT with a BZ ($n = 10$), alprazolam demonstrated no efficacy for core PTSD symptoms.[65] When used in PTSD patients who have problems with substance use, BZs have a high potential for abuse.[19] As with the use of antidepressants in bipolar disorder, the use of BZs in patients with PTSD (with or without substance abuse) represents an area of significant difference between common practice and guideline recommendations.[5,8,66] In both cases, clinicians may perceive that patients improve in the short term while not suspecting placebo effects and without anticipating the potential for harm over the long term. BZs might be considered when a past history of clear response without significant abuse or misuse is present.[4] If the patient has a history of substance abuse, one possibility is to prescribe a small quantity to test the patient's ability to use appropriately.

Recently, eszopiclone, a GABA-A/benzodiazepine receptor agonist, was administered for insomnia associated with PTSD in 24 patients, mostly women with civilian trauma and no history of substance abuse. Efficacy was demonstrated over three weeks in this placebo-controlled RCT. Further research on the use of this class of agents is warranted.[67]

Quetiapine is also widely prescribed for sleep in PTSD. However, a review of reports of using quetiapine for sleep in various patient populations concluded that the benefits did not justify the risks and that it should not be used as a first-line treatment for insomnia.[68] Notably, the weight gain from quetiapine is not dose related and can occur even at low doses.[69,70] A recent observational study mentioned earlier compared results with quetiapine and prazosin for PTSD in a VA setting between 2002 and 2005 ($n = 62$ on prazosin; $n = 175$ on quetiapine).[47] Quetiapine at a low mean dose of 64 mg was much more likely than low-dose prazosin (3 mg) to be discontinued due to intolerable side effects (35% vs. 18%, $p = 0.008$). Sedation and metabolic effects were the most common reasons for discontinuing quetiapine. The authors' concluding recommendation was that "prazosin be used first-line for treating nighttime PTSD symptoms in veterans." One RCT of low to moderate doses of quetiapine monotherapy versus placebo for PTSD with prominent insomnia has been presented in poster format.[71] Some uncontrolled evidence also suggests that quetiapine be added to SSRI therapy after the latter has proved unsatisfactory.[47,72] These reports will be discussed at a later node in the algorithm—in particular, when we consider augmentation strategies for SSRIs.

Other hypnotics (e.g., zolpidem) and other sedating psychotropic agents (e.g., gabapentin) are occasionally used in clinical practice for PTSD-related sleep problems, but the evidence base for them is too small to consider them in this algorithm as options for initial treatment.

NODE 3: HAVE YOU GIVEN A TRIAL OF AN SSRI?

If the patient does not have prominent sleep disturbance, or if prazosin or trazodone was not tolerated or only partially effective for residual PTSD symptoms such as hyperarousal, reexperiencing, and avoidance, the next step in the algorithm would generally be to consider an SSRI trial. The evidence supporting the use of SSRIs is weak, however, which is one reason that they are not at the top of this algorithm for patients with prominent insomnia. Also, as noted earlier, SSRIs often fail to treat insomnia associated with PTSD, can sometimes aggravate it,[59] and can produce intolerable sexual dysfunction.[73]

Several recent comprehensive reviews and meta-analyses focus on using SSRIs for PTSD. The first was a Cochrane Review.[74] Overall, the authors found a number needed to treat (NNT) of about 5, which is reasonable. The calculated NNT was based on the number of patients across all studies found to be "responders" to medication. "Response" was defined for purposes of that review as having either a final rating of "much improved" or "improved" as measured by the Clinical Global Impression of Improvement (CGI-I) or, for a small number of studies, similar outcomes on the Duke Global Rating for PTSD or on other validated scales. The authors noted, however, that many of the studies were flawed because of relatively small numbers, low effect sizes, and short trial periods. Positive clinical outcomes were less convincing because of high dropout rates (27% to 40%).[26,28,75,76] Also, problems were also noted with tolerability. A separate concern was that many trial subjects came from primary care populations that are "less sick" than patients seen in a psychiatric setting.

Another major review of PTSD treatment data, published in 2008, was commissioned by the VA and conducted by an eight-expert panel from the Institute of Medicine of the U.S. National Academy of Sciences.[11] This review examined data from 14 SSRI studies conducted between 1991 and 2007. Seven of these studies were deemed to be "weakly informative with respect to efficacy because of study limitations." The committee reached the overall conclusion that "the evidence is inadequate to determine the efficacy of SSRIs in PTSD."

Another detailed meta-analysis was conducted by the National Institute for Clinical Excellence (NICE), part of the British National Health Service.[7] That review, which employed a more intensive and statistically rigorous analysis than many qualitative reviews of this literature, also raised concern that SSRIs might be significantly less effective than commonly thought for the treatment of PTSD. The NICE analysis examined data for the SSRIs citalopram, fluoxetine, paroxetine, and sertraline, as well as for amitriptyline, brofaromine, imipramine, mirtazapine, olanzapine, phenelzine, risperidone, and venlafaxine. Data from unpublished studies were included when obtainable from pharmaceutical companies.

The NICE guidelines proposed definitions of levels of efficacy that could be considered "clinically meaningful" or "clinically important." Setting a conservative standard, an effect size compared to placebo of a standard mean difference (SMD) of 0.5 or better was considered "clinically meaningful," and an SMD of 0.8 or more was considered "clinically important." They found that none of the SSRIs were beneficial for PTSD symptoms at an effect size of 0.5 and thus that the benefits were not clinically meaningful. Furthermore, reported effect sizes were considered to be overestimated because of the use of intent-to-treat analyses with last-observation-carried-forward in studies that had high dropout rates.

Some details of the NICE data on individual SSRIs will be briefly reviewed.

Paroxetine was evaluated in four RCTs, two of which were unpublished. One was a placebo-controlled study by Marshall and colleagues in 2001 that reported positive outcomes using the Clinician-Administered PTSD Scale (CAPS).[28] The specific PTSD symptom clusters of reexperiencing, hyperarousal, and numbing/avoidance were included. Marshall and colleagues replicated those results in a second RCT in 2007.[31]

The NICE meta-analysis of these paroxetine studies found that efficacy on the CAPS (effect size = 0.42) and on the Davidson Trauma Scale (DTS) (0.41) approached the 0.5 benchmark for clinical meaningfulness. In one *unpublished* study, however—a maintenance trial carried out in patients who responded to paroxetine in a 12-week acute study and then were assigned to either placebo or continuation of paroxetine for 24 weeks—there was no efficacy and actually a trend in favor of placebo on the CAPS (effect size = 0.19). This surprising result suggests that something may have been irregular about the patient sample of this unpublished study.

Sertraline, the other FDA-approved SSRI, was studied in four large RCTs, two with positive results and two showing no efficacy. Three are published. Brady and colleagues[75] showed positive drug-versus-placebo differences for three of four primary outcome measures (CAPS, CGI of change, and CGI of severity) in a population of mostly women with sexual and other civilian trauma. Davidson and colleagues[26] used a similar design and population, and found sertraline to be statistically superior to placebo using four primary outcome measures. In the RCT by Friedman and colleagues,[17] however, which involved chronically ill combat veterans, sertraline produced no efficacy versus placebo as measured by the CAPS, CGI, or Impact of Event Scale. The fourth study, which is unpublished but was included in the NICE meta-analysis discussed earlier,[7] found no efficacy—possibly related, it was speculated, to the chronicity of symptoms, gender, or the type of trauma that subjects endured.

In the NICE meta-analysis of these sertraline data,[7] it was found that sertraline was "unlikely" to be beneficial by self-report measures of the DTS or the Impact of Event Scale, because of very small effect sizes of 0.18 and 0.06, respectively. The effect size on the CAPS (0.26) was rated as "inconclusive."

After evaluating the sertraline studies, licensing authorities in England approved sertraline only for women with PTSD. In the United States the FDA approved sertraline for PTSD patients of both genders. However, the FDA imposed a fine on the corporate sponsor of the trial by Friedman and colleagues[17] for withholding the study's negative data for almost ten years.

Fluoxetine was the subject of three major studies, with mixed results.[77–79] Two of the studies, which involved RCTs of 12 weeks followed by a 24-week maintenance phase, showed fluoxetine to be effective and well tolerated for the initial 12-week period and for the relapse-prevention phase. Subjects were mostly combat veterans, though some had civilian trauma, and the overall effect size for fluoxetine was about 0.4. The largest study, however—involving 411 civilian women—found fluoxetine to be equivalent to placebo on the CAPS.[79] An earlier, smaller study found no efficacy for fluoxetine in older, chronically ill combat veterans.[16] The NICE meta-analysis of fluoxetine, which looked at the above studies and some unpublished data, found the overall evidence for fluoxetine "inconclusive" on the DTS or CAPS (effect size = 0.28). They found no efficacy (effect size = 0.02) on the self-report measure of the Treatment Outcome PTSD Scale.[7]

Citalopram has been employed in one published RCT and several open-label studies. In an open trial (*n* = 38, mostly children and adolescents), citalopram improved total CAPS-2 scores and subscale ratings for reexperiencing, hyperarousal, and avoidance.[80] English and colleagues[81] conducted an eight-week, open-label study of citalopram in eight combat veterans. They found improvement on the CAPS, Hamilton Rating Scale for Anxiety, and CGI (among others) at week 4 but not at week 8. Tucker and colleagues[76] conducted a double-blind study of citalopram versus sertraline versus placebo for PTSD patients (n = 25, 23, and 10, respectively). Using an intent-to-treat analysis, the authors found significant improvement in total symptoms of PTSD measured by the CAPS, as well as for all three symptom clusters and sleep time, in all three groups, including placebo.

Robert and colleagues[82] published an open-label study with *escitalopram* in 25 patients, finding significant improvement for the CAPS-C (avoidance/numbing) and CAPS-D (hyperarousal) subscales, but only trend improvement for the CAPS-B (reexperiencing) subscale.

Alternatives to SSRIs at Node 3

As noted, side effects such as sexual dysfunction may make SSRIs unacceptable to some patients. Options that might be considered at node 3 include bupropion, mirtazapine, and certain antipsychotics. Nefazodone also has few sexual side effects and some evidence of efficacy in PTSD, but due to the risk of liver toxicity, it is not considered until later in the algorithm. Venlafaxine has efficacy for PTSD, but it has sexual side effects, and for other reasons (to be discussed) it seems better as a second-line option.

Bupropion showed some promise in an open-label trial in 17 combat veterans, but those results were not confirmed in an eight-week, placebo-controlled RCT in 30 patients with mixed civilian and military trauma.[83,84] Some patients had bupropion added to an SSRI. A trend toward better outcomes was evident in younger patients and those on monotherapy. More research is needed to determine if bupropion is effective for PTSD.

The evidence for using mirtazapine is more favorable, although its desirability is limited by the risk of weight gain. Bahk and colleagues[85] published a small study (n = 15) of the effectiveness and tolerability of mirtazapine in an eight-week trial in Korean patients with chronic PTSD. The dosing regimen was flexible, and patients were evaluated at four and eight weeks on several rating scales. At eight weeks, scores on all scales showed significant improvement. The medication was well tolerated. An open-label study by Chung and colleagues in 2004,[86] also in Korean veterans, compared mirtazapine to sertraline. Both were well tolerated and seemed effective.

Davidson and colleagues[87] conducted a placebo-controlled, double-blind RCT of mirtazapine in 29 patients, with impressive results. The dose ranged up to 45 mg per day for eight weeks, with the DTS used as the primary outcome measure. Rates of response were 65% and 20% for mirtazapine and placebo, respectively (NNT = 2.2). The medication was well tolerated.

A long-term (24-week) study of mirtazapine was published by Kim and colleagues in 2005.[88] Twelve of 15 participants completed the study. The results suggested that mirtazapine might be effective for continuation treatment.

Certain antipsychotics are another alternative to SSRIs at node 3. For example, as noted at node 2, some clinicians use quetiapine as a monotherapy, first-line treatment for the global symptoms of PTSD, although the published evidence to support this practice is minimal. As noted earlier, the side effect risks are considerable, making the product appear unsuitable for early selection in the algorithm.

Node 3 Conclusion

The FDA has approved the SSRIs sertraline and paroxetine for the treatment of PTSD. Paroxetine has the best evidence of efficacy but has more problems with sexual dysfunction, constipation, sedation, drug interactions, withdrawal syndrome, and weight gain than the other SSRIs.[66] The pregnancy risk rating of D is an issue with women of childbearing potential. Though the evidence supporting sertraline is weaker, especially in male combat veterans, it has fewer side effects than paroxetine. It may be reasonable to consider non-FDA-approved citalopram: although the subject of fewer and less rigorous studies in relation to PTSD, citalopram's efficacy in other anxiety disorders and in major depression suggests that its benefit in treating PTSD might be comparable to that of other SSRIs. It was thought to have the fewest side effects within the SSRI class.[89] However, the FDA just issued a Drug Safety Communication saying that the dose should not exceed 40 mg daily due to QTc prolongation risks.

According to most sources, an adequate trial of an SSRI for treating a PTSD patient would run 4 to 6 weeks, although sometimes up to 12 weeks are required.

Some patients show a partial response to SSRIs or a response that is limited to certain symptom domains in PTSD. Patients who partially respond but are still improving should be continued until the benefits reach a plateau. If improvement stalls for two or three weeks, consider raising the dose or switching to another option (see node 4). Augmentation may be considered (see nodes 3a and 5a) if both clinician and patient are convinced that the partial improvement was not a placebo effect and not attributable to other aspects of the treatment such as psychotherapy—which can be difficult to evaluate. Before proceeding with augmentation, keep in mind the preceding discussion indicating that SSRIs outperform placebo in controlled trials much less than generally assumed. "Augmenting" a likely placebo effect with another medication should be avoided. Also, augmentation introduces risks of increased side effects and drug interactions, reduced compliance due to complexity of regimens, and increased cost. In this algorithm, augmentation for partial response is considered most appropriate at nodes 3a and 5a. A switch is considered at node 4. See Figure 1.

Node 3a: Does the Patient Have PTSD-Related Psychosis?

PTSD-related psychotic symptoms are often present in PTSD patients.[90] Symptoms include phenomena referable to the original trauma—for example, hearing soldiers scream, experiencing visual hallucinations of an enemy, or other combat-related themes. Unrelated—for example, paranoid—delusions can also occur. Delusions related to PTSD are non-bizarre and not associated with disorganized thought or flat or inappropriate affect, and are not related to substance abuse or withdrawal. They do not occur only during dissociative flashbacks.[91] Patients with these psychotic symptoms can be considered one subgroup of PTSD patients for whom early augmentation may be justified. For this purpose, atypical antipsychotics are the medication of choice.

A preliminary study of risperidone (mean dose = 2.5 ± 1.25 mg/day) as an augmentation of antidepressants in 40 combat veterans with chronic PTSD-related psychotic symptoms demonstrated a significant decrease in psychotic symptoms and an improvement in reexperiencing symptoms.[92] A more recent, placebo-controlled RCT of risperidone augmentation for SSRI-resistant civilians with psychotic PTSD found improvement in the positive symptoms and paranoia subscales of the Positive and Negative Symptom Scale.[93]

Open-label studies support the addition of quetiapine and olanzapine, but not the first-generation neuroleptic fluphenazine, for antidepressant-resistant psychotic combat veterans with PTSD.[22,94,95] The quetiapine study involved patients resistant to SSRIs and other medications who were admitted to an inpatient unit for the trial.[22] Without a placebo control it is impossible to exclude that the positive outcome (on all three dimensions of PTSD symptoms) was due to the effects of hospitalization. We could not find any reports of aripiprazole augmentation in patients with PTSD-related psychosis.

Thus, if the patient does not respond satisfactorily to an antidepressant and has PTSD-related psychosis, it seems reasonable to add an antipsychotic. The evidence base points to risperidone since it has one published, placebo-controlled RCT with favorable results. Quetiapine is widely used, has some evidence as an augmentation in nonpsychotic PTSD,[96] and might also be tried here. If the patient responds well to addition of an antipsychotic, and the SSRI had minimal benefit, gradually removing the SSRI should be considered to determine if it was necessary for the improvement.

NODE 4: HAVE YOU TRIED A SECOND SSRI, SNRI, OR MIRTAZAPINE?

If the patient is not psychotic and was nonresponsive to the initial SSRI chosen in node 3, several prime options are available: trying a different SSRI, an SNRI (especially venlafaxine), or an antidepressant with different dual actions (mirtazapine, evidence for which was discussed under node 3).

Venlafaxine was initially thought less likely to be effective in PTSD because of its noradrenergic component, given that PTSD is characterized by excessive noradrenergic activity.[97,98] An early RCT in combat veterans employing the strong norepinephrine reuptake-blocking tricyclic desipramine ($n = 18$) found no efficacy.[99] However, two large, placebo-controlled RCTs have been conducted to evaluate the efficacy of venlafaxine ER in PTSD, and both demonstrated some efficacy.

One of these venlafaxine studies involved 329 outpatients, mostly female, from international sites.[100] Only 12% had combat-related trauma. In this 24-week trial, CAPS scores improved five points more on venlafaxine than on placebo ($p = 0.06$). Mean daily maximum dose of venlafaxine ER was 222 mg. Reexperiencing and avoidance symptoms improved, but hyperarousal did not, possibly due to the impact of the noradrenergic component of venlafaxine. Overall effect sizes were small and similar to those found in the short-term SSRI studies even after almost six months of treatment.

The second study was a 12-week comparison of venlafaxine ER, sertraline, and placebo in a similar population of 538 patients, with CAPS scores again used as the primary outcome measure.[101] Remission rates at week 12 were 30% with venlafaxine, 24% with sertraline, and 20% with placebo. Mean daily maximum doses with venlafaxine and sertraline were 225 mg and 151 mg, respectively. Venlafaxine demonstrated statistically significant benefits over placebo ($p < 0.05$), but again, effect sizes were generally small on secondary outcome measures (particularly patient satisfaction and quality of life). Sertraline response did not differ from placebo on most measures, consistent with the unimpressive results with sertraline discussed earlier, in node 3. Both medications were similarly tolerated, with 10% attrition from side effects.

In a separate pooled analysis, the authors of these two studies attempted to differentiate response by gender and by trauma type.[102] No consistent predictors were found despite the opportunity presented by the large number of subjects. Venlafaxine offered no benefit for insomnia or nightmares.[103]

Thus, venlafaxine is a reasonable option as a second-choice pharmacotherapy, but the evidence base (despite the better response rate than sertraline in one study) seems to suggest no reason to prefer it to SSRIs for first-line use. It was ineffective for hyperarousal and sleep disturbance. Cardiovascular safety issues might affect certain vulnerable patients.[101]

NODE 5: HAVE YOU TRIED A THIRD MEDICATION AMONG SSRIS, SNRIS, MIRTAZAPINE, OR NEFAZODONE?

If two adequate monotherapy regimens among the SSRIs, SNRIs, or mirtazapine have been tried with no response to either, a third trial seems reasonable. The options may now include nefazodone, which is limited to third-line due to its liver toxicity. Fatal hepatotoxicity has been estimated to occur in about one in 250,000 patients.[104] Despite the rarity of this complication, nefazodone was removed from European formularies in 2003 but remains available in the United States as a generic. The usual side-effect profile of nefazodone actually makes it rather desirable, given the lack of weight gain or sexual side effects, less sedation than trazodone, and low risk of priapism.

Evidence to support the efficacy of nefazodone for PTSD includes two RCTs (one placebo-controlled) and several open-label trials.[105-107] The placebo-controlled RCT, with 41 patients, found benefits on the CAPS, with an impressive effect size of 0.6 ($p = 0.04$).[107] The other RCT was less impressive: it was a comparator study of the effectiveness of nefazodone and sertraline in a 12-week, randomized, double-blind study involving 37 patients, using the CAPS, CGI, and DTS measures.[108] It found no significant difference between groups on any outcome measure, including PTSD cluster symptoms, depression, sleep, and quality of life over time. In an analysis of six open-label trials involving 105 patients, Hidalgo and colleagues[109] found that 46% had an improvement of at least 30% on the CAPS.

Although small ($n = 10$), a nefazodone study conducted by Hertzberg and colleagues[110,111] is of interest because subjects were followed for three to four years. Originally conducted as a 12-week study,[110] long-term follow-up was described in 2002.[111] The dose was 400–600 mg, and ten of ten participants were rated as "much improved" on the CGI at 12 weeks. After three years of monitoring, seven of ten were still "much improved," while two were minimally improved and one was worse than his original baseline.

Another interesting nefazodone case series involved 19 treatment-resistant combat veterans with PTSD. Zisook and colleagues[112] administered doses of 100–600 mg per day for 12 weeks to patients who had failed three previous medication trials. Improvements were noted in intrusive thoughts, avoidance, hyperarousal, sleep, sexual function, and depression. The reduction in PTSD symptoms, as measured by the CAPS, was 32%. Side effects were typically mild and included headaches, dry mouth, and gastrointestinal disturbance.

Node 5a: If No Response or Partial Response, Consider Augmentation (Depending on Residual Symptoms) or Try Other Monotherapies

If the patient failed to respond to the previous interventions, or if the response was partial, not explained by placebo effect, and still unsatisfactory in some respects, various options are available: mood stabilizers (gabapentin, lamotrigine, levetiracetam, tiagabine, topiramate, and valproate), antipsychotics (aripiprazole, olanzapine, quetiapine, risperidone, and ziprasidone), anti-adrenergic agents (alpha-1 antagonists, alpha-2 blockers, and beta-blockers), and monoamine oxidase inhibitors (MAOIs). The supporting evidence ranges from unconvincing to fairly robust.

Some of these treatments appear useful for all of the symptom clusters of PTSD (avoidance, hyperarousal, reexperiencing), whereas others have evidence that they target one or more clusters. As noted earlier, the general principle is that one should try to minimize polypharmacy by critically evaluating partial response and determining if improvement was due to real effects of the medication or to a nonspecific response to other concomitantly administered treatments (including psychotherapy) or to changed circumstances (including hospitalization). If either of the latter is suspected, consider switching rather than augmenting. It must be kept in mind, however, that the constellation of PTSD manifestations is currently thought to include multiple symptom domains with potentially different responses to medication, suggesting that some patients will need more than one agent. We will briefly review some of the options, considering strength of evidence and how the choice might be influenced by comorbid psychiatric or medical problems. Patient preference and formulary availability/cost will also affect choice. Medications are not listed in order of preference, and the list is not complete. The flowchart in Figure 1 organizes these medications by their target symptom clusters, consistent with the evidence to be described below.

Anticonvulsants. In a 1991, open-label trial of *valproic acid* conducted at the Seattle Veterans Affairs Medical Center involving 16 Vietnam veterans with PTSD, 10 improved, mainly in symptoms of hyperarousal.[113] More recently, two placebo-controlled RCTs of divalproex have been reported. The larger study, published in 2008, involved 85 U.S. military veterans. It was conducted at the Tuscaloosa Veterans Affairs Medical Center and supported by the manufacturer. The subjects received a mean dose of 2,300 mg daily, which produced a mean average plasma level of 82 mg/L.[114] For total CAPS scores and for two of the CAPS symptom clusters (reexperiencing, avoidance), the divalproex group showed slightly less improvement than the placebo group. For the hyperarousal cluster, the study and control groups had the same final scores. Depression, anxiety, and CGI of severity likewise showed no differentiation between the study and control groups, with the quantity of improvement similar to that seen in the open-label trial. The other RCT, published in 2009 and conducted at the Ralph A. Johnson VA Medical Center in Charleston, South Carolina, randomized 29 combat veterans to divalproex or placebo and also found no advantages for divalproex. In fact, the placebo group did significantly better for the avoidance symptom cluster and on changes in CGI of severity. Given that all three of these studies involved monotherapy with male combat veterans, it remains to be seen whether this drug might prove more effective for use with veterans in an adjunctive role or when used either as monotherapy or adjunctive therapy for civilian males or for females.

In a double-blind, placebo-controlled study of *lamotrigine* for PTSD, 14 patients with different kinds of trauma were randomized 2:1 to either lamotrigine or placebo.[115] Over eight weeks the medication was titrated to a maximum of 500 mg per day (as tolerated). The study found nonsignificant, but possibly promising, improvement in reexperiencing and avoidance/numbing symptoms with lamotrigine in comparison to placebo.

Two negative studies of *topiramate* for PTSD have been published. In a double-blind, placebo-controlled RCT, 38 subjects with non-combat-related PTSD were studied on doses up to 400 mg per day.[116] Overall results showed a nonsignificant decrease in total CAPS scores. However, the treatment group did have significant reductions in symptoms of reexperiencing and on a secondary global outcome measure. The second study was a seven-week, double-blind, placebo-controlled RCT in 40 subjects, all male veterans in a residential PTSD treatment program.[117] The experimental group received flexible-dose topiramate and had a high dropout rate (40% vs. 10% for placebo recipients). The authors found no significant treatment effects, but the high dropout rate may have been a factor in this outcome.

In an observational study, *levetiracetam* was administered to 23 civilian patients with treatment-resistant PTSD, with the medication used adjunctively in 19 of those cases.[118] Outcome was evaluated retrospectively with several rating instruments, including the CGI. At a mean dose of 2000 mg for 10 weeks, patients improved significantly on all measures. Fifty-six percent responded, 26% remitted, and the medication was well tolerated.

One small, open-label study and one large, multicenter, double-blind RCT of *tiagabine* have been published. In the former, 29 outpatients were treated for 12 weeks.[119] Responders ($n = 18$) were later entered into a double-blind maintenance study and randomly assigned to continue on tiagabine or placebo. During the extension phase, the placebo-treated patients did not relapse, but the tiagabine patients made further improvements. In the RCT, 232 patients were randomized to tiagabine or placebo for 12 weeks.[120] The experimental group received up to 16 mg daily of tiagabine. No efficacy was found for the anticonvulsant.

Antipsychotics. *Risperidone* has been evaluated in four small, placebo-controlled RCTs in nonpsychotic patients (civilians and veterans) with PTSD[121,122] and in a recent, larger-scale, placebo-controlled RCT studying 247 veterans who had served in combat zones.[123] Many of these patients were "treatment-resistant," and in most, the risperidone was added to other medications. It seemed to have some efficacy on the reexperiencing and hyperarousal symptom clusters, although the effects were small. There was no effect shown for avoidance.

In two open-label trials, *quetiapine* administered as an adjuvant was shown to improve all three clusters of PTSD symptoms and also sleep disturbance.[72,124] One double-blind, placebo-controlled RCT of quetiapine monotherapy in 80 patients with "chronic PTSD" (94% male, mean age = 52) has been completed and is under review, but some results were provided in a poster.[96] Patients were all U.S. combat veterans, and 30% had PTSD-related psychotic features. The doses ranged from 50 to 800 mg per day, with a mean of 258 mg. Reexperiencing and hyperarousal improved significantly (p = 0.002 and p = 0.03, respectively), but as with risperidone, the avoidance symptom cluster did not (p = 0.56). A separate analysis was not provided for the psychotic and nonpsychotic patients. Thus, it is unclear if these results best apply here or at node 3a.

Aripiprazole has been investigated in three uncontrolled studies of PTSD patients from mixed populations, including civilians and veterans. Medication was used as monotherapy in two of these studies[125,126] and as an adjunct to various other treatments in the third.[95] Aripiprazole monotherapy was found effective over 12 weeks in an open-label trial in 22 combat veterans at a mean dose of 13 mg.[125] CAPS scores improved (p = .01). Another case series of 32 civilian patients from Brazil experienced good results at a mean dose of 10 mg daily.[126] CAPS scores improved from a mean of 83 at baseline to 51 at the endpoint 16 weeks later (p = .001). All studies reported significant improvement in reexperiencing and avoidance/numbing, but marginal benefit for hyperarousal. Doses generally started at 5 mg.

Based on two small studies, the use of *olanzapine* has minimal support.[127,128] In a case series *ziprasidone* was reported to be effective in nonpsychotic PTSD.[129]

The benefits of atypical antipsychotics must be weighed against their side effects, including weight gain, metabolic syndrome, and cardiac risk.[69] Ray and colleagues,[130] in a large epidemiological survey, found that patients treated with antipsychotics had about double the rate of sudden cardiac death compared to non-treated controls who had similar psychiatric diagnoses and metabolic syndrome symptoms. The relative risk ratio of death was 2.26 (95% CI, 1.88–2.72) with atypical antipsychotics, and it was dose related.[130] The mechanism of death was thought likely to be arrhythmias, perhaps involving QTc prolongations. The authors of this study advised a "sharp reduction" in using these agents in populations for which the evidence of efficacy is limited. There is growing concern that antipsychotics should not be used as primary or adjunctive agents in treating PTSD unless other options with comparable effectiveness and better safety have already been tried.[131]

Medications Targeting Central Noradrenergic Dysregluation. Studies with the alpha-1 adrenergic antagonist prazosin were reviewed earlier. Alpha-2 agonists (clonidine and guanfacine) and beta-adrenergic antagonists have also been used for PTSD, with mixed results.

Two studies, one a placebo-controlled RCT, investigated *clonidine*. Kinzie[132] studied the combination of imipramine and clonidine in 9 traumatized Cambodian refugees with concurrent PTSD and major depression. PTSD global symptoms (CAPS) improved in 6 patients, nightmares improved in 7 patients, and hyperarousal in 4 patients. Avoidance behavior showed no improvement. In the RCT, 18 patients (17 female) with borderline personality disorder, all of whom had prominent hyperarousal symptoms on the CAPS, were treated with clonidine, up to 0.45 mg in divided doses, for two weeks.[133] Most were on other medications, which were maintained, but benzodiazepines were not allowed. Hyperarousal improved significantly versus placebo ($p = 0.003$), irrespective of PTSD comorbidity. Sleep also improved across all subjects.

Guanfacine, a longer-acting alpha-2 agonist, was administered in two recent RCTs, both with negative outcomes. Neylan and colleagues[134] treated 63 chronically ill U.S. veterans with guanfacine at a mean daily dose of 2.4 mg at bedtime (achieved with weekly 0.5 mg increases) or placebo for eight weeks. Most were on one or more other medications. Analysis showed no separation of guanfacine and placebo on the CAPS, the Impact of Events Scale, general mood, or subjective quality of sleep. In a smaller study, Davis and colleagues[135] administered guanfacine or placebo to combat veterans for eight weeks while continuing their antidepressants. No improvement was shown on the CAPS or DTS.

Beta-blockers have not received substantial study in chronic PTSD. Several studies have explored the use of propranolol immediately after a trauma to prevent the onset of PTSD.[136–139] The findings are variable, and more research is needed before this treatment can be recommended.

Four RCTs have examined the short-term benefits of *monoamine-oxidase inhibitors* in PTSD due to a variety of traumas. Two involved phenelzine.[62,140] In the first, a comparison of phenelzine ($n = 19$), imipramine ($n = 23$), and placebo ($n = 18$), there was significant improvement with both antidepressants compared to placebo, but more so with the MAOI.[62] The dropout rate was about 50%, however, making interpretation difficult. The other phenelzine study was small and showed no benefit.[140] The other two MAOI trials involved brofaromine, a non-selective MAOI not available in the United States.[141,142] Both found no efficacy.

COMPARISON TO OTHER ALGORITHMS AND GUIDELINE RECOMMENDATIONS:

The present algorithm for selecting psychopharmacology treatment for PTSD differs in some respects from earlier versions of the PAPHSS algorithm and other published algorithms and guidelines. The 1999 version of the PAPHSS algorithm recommended initial use of trazodone for managing sleep disturbance, including nightmares, with low-dose doxepin a second choice for patients not at high risk for suicide, seizures, or cardiac events.[4] That algorithm was similar to the present version (and different from other guidelines at that time) in proposing efforts to manage PTSD-related sleep problems before the introduction of an SSRI or other antidepressants. The most recent (2005) NICE guidelines recommended paroxetine and mirtazapine as first-line pharmacotherapy and discouraged sertraline.[7] Similarly, the International Psychopharmacology Algorithm Project's 2005 algorithm recommended an SSRI, SNRI, or mirtazapine, whereas the American Psychiatric Association practice guideline (2004) also endorsed SSRIs as first-line treatment.[5,143] However, the association's March 2009 "Guideline Watch" for PTSD noted that more recent studies "suggest that SSRIs may no longer be recommended with the same level of confidence for veterans with combat-related PTSD."[10] It was also noted that prazosin is "among the most promising advances," though without any indication as to when it should be used.

Table 3 | Characteristics of Other Algorithms and Guidelines for the Treatment of PTSD		
Algorithm/guideline	Year	Comments
Expert consensus guidelines[144]	1999	First-line: SSRIs, venlafaxine, & nefazodone Second-line: TCAs
Psychopharmacology Algorithm Project at Harvard South Shore Program[4]	1999	Early use of hypnotic agent for sleep, trazodone first-line, followed by SSRI for persistent daytime PTSD symptoms
The United Kingdom's National Institute for Clinical Excellence[7]	2005	SSRIs in PTSD are reviewed & shown to have a more modest effect size then commonly considered Psychotherapy recommended as first-line treatment
Canadian clinical practice guidelines[145]	2005	First-line: one agent among fluoxetine, paroxetine, sertraline, & venlafaxine XR Second-line: mirtazapine, fluvoxamine, phenelzine, & moclobemide, plus adjunctive olanzapine or risperidone
The International Psychopharmacology Algorithm Project[5]	2005	Once diagnosis of PTSD established, SSRI trial recommended as first-line pharmacological intervention, followed by venlafaxine & mirtazapine trials
The International Society of Traumatic Stress Studies[6]	2008	SSRIs recommended as first-line intervention, followed by augmentation with atypical antipsychotics Prazosin considered "promising"
APA Guidelines Watch[10]	2009	Concludes new studies suggest SSRIs are less effective than previously assumed Prazosin considered a promising option for sleep disturbance in PTSD
VA/DoD clinical practice guideline for managing posttraumatic stress[146]	2010	Strongest recommendation is for SSRIs & SNRIs but suggests "some benefit" for prazosin, mirtazapine, & adjunctive atypical antipsychotics Recommends consideration of prazosin for nightmares as adjunctive treatment if trazodone & other hypnotics are insufficient

APA, American Psychiatric Association; DoD, Department of Defense; SNRI, serotonin-norepinephrine reuptake inhibitor; SSRI, selective serotonin reuptake inhibitor; TCA, tricyclic antidepressant; VA, Veterans Administration.

The 2008 assessment by the National Academy of Sciences made no psychopharmacology recommendations; it found the evidence "inadequate to determine efficacy" for all classes of drugs reviewed.[11] See Table 3 for a summary of these and other algorithms and guidelines, with comments on their essential features.

FINAL COMMENT

This heuristic will serve clinicians by offering a summary and interpretation of the current evidence base pertinent to psychopharmacological practice. Nevertheless, despite development of this and other algorithms and guidelines, the treatment of PTSD remains a challenge for physicians and patients. More needs to be learned about the pathophysiology of this chronic, disabling condition and about the comorbidities with which it often presents. Improvements in our understanding of genetics, the neurobiological underpinnings of PTSD, and mechanisms related to each symptom cluster promise to add refinements to the current treatment strategy.

Declaration of interest: The authors report no conflicts of interest. The authors alone are responsible for the content and writing of the article.

REFERENCES

1. Germain A, Buysse DJ, Nofzinger E. Sleep-specific mechanisms underlying posttraumatic stress disorder: integrative review and neurobiological hypotheses. Sleep Med Rev 2008;12:185–95.
2. Rasmusson AM, Vythilingam M, Morgan CA 3rd. The neuroendocrinology of posttraumatic stress disorder: new directions. CNS Spectr 2003;8:651–6, 665–7.
3. Wang Z, Neylan TC, Mueller SG, et al. Magnetic resonance imaging of hippocampal subfields in posttraumatic stress disorder. Arch Gen Psychiatry 2010;67:296–303.
4. Osser DN, Renner JA, Bayog R. Algorithms for the pharmacotherapy of anxiety disorders in patients with chemical abuse and dependence. Psychiatr Ann 1999;29:285–301.
5. Davidson J, Bernik M, Connor KM, Friedman MJ, Jobson KO, Yoshiharo K. A new treatment algorithm for posttraumatic stress disorder. Psychiatr Ann 2005;35:887–98.
6. Foa EB, Keane TM, Friedman MJ, Cohen JA. Effective treatments for PTSD: practice guidelines from the International Society for Traumatic Stress Studies. 2nd ed. New York: Guilford, 2008.
7. National Collaborating Centre for Mental Health. Post-traumatic stress disorder: the management of PTSD in adults and children in primary and secondary care. London; Leicester, UK: Gaskell and the British Psychological Society, 2005.
8. Bisson JI. Post-traumatic stress disorder. Clin Evid (Online). 2007 Aug 1; 2007. pii:1005.
9. Bisson J, Andrew M. Psychological treatment of post-traumatic stress disorder (PTSD). Cochrane Database Syst Rev 2005;(2):CD003388.
10. Benedek DM, Friedman MJ, Zatzick D, Ursano RJ. Practice guideline for the treatment of patients with acute stress disorder and post-traumatic stress disorder. Arlington, VA: American Psychiatric Publishing, 2009.
11. Committee on Treatment of Post-traumatic Stress Disorder, Institute of Medicine. Treatment of post-traumatic stress disorder: an assessment of the evidence. Washington, DC: National Academies, 2008.
12. Hamoda HM, Osser DN. The Psychopharmacology Algorithm Project at the Harvard South Shore Program: an update on psychotic depression. Harv Rev Psychiatry 2008;16: 235–47.

13. Ansari A, Osser DN. The Psychopharmacology Algorithm Project at the Harvard South Shore Program: an update on bipolar depression. Harv Rev Psychiatry 2010;18:36–55.

14. Osser DN, Dunlop LR. The Psychopharmacology Algorithm Project at the Harvard South Shore Program: an update on generalized social anxiety disorder. Psychopharm Rev 2010;45:91–8.

15. American Psychiatric Association. Diagnostic and statistical manual of mental disorders. 4th ed., text rev. Washington, DC: American Psychiatric Press, 2000.

16. van der Kolk BA, Dreyfuss D, Michaels M, et al. Fluoxetine in posttraumatic stress disorder. J Clin Psychiatry 1994;55:517–22.

17. Friedman MJ, Marmar CR, Baker DG, Sikes CR, Farfel GM. Randomized, double-blind comparison of sertraline and placebo for posttraumatic stress disorder in a Department of Veterans Affairs setting. J Clin Psychiatry 2007;68:711–20.

18. Strawn JR, Geracioti TD Jr. Noradrenergic dysfunction and the psychopharmacology of posttraumatic stress disorder. Depress Anxiety 2008;25:260–71.

19. Chilcoat HD, Breslau N. Posttraumatic stress disorder and drug disorders: testing causal pathways. Arch Gen Psychiatry 1998;55:913–7.

20. Mason BJ, Kocsis JH, Ritvo EC, Cutler RB. A double-blind, placebo-controlled trial of desipramine for primary alcohol dependence stratified on the presence or absence of major depression. JAMA 1996;275:761–7.

21. Otto MW, Perlman CA, Wernicke R, Reese HE, Bauer MS, Pollack MH. Posttraumatic stress disorder in patients with bipolar disorder: a review of prevalence, correlates, and treatment strategies. Bipolar Disord 2004;6:470–9.

22. Kozaric-Kovacic D, Pivac N. Quetiapine treatment in an open trial in combat-related post-traumatic stress disorder with psychotic features. Int J Neuropsychopharmacol 2007;10:253–61.

23. Breslau N, Davis GC, Peterson EL, Schultz LR. A second look at comorbidity in victims of trauma: the posttraumatic stress disorder-major depression connection. Biol Psychiatry 2000;48:902–9.

24. Gill J, Vythilingam M, Page GG. Low cortisol, high DHEA, and high levels of stimulated TNF-alpha, and IL-6 in women with PTSD. J Trauma Stress 2008;21:530–9.

25. Rasmusson AM, Wu R, Paliwal P, Anderson GM, Krishnan-Sarin S. A decrease in the plasma DHEA to cortisol ratio during smoking abstinence may predict relapse: a preliminary study. Psychopharmacology (Berl) 2006;186:473–80.

26. Davidson JR, Rothbaum BO, van der Kolk BA, Sikes CR, Farfel GM. Multicenter, double-blind comparison of sertraline and placebo in the treatment of posttraumatic stress disorder. Arch Gen Psychiatry 2001;58:485–92.

27. Brady KT, Clary CM. Affective and anxiety comorbidity in post-traumatic stress disorder treatment trials of sertraline. Compr Psychiatry 2003;44:360–9.

28. Marshall RD, Beebe KL, Oldham M, Zaninelli R. Efficacy and safety of paroxetine treatment for chronic PTSD: a fixed-dose, placebo-controlled study. Am J Psychiatry 2001;158:1982–8.

29. Lewis CC, Simons AD, Nguyen LJ. Impact of childhood trauma on treatment outcome in the treatment for adolescents with depression study (TADS). J Am Acad Child Adolesc Psychiatry 2010;49:132–40.

30. Brand BL, Classen CC, McNary SW, Zaveri P. A review of dissociative disorders treatment studies. J Nerv Ment Dis 2009;197:646–54.

31. Marshall RD, Lewis-Fernandez R, Blanco C, et al. A controlled trial of paroxetine for chronic PTSD, dissociation, and interpersonal problems in mostly minority adults. Depress Anxiety 2007;24:77–84.

32. Steiner H, Carrion V, Plattner B, Koopman C. Dissociative symptoms in posttraumatic stress disorder: diagnosis and treatment. Child Adolesc Psychiatr Clin N Am 2003;12:231–49, viii.

33. Menon SJ. Psychotropic medication during pregnancy and lactation. Arch Gynecol Obstet 2008;277:1–13.

34. Kirby AC, Hertzberg BP, Collie CF, et al. Smoking in help seeking veterans with PTSD returning from Afghanistan and Iraq. Addict Behav 2008;33:1448–53.

35. Cook J, Jakupcak M, Rosenheck R, Fontana A, McFall M. Influence of PTSD symptom clusters on smoking status among help-seeking Iraq and Afghanistan veterans. Nicotine Tob Res 2009;11:1189–95.

36. Hertzberg MA, Moore SD, Feldman ME, Beckham JC. A preliminary study of bupropion sustained-release for smoking cessation in patients with chronic posttraumatic stress disorder. J Clin Psychopharmacol 2001;21:94–8.

37. Spoormaker VI, Montgomery P. Disturbed sleep in posttraumatic stress disorder: secondary symptom or core feature? Sleep Med Rev 2008;12:169–84.

38. Belleville G, Guay S, Marchand A. Impact of sleep disturbances on PTSD symptoms and perceived health. J Nerv Ment Dis 2009;197:126–32.

39. Thompson CE, Taylor FB, McFall ME, Barnes RF, Raskind MA. Nonnightmare distressed awakenings in veterans with posttraumatic stress disorder: response to prazosin. J Trauma Stress 2008;21:417–20.

40. Neylan TC, Marmar CR, Metzler TJ, et al. Sleep disturbances in the Vietnam generation: findings from a nationally representative sample of male Vietnam veterans. Am J Psychiatry 1998;155:929–33.

41. Mellman TA, Knorr BR, Pigeon WR, Leiter JC, Akay M. Heart rate variability during sleep and the early development of posttraumatic stress disorder. Biol Psychiatry 2004;55: 953–6.

42. Raskind MA, Peskind ER, Kanter ED, et al. Reduction of nightmares and other PTSD symptoms in combat veterans by prazosin: a placebo-controlled study. Am J Psychiatry 2003;160:371–3.

43. Raskind MA, Peskind ER, Hoff DJ, et al. A parallel group placebo controlled study of prazosin for trauma nightmares and sleep disturbance in combat veterans with post-traumatic stress disorder. Biol Psychiatry 2007;61:928–34.

44. Lamarche LJ, De Koninck J. Sleep disturbance in adults with posttraumatic stress disorder: a review. J Clin Psychiatry 2007;68:1257–70.

45. Kobayashi I, Boarts JM, Delahanty DL. Polysomnographically measured sleep abnormalities in PTSD: a meta-analytic review. Psychophysiology 2007;44:660–9.

46. Taylor FB, Martin P, Thompson C, et al. Prazosin effects on objective sleep measures and clinical symptoms in civilian trauma posttraumatic stress disorder: a placebo-controlled study. Biol Psychiatry 2008;63:629–32.

47. Byers MG, Allison KM, Wendel CS, Lee JK. Prazosin versus quetiapine for nighttime posttraumatic stress disorder symptoms in veterans: an assessment of long-term comparative effectiveness and safety. J Clin Psychopharmacol 2010;30:225–9.

48. Nuzhat SS, Osser DN. Chest pain in a young patient treated with prazosin for PTSD. Am J Psychiatry 2009;166: 618–9.

49. Contopoulos-Ioannidis DC, Gilbody SM, Trikalinos TA, Churchill R, Wahlbeck K, Ioannidis J. Comparison of large versus smaller trials for mental-health interventions. Am J Psychiatry 2005;162: 578–84.

50. Troxel WM, Buysse DJ, Matthews KA, et al. Sleep symptoms predict the development of the metabolic syndrome. Sleep 2010;33:1633–40.

51. Chung. Effect of terazosin on posttraumatic nightmares. Poster (No. 356) presented at the annual meeting of the American Psychiatric Association, San Diego, CA, May 2007.

52. De Jong J, Wauben P, Huijbrechts I, Oolders H, Haffmans J. Doxazosin treatment for posttraumatic stress disorder. J Clin Psychopharmacol 2010;30:84–5.

53. Hertzberg MA, Feldman ME, Beckham JC, Davidson JR. Trial of trazodone for posttraumatic stress disorder using a multiple baseline group design. J Clin Psychopharmacol 1996;16:294–8.

54. Leshner HI, Bagdhoyan HA, Bennett SJ, Caples SM, DeRubeis RJ, Glynn RJ. NIH State-of-the-Science Conference Statement on manifestations and management of chronic insomnia in adults. NIH Consens State Sci Statements 2005;22(2):1–30.

55. Warner MD, Dorn MR, Peabody CA. Survey on the usefulness of trazodone in patients with PTSD with insomnia or nightmares. Pharmacopsychiatry 2001;34:128–31.

56. Sadock BJ, Sadock VA. Trazodone. In: Kaplan and Sadock's pocket handbook of psychiatric drug treatment. New York: Lippincott Williams & Wilkins, 2001:237–40.

57. Stahl SM. Mechanism of action of trazodone: a multifunctional drug. CNS Spectr 2009;14:536–46.

58. Walsh JK. Subjective hypnotic efficacy of trazodone and zolpidem in DSM III-R primary insomnia. Hum Psychopharmacol 1998;13:191–8.

59. Kaynak H, Kaynak D, Gozukirmizi E, Guilleminault C. The effects of trazodone on sleep in patients treated with stimulant antidepressants. Sleep Med 2004;5:15–20.

60. Nierenberg AA, Adler LA, Peselow E, Zornberg G, Rosenthal M. Trazodone for antidepressant-associated insomnia. Am J Psychiatry 1994;151:1069–72.

61. Davidson J, Kudler H, Smith R, et al. Treatment of posttraumatic stress disorder with amitriptyline and placebo. Arch Gen Psychiatry 1990;47:259–66.

62. Kosten TR, Frank JB, Dan E, McDougle CJ, Giller EL Jr. Pharmacotherapy for post-traumatic stress disorder using phenelzine or imipramine. J Nerv Ment Dis 1991;179:366–70.

63. Scharf M, Rogowski R, Hull S, et al. Efficacy and safety of doxepin 1 mg, 3 mg, and 6 mg in elderly patients with primary insomnia: a randomized, double-blind, placebo-controlled crossover study. J Clin Psychiatry 2008;69:1557–64.

64. Richardson GS, Roehrs TA, Rosenthal L, Koshorek G, Roth T. Tolerance to daytime sedative effects of H1 antihistamines. J Clin Psychopharmacol 2002;22:511–5.

65. Braun P, Greenberg D, Dasberg H, Lerer B. Core symptoms of posttraumatic stress disorder unimproved by alprazolam treatment. J Clin Psychiatry 1990;51:236–8.

66. Baker DG, Nievergelt CM, Risbrough VB. Post-traumatic stress disorder: emerging concepts of pharmacotherapy. Expert Opin Emerg Drugs 2009;14:251–72.

67. Pollack MH, Hoge EA, Worthington JJ. Eszopiclone for the treatment of posttraumatic stress disorder and associated insomnia: a randomized, double-blind, placebo-controlled trial. J Clin Psychiatry 2011;72:892–7.

68. Wine JN, Sanda C, Caballero J. Effects of quetiapine on sleep in nonpsychiatric and psychiatric conditions. Ann Pharmacother 2009;43:707–13.

69. Simon V, van Winkel R, De Hert M. Are weight gain and metabolic side effects of atypical antipsychotics dose dependent? A literature review. J Clin Psychiatry 2009;70:1041–50.

70. Williams SG, Alinejad NA, Williams JA, Cruess DF. Statistically significant increase in weight caused by low-dose quetiapine. Pharmacotherapy 2010;30:1011–5.

71. Hamner MB, Canive J, Robert S, Calais LA, Villarreal G, Durkalski V. Quetiapine monotherapy in chronic posttraumatic stress disorder: a randomized, double-blind, placebo-controlled trial. Paper presented at the annual meeting of the American Psychiatric Association, San Francisco, CA, May 2009.

72. Hamner MB, Deitsch SE, Brodrick PS, Ulmer HG, Lorberbaum JP. Quetiapine treatment in patients with posttraumatic stress disorder: an open trial of adjunctive therapy. J Clin Psychopharmacol 2003;23:15–20.

73. Cascade E, Kalali AH, Kennedy SH. Real-world data on SSRI antidepressant side effects. Psychiatry (Edgmont) 2009;6:16–8.

74. Stein DJ, Ipser J, McAnda N. Pharmacotherapy of posttraumatic stress disorder: a review of meta-analyses and treatment guidelines. CNS Spectr 2009;14:25–31.

75. Brady K, Pearlstein T, Asnis GM, et al. Efficacy and safety of sertraline treatment of posttraumatic stress disorder: a randomized controlled trial. JAMA 2000;283:1837–44.

76. Tucker P, Potter-Kimball R, Wyatt DB, et al. Can physiologic assessment and side effects tease out differences in PTSD trials? A double-blind comparison of citalopram, sertraline, and placebo. Psychopharmacol Bull 2003;37:135–49.

77. Martenyi F, Brown EB, Zhang H, Prakash A, Koke SC. Fluoxetine versus placebo in posttraumatic stress disorder. J Clin Psychiatry 2002;63:199–206.

78. Martenyi F, Soldatenkova V. Fluoxetine in the acute treatment and relapse prevention of combat-related post-traumatic stress disorder: analysis of the veteran group of a placebo-controlled, randomized clinical trial. Eur Neuropsychopharmacol 2006;16:340–9.

79. Martenyi F, Brown EB, Caldwell CD. Failed efficacy of fluoxetine in the treatment of posttraumatic stress disorder: results of a fixed-dose, placebo-controlled study. J Clin Psychopharmacol 2007;27:166–70.

80. Seedat S, Stein DJ, Emsley RA. Open trial of citalopram in adults with post-traumatic stress disorder. Int J Neuropsychopharmacol 2000;3:135–40.

81. English BA, Jewell M, Jewell G, Ambrose S, Davis LL. Treatment of chronic posttraumatic stress disorder in combat veterans with citalopram: an open trial. J Clin Psychopharmacol 2006;26:84–8.

82. Robert S, Hamner MB, Ulmer HG, Lorberbaum JP, Durkalski VL. Open-label trial of escitalopram in the treatment of posttraumatic stress disorder. J Clin Psychiatry 2006;67: 1522–6.

83. Canive JM, Clark RD, Calais LA, Qualls C, Tuason VB. Bupropion treatment in veterans with post-traumatic stress disorder: an open study. J Clin Psychopharmacol 1998;18:379–83.

84. Becker ME, Hertzberg MA, Moore SD, Dennis MF, Bukenya DS, Beckham JC. A placebo-controlled trial of bupropion SR in the treatment of chronic posttraumatic stress disorder. J Clin Psychopharmacol 2007;27:193–7.

85. Bahk WM, Pae CU, Tsoh J, et al. Effects of mirtazapine in patients with post-traumatic stress disorder in Korea: a pilot study. Hum Psychopharmacol 2002;17:341–4.

86. Chung MY, Min KH, Jun YJ, Kim SS, Kim WC, Jun EM. Efficacy and tolerability of mirtazapine and sertraline in Korean veterans with posttraumatic stress disorder: a randomized open label trial. Hum Psychopharmacol 2004;19:489–94.

87. Davidson JR, Weisler RH, Butterfield MI, et al. Mirtazapine vs. placebo in posttraumatic stress disorder: a pilot trial. Biol Psychiatry 2003;53:188–91.

88. Kim W, Pae CU, Chae JH, Jun TY, Bahk WM. The effectiveness of mirtazapine in the treatment of post-traumatic stress disorder: a 24-week continuation therapy. Psychiatry Clin Neurosci 2005;59:743–7.

89. Preskorn SH. Outpatient management of depression: a guide for the practitioner. 3rd ed. West Islip, NY: Professional Communications, 2009.

90. David D, Kutcher GS, Jackson EI, Mellman TA. Psychotic symptoms in combat-related posttraumatic stress disorder. J Clin Psychiatry 1999;60:29–32.

91. Moskowitz A, ed. Psychosis, trauma, and dissociation. Oxford: Wiley & Sons, 2009.

92. Hamner MB, Faldowski RA, Ulmer HG, Frueh BC, Huber MG, Arana GW. Adjunctive risperidone treatment in posttraumatic stress disorder: a preliminary controlled trial of effects on comorbid psychotic symptoms. Int Clin Psychopharmacol 2003;18:1–8.

93. Rothbaum BO, Killeen TK, Davidson JR, Brady KT, Connor KM, Heekin MH. Placebo-controlled trial of risperidone augmentation for selective serotonin reuptake inhibitor resistant civilian posttraumatic stress disorder. J Clin Psychiatry 2008;69:520–5.

94. Pivac N, Kozaric-Kovacic D, Muck-Seler D. Olanzapine versus fluphenazine in an open trial in patients with psychotic combat-related post-traumatic stress disorder. Psychopharmacology (Berl) 2004;175:451–6.

95. Robert S, Hamner MB, Durkalski VL, Brown MW, Ulmer HG. An open-label assessment of aripiprazole in the treatment of PTSD. Psychopharmacol Bull 2009;42:69–80.

96. Hamner MB, Canive J, Robert S, Calais LA, Villarreal G, Durkalski V. Quetiapine monotherapy in chronic posttraumatic stress disorder: a randomized, double-blind, placebo-controlled trial. Paper presented at the annual meeting of the American Psychiatric Association, San Francisco, CA, May 2009.

97. Southwick SM. Noradrenergic alterations in posttraumatic stress disorder. Ann N Y Acad Sci 1997;821:125–41.

98. Murphy SE, Yiend J, Lester KJ, Cowen PJ, Harmer CJ. Short term serotonergic but not noradrenergic antidepressant administration reduces attentional vigilance to threat in healthy volunteers. Int J Neuropsychopharmacol 2009;12:169–79.

99. Reist C, Kauffmann CD, Haier RJ, et al. A controlled trial of desipramine in 18 men with posttraumatic stress disorder. Am J Psychiatry 1989;146:513–6.

100. Davidson J, Baldwin D, Stein DJ, et al. Treatment of posttraumatic stress disorder with venlafaxine extended release: a 6-month randomized controlled trial. Arch Gen Psychiatry 2006;63:1158–65.

101. Davidson J, Rothbaum BO, Tucker P, Asnis G, Benattia I, Musgnung JJ. Venlafaxine extended release in posttraumatic stress disorder: a sertraline- and placebo-controlled study. J Clin Psychopharmacol 2006;26:259–67.

102. Rothbaum BO, Davidson JR, Stein DJ, et al. A pooled analysis of gender and trauma-type effects on responsiveness to treatment of PTSD with venlafaxine extended release or placebo. J Clin Psychiatry 2008;69:1529–39.

103. Stein DJ, Pedersen R. Onset of activity and time to response on individual CAPS-SX17 items in patients treated for posttraumatic stress disorder with venlafaxine ER: a pooled analysis. Int J Neuropsychopharmacol 2009;12:23–31.

104. Gelenberg AJ. Nefazedone hepatotoxicity: black box warning. Biol Ther Psychiatry 2002;25:2.

105. Davis LL, Nugent AL, Murray J, Kramer GL, Petty F. Nefazodone treatment for chronic posttraumatic stress disorder: an open trial. J Clin Psychopharmacol 2000;20:159–64.

106. Garfield DA, Fichtner CG, Leveroni C, Mahableshwarkar A. Open trial of nefazodone for combat veterans with posttraumatic stress disorder. J Trauma Stress 2001;14:453–60.

107. Davis LL, Jewell ME, Ambrose S, et al. A placebo-controlled study of nefazodone for the treatment of chronic posttraumatic stress disorder: a preliminary study. J Clin Psychopharmacol 2004;24:291–7.

108. McRae AL, Brady KT, Mellman TA, et al. Comparison of nefazodone and sertraline for the treatment of posttraumatic stress disorder. Depress Anxiety 2004;19:190–6.

109. Hidalgo R, Hertzberg MA, Mellman T, et al. Nefazodone in post-traumatic stress disorder: results from six open-label trials. Int Clin Psychopharmacol 1999;14:61–8.

110. Hertzberg MA, Feldman ME, Beckham JC, Moore SD, Davidson JR. Open trial of nefazodone for combat-related posttraumatic stress disorder. J Clin Psychiatry 1998;59:460–4.

111. Hertzberg MA, Feldman ME, Beckham JC, Moore SD, Davidson JR. Three- to four-year follow-up to an open trial of nefazodone for combat-related posttraumatic stress disorder. Ann Clin Psychiatry 2002;14:215–21.

112. Zisook S, Chentsova-Dutton YE, Smith-Vaniz A, et al. Nefazodone in patients with treatment-refractory posttraumatic stress disorder. J Clin Psychiatry 2000;61:203–8.

113. Fesler FA. Valproate in combat-related posttraumatic stress disorder. J Clin Psychiatry 1991;52:361–4.

114. Davis LL, Davidson JR, Ward LC, Bartolucci A, Bowden CL, Petty F. Divalproex in the treatment of posttraumatic stress disorder: a randomized, double-blind, placebo-controlled trial in a veteran population. J Clin Psychopharmacol 2008;28:84–8.

115. Hertzberg MA, Butterfield MI, Feldman ME, et al. A preliminary study of lamotrigine for the treatment of posttraumatic stress disorder. Biol Psychiatry 1999;45:1226–9.

116. Tucker P, Trautman RP, Wyatt DB, et al. Efficacy and safety of topiramate monotherapy in civilian posttraumatic stress disorder: a randomized, double-blind, placebo-controlled study. J Clin Psychiatry 2007;68:201–6.

117. Lindley SE, Carlson EB, Hill K. A randomized, double blind, placebo-controlled trial of augmentation topiramate for chronic combat-related posttraumatic stress disorder. J Clin Psychopharmacol 2007;27:677–81.

118. Kinrys G, Wygant L, Pardo T, Melo M. Levetiracetam for treatment-refractory posttraumatic stress disorder. J Clin Psychiatry 2006;67:211–4.

119. Connor KM, Davidson JR, Weisler RH, Zhang W, Abraham K. Tiagabine for posttraumatic stress disorder: effects of open-label and double-blind discontinuation treatment. Psychopharmacology (Berl) 2006;184:21–5.

120. Davidson JR, Brady K, Mellman TA, Stein MB, Pollack MH. The efficacy and tolerability of tiagabine in adult patients with post-traumatic stress disorder. J Clin Psychopharmacol 2007;27:85–8.

121. Pae CU, Lim HK, Peindl K, et al. The atypical antipsychotics olanzapine and risperidone in the treatment of posttraumatic stress disorder: a meta-analysis of randomized, double-blind, placebo-controlled clinical trials. Int Clin Psychopharmacol 2008;23:1–8.

122. Monnelly EP, Ciraulo DA, Knapp C, Keane T. Low-dose risperidone as adjunctive therapy for irritable aggression in posttraumatic stress disorder. J Clin Psychopharmacol 2003;23:193–6.

123. Krystal J, Rosenheck R, Cramer J. Adjunctive risperidone treatment for antidepressant-resistant symptoms of chronic military service-related PTSD. JAMA 2011;306: 493–502.

124. Ahearn EP, Mussey M, Johnson C, Krohn A, Krahn D. Quetiapine as an adjunctive treatment for post-traumatic stress disorder: an 8-week open-label study. Int Clin Psychopharmacol 2006;21:29–33.

125. Villarreal G, Calais LA, Canive JM, Lundy SL, Pickard J, Toney G. Prospective study to evaluate the efficacy of aripiprazole as a monotherapy in patients with severe chronic posttraumatic stress disorder: an open trial. Psychopharmacol Bull 2007;40:6–18.

126. Mello MF, Costa MC, Schoedl AF, Fiks JP. Aripiprazole in the treatment of posttraumatic stress disorder: an open-label trial. Rev Bras Psiquiatr 2008;30:358–61.

127. Butterfield MI, Becker ME, Connor KM, Sutherland S, Churchill LE, Davidson JR. Olanzapine in the treatment of post-traumatic stress disorder: a pilot study. Int Clin Psychopharmacol 2001;16:197–203.

128. Stein MB, Kline NA, Matloff JL. Adjunctive olanzapine for SSRI-resistant combat-related PTSD: a double-blind, placebo-controlled study. Am J Psychiatry 2002;159:1777–9.

129. Siddiqui Z, Marcil WA, Bhatia SC, Ramaswamy S, Petty F. Ziprasidone therapy for post-traumatic stress disorder. J Psychiatry Neurosci 2005;30:430–1.

130. Ray WA, Chung CP, Murray KT, Hall K, Stein CM. Atypical antipsychotic drugs and the risk of sudden cardiac death. N Engl J Med 2009;360:225–35.

131. Pies R. Should psychiatrists use atypical antipsychotics to treat nonpsychotic anxiety? Psychiatry (Edgmont) 2009;6:29–37.

132. Kinzie JD, Leung P. Clonidine in Cambodian patients with posttraumatic stress disorder. J Nerv Ment Dis 1989;177:546–50.

133. Ziegenhorn AA, Roepke S, Schommer NC, et al. Clonidine improves hyperarousal in borderline personality disorder with or without comorbid posttraumatic stress disorder: a randomized, double-blind, placebo-controlled trial. J Clin Psychopharmacol 2009;29:170–3.

134. Neylan TC, Lenoci M, Samuelson KW, et al. No improvement of posttraumatic stress disorder symptoms with guanfacine treatment. Am J Psychiatry 2006;163:2186–8.

135. Davis LL, Ward C, Rasmusson A, Newell JM, Frazier E, Southwick SM. A placebo-controlled trial of guanfacine for the treatment of posttraumatic stress disorder in veterans. Psychopharmacol Bull 2008;41:8–18.

136. Pitman RK, Sanders KM, Zusman RM, et al. Pilot study of secondary prevention of posttraumatic stress disorder with propranolol. Biol Psychiatry 2002;51:189–92.

137. Vaiva G, Ducrocq F, Jezequel K, et al. Immediate treatment with propranolol decreases posttraumatic stress disorder two months after trauma. Biol Psychiatry 2003;54:947–9.

138. Stein MB, Kerridge C, Dimsdale JE, Hoyt DB. Pharmacotherapy to prevent PTSD: results from a randomized controlled proof-of-concept trial in physically injured patients. J Trauma Stress 2007;20:923–32.

139. Brunet A, Orr SP, Tremblay J, Robertson K, Nader K, Pitman RK. Effect of post-retrieval propranolol on psychophysiologic responding during subsequent script-driven traumatic imagery in post-traumatic stress disorder. J Psychiatr Res 2008;42:503–6.

140. Shestatzky M, Greenberg D, Lerer B. A controlled trial of phenelzine in posttraumatic stress disorder. Psychiatry Res 1988;24:149–55.

141. Baker DG, Diamond BI, Gillette G, et al. A double-blind, randomized, placebo-controlled, multi-center study of brofaromine in the treatment of post-traumatic stress disorder. Psychopharmacology (Berl) 1995;122:386–9.

142. Katz RJ, Lott MH, Arbus P, et al. Pharmacotherapy of posttraumatic stress disorder with a novel psychotropic. Anxiety 1994;1:169–74.

143. American Psychiatric Association. Practice guideline for the treatment of patients with acute stress disorder and posttraumatic stress disorder. Arlington, VA: APA, 2004.

144. Foa EB, Davidson JR, Frances A. The expert consensus guidelines: treatment of posttraumatic stress disorder. J Clin Psychiatry 1999;60 (suppl 16).

145. Canadian Psychiatric Association. Clinical practice guidelines. Management of anxiety disorders. Can J Psychiatry 2006; 51(8 suppl 2):9S–91S.

146. United States Department of Veterans Affairs; United States Department of Defense. Clinical practice guideline for management of post-traumatic stress. Washington, DC: Veterans Health Administration, DoD, 2010.

UPDATE

POSTTRAUMATIC STRESS DISORDER*

Prazosin: Still First Line for PTSD Patients With Prominent Insomnia

Since the publication of the algorithm, there have been two more studies of prazosin versus placebo for veterans with combat-related trauma and posttraumatic stress disorder (PTSD).[1,2] One of these (n = 67) showed a robust advantage of prazosin over placebo, and the second, larger and multicentered, (n = 304 distributed over 13 Veterans Hospital sites) found no advantage for prazosin. There was also a small placebo-controlled study with 20 subjects in a civilian population, 85% female, with mild-to-moderate levels of suicidality, and half of the patients had comorbid major depression. This study found an advantage for placebo over prazosin for insomnia and nightmares.[3] Added to the three small placebo-controlled studies reviewed in the algorithm paper, there are, therefore, now six studies, four in veterans or soldiers of which three were positive and two among civilians of which one was positive.

In the 2013 Department of Veterans Affairs (VA) study, subjects took prazosin at night and in the morning, and there was robust improvement on all primary and secondary outcome measures on sleep, nightmares, global functioning, and hyperarousal—similar to the previous three studies from Raskind et al. A total of 64% responded to prazosin versus 27% on placebo, a number needed to treat (NNT) of 2.7. However, in the much larger 2018 study, there were no differences from placebo despite similar dosing to the 2013 study. The authors and editorialists discussed possible explanations for these negative results. Subjects were relatively stable socially, economically, and clinically compared to those in previous studies. None of the previous studies excluded patients who were unstable in these respects. If patients were on trazodone and getting some benefit from it, they could not participate unless they were willing to stop it. Trazodone helps many PTSD patients fall asleep even if it is not as helpful for staying asleep and preventing nightmares, while prazosin (a nonsedative) is not particularly helpful for initial insomnia. It should also be noted that prazosin had been prescribed in these VA hospitals for years, and perhaps the best candidates for it had already been treated. It was also noted that patients had low baseline blood pressure, suggesting they had a PTSD subtype that was less adrenergically driven. A study of previous patient samples found that higher pretreatment blood pressure was associated with greater PTSD symptom reduction with prazosin.[4] Clinicians are advised to pay attention to this possible predictor.

*I thank Laura A. Bajor, D.O. for her contributions to this update on the PTSD algorithm.

It seems reasonable to conclude that response to prazosin is heterogeneous and precision medicine needs to be elaborated by future studies to enable prediction of responders. However, meanwhile, the medication had four positive studies with robust effect sizes. There clearly are responders out there and it seems an important contributor to the armamentarium of medications that could be considered. The evidence base on prazosin may be contrasted with that of sertraline, a Food and Drug Administration (FDA)-approved medication treatment for PTSD commonly recommended at the top of guidelines, such as those of the Veterans Administration.[5] This medication has had at least seven placebo-controlled studies in PTSD, several of them unpublished but discussed in a National Institute of Clinical Excellence (NICE) review,[6] but only two have been positive. As we indicated in the 2011 review, the licensing agency in England approved sertraline only for women with PTSD due to unsatisfactory results in male veterans. Also, even in the best sertraline studies, it had a small effect size—much smaller than what was found in the positive prazosin studies.[6] A recent review of PTSD psychopharmacology concluded that sertraline is "best avoided" in combat veterans.[7] Also, there has been much discussion of a 2019 study in veterans comparing sertraline to prolonged exposure therapy and to their combination.[8] All groups improved equally, but there was no control group on just placebo and some nonspecific supportive therapy. Given, as noted above, that previous studies have not found efficacy versus placebo for sertraline in this population, this study raises more questions than provides answers about treatment choices. Another large 2019 study in a civilian population compared sertraline and prolonged exposure (again, without placebo control), and there were advantages found for the exposure therapy.[9]

How should the aggregate evidence on prazosin, including the clinical experience of many prescribers, be interpreted, in comparison with the evidence on selective serotonin reuptake inhibitors (SSRIs)? We think it favors prazosin despite the small numbers of patients studied, and we are retaining prazosin at the top of the algorithm for patients with prominent insomnia. This includes the great majority of patients with PTSD. The sleep disturbances typically involve nightmares, but some patients have disturbed awakenings without recalling nightmares, and clinicians should be sure to ask about those. They may wake up one or more times a night feeling anxious, perspiring profusely, hyperventilating, or experiencing tachycardia. It is usually difficult to return to sleep and they may have to get up and pace about, watch TV, play video games, or otherwise distract themselves to calm down before they can return to sleep. Also, many patients have night terrors (phenomena witnessed by a bed partner or roommate during which the patient is talking, yelling, fighting, kicking, or otherwise appearing to be in distress—but nothing is recalled by the patient upon awakening). All of these are candidates for treatment with prazosin and related medications targeting alpha adrenergic mechanisms.

Prazosin is often underdosed, resulting in a negative outcome.[10] It seems reasonable to use the dosing in the largest study with a positive outcome.[1] The dosing protocol was somewhat complex, and it takes time and, often, a series of outpatient visits to administer effectively and address side effects. For example, the patient may already be on one or more antihypertensives, and introducing prazosin may bring on light-headedness or low blood pressure. Negotiation with the prescriber of the antihypertensive regimen is advised to determine which agent should be lowered or eliminated to allow for the titration of the prazosin.

The dosing protocol for men was:

1 mg HS × 2 nights
2 mg for 5 nights
4 mg for 7 nights
6 mg for 7 nights
10 mg for 7 nights
15 mg for 7 nights
20 mg maximum at bedtime

Median final bedtime dose was 15.6 mg.

The day dose was: (usually taken about 10 AM to avoid any overlap with night dose—use cell phone to set up reminder)

Week 2: 1 mg
Weeks 3–4: 2 mg
Weeks 5–6: 5 mg

Women seem to need lower doses, for reasons that have not been fully explained. For women, the protocol was:

1 mg at bedtime for 2 nights
2 mg for 12 nights
4 mg for 7 nights
6 mg for 7 nights
10 mg maximum at bedtime

Median final bedtime dose was 7 mg

Midmorning dose
Weeks 2–3: 1 mg
Weeks 4–5: 2 mg

These increases may need to be slowed or modified depending on side effects. One should not prescribe this protocol and expect the patient to follow it precisely without consultation along the way. A check-in with the patient is advised every week or two. To get the most out of prazosin, it is very important to begin with a discussion about expectations. The person with nightmares every night and who gets 3 hours of sleep a night is not going to transition to no nightmares and 7–8 hours of restful, restorative sleep in a week or two. The process will be gradual and may take weeks or months as the dose is slowly increased as tolerated. Some patients experience worsening of nightmares after the first few doses, though this could be due to traumatic triggers coincidentally occurring at this point rather than a medication effect. The patient should be prepared for this possibility and urged to keep taking it and (if otherwise tolerated) progress to the higher doses, at which point usually this problem will fade. The first sign of actual improvement may be that the nightmares will become less severe or the time required to recover from them and return to sleep will shorten. Next, the frequency of nightmares should reduce, though disturbed awakenings without nightmare recollection may continue even when patients no longer remember any nightmares. The doses of prazosin should still be increased as in the protocols, attempting to reach goals of no nightmares or disturbed awakenings and longer total sleep time. It can be very helpful to give patients a handout with these instructions or a copy of the Raskind et al. study.[1]

Some patients may need, and tolerate, doses higher than in the Raskind and colleagues. protocol. There are case reports in the literature of patients being raised to 30 and even 45 mg at bedtime safely with good outcome.[11]

Since the 2011 PTSD algorithm publication, there is the first placebo-controlled trial of doxazosin XL as an alternative to prazosin.[12] We had mentioned an open-label trial suggesting effectiveness, but in this study with crossover design, eight patients had trials on placebo and on active medication. Results were positive on one of the two primary outcome measures (the PTSD Checklist—Military version). Like prazosin, doxazosin is an alpha-1 adrenergic antagonist, but its half-life is 15–19 hours compared to the 2–3 hours half-life of prazosin. These properties may render it less prone to hypotensive and other side effects. Previous studies suggested that doxazosin does not cross the blood–brain barrier, or does so only minimally. However, the authors provided evidence that it does have central effects.[12] Clinical experience has been accumulating with doxazosin for PTSD, and some clinicians prefer it over prazosin because of impressions of better tolerability. Dosing is similar.

Comorbidities and How They Affect the Algorithm

There is one pertinent new study that may be relevant for patients with comorbid alcohol use disorder and PTSD.[13] At doses up to 300 mg daily, topiramate reduced alcohol cravings, alcohol consumption, and also PTSD symptoms, especially hyperarousal complaints. However, patients should be warned about the significant risk of symptomatic kidney stones, which is about 2.1%, with the highest rates occurring in patients on 300 mg daily or more or who have a previous history of kidney stones.[14]

Under the heading of women of child-bearing potential, a new large study confirms that paroxetine deserves the D rating it had from the FDA because of atrial septal defects.[15] Fluoxetine also turned up as having a similar rate in this observational study.

Many patients with PTSD report anxiety. Clinicians may diagnose this anxiety as coming from comorbid anxiety disorders like generalized anxiety disorder, social anxiety disorder, or panic disorder. Medications with an evidence base for treating those disorders may therefore be tried. However, more careful evaluation often reveals that these apparent comorbid anxiety symptoms are actually coming from the PTSD. The triggers for these anxiety symptoms may be events that are similar to or remind the patient of previous traumatic experiences. Often one finds PTSD patients who are on medications such as benzodiazepines, hydroxyzine, gabapentin, and buspirone. They were put on these medications to treat anxiety symptoms. But if the symptoms are coming from PTSD, one may not see significant benefit: none of these has any important evidence base supporting effectiveness in PTSD.

Considerations for Helping Patients With Initial Insomnia

The discussion in the original paper still holds. Quetiapine, benzodiazepines, and sedating tricyclics are not recommended. A newer study adds to the reasons to avoid benzodiazepines: they may reduce the short- and long-term effectiveness of exposure-mediated psychotherapies commonly used for PTSD.[16]

Considerations for First- and Second-Line Pharmacotherapy Choices if Symptoms Remain Significant After Addressing Sleep Disturbance

The discussion and recommendations in the original paper still hold. There have been some new data on mirtazapine usage. There has been one randomized controlled trial in mostly civilian subjects (N-29) and five open-label studies, recently summarized in a critical review.[17] The potential advantages of mirtazapine are that it could be more sedating than SSRIs and it has low sexual side effects. The disadvantage is the weight gain, and also since it has alpha-adrenergic stimulating properties it might, like venlafaxine, also not be beneficial for (or might worsen) hyperarousal symptoms of PTSD. The studies to date have not evaluated this. There is also one study of mirtazapine as an augmentation strategy in 36 civilian patients with PTSD, added to sertraline (mean dose 120 mg).[18] There was no difference from adding placebo in the primary outcome measures, and sexual side effects were not reduced. However, a secondary outcome showed that at 24-week follow-up, 39% of the mirtazapine patients remitted versus only 11% of those with added placebo. It seems that mirtazapine should stay where it is as a second-line option and could be considered to be somewhat promising as an augmentation.

Recommendations for Treatment-Resistant Patients (Node 5a of the Algorithm)

These, as well, appear reasonably current as written. There was a new placebo-controlled study of topiramate that was positive.[19] The two previous randomized trials, from 2007, were not impressive. However, Yeh and colleagues treated 70 civilian patients in Brazil for 12 weeks and the reduction on the Clinician-Administered PTSD Scale (CAPS) in the topiramate group was 58 points versus a 32-point improvement on placebo ($p = 0.008$). There was improvement in reexperiencing (which is where we recommended it) and also in avoidance symptoms. Hence topiramate may be **added to the options for prominent avoidance symptoms** though with consideration of the side-effect risks including kidney stones, mentioned earlier.

Regarding the use of second-generation antipsychotics (SGAs) as augmentations or monotherapies for PTSD at node 5a, there are some new studies. Some had thought that the large 2011 VA Cooperative study of risperidone as adjunctive therapy to SSRIs, discussed in the algorithm publication, which did not find any benefit on global severity of PTSD, was the "nail in the coffin"[20] for a major role for SGAs. There was actually a small effect on hyperarousal, and this is why we listed risperidone as an option for residual symptoms in this domain. However, a new study of the SGA quetiapine as monotherapy versus placebo for PTSD appeared in 2016.[21] A total of 80 subjects were randomized for 12 weeks, and there were positive results for both hyperarousal and reexperiencing symptoms, and in multiple other domains of secondary outcomes. Doses could be titrated up to 800 mg daily, and the mean dose was about 250 mg. Improvement at end point, though greater than placebo, was modest, and patients were left with significant residual symptoms and "additional psychopharmacological or psychotherapeutic interventions would need to be considered."[21] One always has to wonder, in quetiapine placebo-controlled studies, if the blind was successful; it might be very easy for patients to guess if they were randomized to quetiapine because of the strong sedative effects and the appetite stimulation. Metabolic side effects, though not thoroughly measured in this short-term study, did seem modest. However, considering benefits and risks, it would seem that this study would not justify changing the previous placement of quetiapine in the algorithm, namely as a third-line option at node 5a, in the list of choices to consider for patients with residual hyperarousal or reexperiencing symptoms.

There was also a recent small placebo-controlled trial of ziprasidone as an augmentation of SSRIs in PTSD.[22] After unsatisfactory response to sertraline or paroxetine, 24 patients were randomized for 8 weeks. About 44% completed the ziprasidone trial while 64% completed the placebo treatment. There were no efficacy differences.

In conclusion, SGAs still deserve to be at node 5a as a third-line option because of their modest effectiveness and significant side effects, compared to the antidepressants.

Are There Any New Options to Be Considered That Were Not Reviewed in 2011?

Cannabis and derivatives (e.g., cannabidiol) have received much publicity as possible treatments for PTSD. It is one of more than 50 indications for "medical marijuana" that are approved by various State governments. Cannabis is legal in 36 states and 10 states allow recreational use, but there is no regulation of the quality or purity of these products. Patients are vocal in reporting that they feel more relaxed or may sleep better after taking these products. Many report that it is the only thing that is reliably helpful for their sleep and anxiety symptoms, compared with what we prescribe. Notably, nicotine users say the similar things: it is their coping strategy of choice for just about every stress, or even their "only pleasure in life." Others say the same things about benzodiazepines. So, here is a rhetorical question: What do these substances have in common? What PTSD patients do not seem to appreciate is that after the relaxation wears off, they need it again and again, and overall the course of their PTSD seems adversely effected, especially anger management, according to limited evidence that is available.[23] More research is needed.

Transcranial magnetic stimulation (TMS) has received considerable interest as a treatment for PTSD. A meta-analysis of nine studies found an impressive effect size of -0.88 on reducing PTSD symptoms using high-frequency application of the magnet over the right dorsolateral prefrontal cortex.[24] More recent TMS work has focused on the theta-burst technique (iTMS) that delivers intensive pulses for 3 minutes over 10 days rather than the 37 minutes over 6 weeks in the standard TMS protocol, but iTMS is hard to deliver accurately to the desired areas.[25] A recent study with iTMS in 50 PTSD subjects found no statistical improvement versus sham at 2 weeks, though the difference appeared clinically meaningful.[26] One-month (unblinded) outcomes were better, with effect size on improvement in social and occupational functioning reaching 0.93. TMS delivered by evolving devices and techniques is among the most promising new treatments for PTSD, but further studies are needed before enough is known to propose it as a standard recommendation.

REFERENCES

1. Raskind MA, Peterson K, Williams T, et al. A trial of prazosin for combat trauma PTSD with nightmares in active-duty soldiers returned from Iraq and Afghanistan. Am J Psychiatry 2013;170:1003–10.
2. Raskind MA, Peskind ER, Chow B, et al. Trial of prazosin for post-traumatic stress disorder in military veterans. N Engl J Med 2018;378:507–17.
3. McCall WV, Pillai A, Case D, et al. A pilot, randomized clinical trial of bedtime doses of prazosin versus placebo in suicidal posttraumatic stress disorder patients with nightmares. J Clin Psychopharmacol 2018;38:618–21.
4. Raskind MA, Millard SP, Petrie EC, et al. Higher pretreatment blood pressure is associated with greater posttraumatic stress disorder symptom reduction in soldiers treated with prazosin. Biol Psychiatry 2016;80:736–42.
5. Ostacher MJ, Cifu AS. Management of posttraumatic stress disorder. JAMA 2019;321:200–1.
6. National Institute for Clinical Excellence. Post-traumatic stress disorder: the management of PTSD in adults and children and secondary care. London, UK: Gaskell and the British Psychological Society, 2005.
7. Akiki TJ, Abdallah CG. Are there effective psychopharmacologic treatments for PTSD? J Clin Psychiatry 2018;80.
8. Rauch SAM, Kim HM, Powell C, et al. Efficacy of prolonged exposure therapy, sertraline hydrochloride, and their combination among combat veterans with posttraumatic stress disorder: a randomized clinical trial. JAMA Psychiatry 2019;76:117–26.
9. Zoellner LA, Roy-Byrne PP, Mavissakalian M, Feeny NC. Doubly randomized preference trial of prolonged exposure versus sertraline for treatment of PTSD. Am J Psychiatry 2019;176:287–96.
10. Alexander B, Lund BC, Bernardy NC, Christopher ML, Friedman MJ. Early discontinuation and suboptimal dosing of prazosin: a potential missed opportunity for veterans with posttraumatic stress disorder. J Clin Psychiatry 2015;76:e639–44.
11. Koola MM, Varghese SP, Fawcett JA. High-dose prazosin for the treatment of post-traumatic stress disorder. Ther Adv Psychopharmacol 2014;4:43–7.
12. Rodgman C, Verrico CD, Holst M, et al. Doxazosin XL reduces symptoms of posttraumatic stress disorder in veterans with PTSD: a pilot clinical trial. J Clin Psychiatry 2016;77:e561–5.
13. Batki SL, Pennington DL, Lasher B, et al. Topiramate treatment of alcohol use disorder in veterans with posttraumatic stress disorder: a randomized controlled pilot trial. Alcohol Clin Exp Res 2014;38:2169–77.
14. Dell'Orto VG, Belotti EA, Goeggel-Simonetti B, et al. Metabolic disturbances and renal stone promotion on treatment with topiramate: a systematic review. Br J Clin Pharmacol 2014;77:958–64.
15. Reefhuis J, Devine O, Friedman JM, Louik C, Honein MA. Specific SSRIs and birth defects: Bayesian analysis to interpret new data in the context of previous reports. BMJ (Clinical Research Ed) 2015;351:h3190.

16. Rosen CS, Greenbaum MA, Schnurr PP, Holmes TH, Brennan PL, Friedman MJ. Do benzodiazepines reduce the effectiveness of exposure therapy for posttraumatic stress disorder? J Clin Psychiatry 2013;74:1241–8.

17. McGrane IR, Shuman MD. Mirtazapine therapy for posttraumatic stress disorder: implications of alpha-adrenergic pharmacology on the startle response. Harv Rev Psychiatry 2018;26:36–41.

18. Schneier FR, Campeas R, Carcamo J, et al. Combined mirtazapine and SSRI treatment of PTSD: a placebo-controlled trial. Depress Anxiety 2015;32:570–9.

19. Yeh MS, Mari JJ, Costa MC, Andreoli SB, Bressan RA, Mello MF. A double-blind randomized controlled trial to study the efficacy of topiramate in a civilian sample of PTSD. CNS Neurosci Ther 2011;17:305–10.

20. Stein MB. Adjusting to traumatic stress research. Am J Psychiatry 2016;173:1165–6.

21. Villarreal G, Hamner MB, Canive JM, et al. Efficacy of quetiapine monotherapy in posttraumatic stress disorder: a randomized, placebo-controlled trial. Am J Psychiatry 2016;173:1205–12.

22. Hamner MB, Hernandez-Tejada MA, Zuschlag ZD, Agbor-Tabi D, Huber M, Wang Z. Ziprasidone augmentation of SSRI antidepressants in posttraumatic stress disorder: a randomized, placebo-controlled pilot study of augmentation therapy. J Clin Psychopharmacol 2019;39:153–7.

23. Mammen G, Rueda S, Roerecke M, Bonato S, Lev-Ran S, Rehm J. Association of cannabis with long-term clinical symptoms in anxiety and mood disorders: a systematic review of prospective studies. J Clin Psychiatry 2018;79.

24. Cirillo P, Gold AK, Nardi AE, et al. Transcranial magnetic stimulation in anxiety and trauma-related disorders: a systematic review and meta-analysis. Brain Behav 2019;9:e01284.

25. McDonald WM, van Rooij SJH. Targeting PTSD. Am J Psychiatry 2019;176:894–6.

26. Philip NS, Barredo J, Aiken E, et al. Theta-burst transcranial magnetic stimulation for posttraumatic stress disorder. Am J Psychiatry 2019;176:939–48.

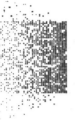

The Psychopharmacology Algorithm Project at the Harvard South Shore Program: An Algorithm for Adults with Obsessive-Compulsive Disorder

Ashley M. Beaulieu, DO[a], Edward Tabasky, MD[b], and
David N. Osser, MD[a],*

Abstract: *A previous algorithm for the pharmacological treatment of obsessive-compulsive disorder was published in 2012. Developments over the past 7 years suggest an update is needed. The authors conducted searches in PubMed, focusing on new studies and reviews since 2012 that would support or change previous recommendations. We identified exceptions to the main algorithm, including pregnant women and women of child-bearing potential, the elderly, and patients with common medical and psychiatric co-morbidities. Selective serotonin reuptake inhibitors (SSRIs) are still first-line. An adequate trial requires a period at typical antidepressant doses and dose adjustments guided by a plasma level to evaluate for poor adherence or ultra-rapid metabolism. If the response is inadequate, consider a trial of another SSRI this time possibly taken to a very high dose. Clomipramine could be an alternative. If the response to the second trial remains inadequate, the next recommendation is to augment with aripiprazole or risperidone. Alternatively, augmentation with novel agents could be selected, including glutamatergic (memantine, riluzole, topiramate, n-acetylcysteine, lamotrigine), serotonergic (ondansetron), and anti-inflammatory (minocycline, celecoxib) agents. A third option could be transcranial magnetic stimulation. Lastly, after several of these trials, deep brain stimulation and cingulotomy have evidence for a role in the most treatment-refractory patients.*

INTRODUCTION

Obsessive-compulsive disorder (OCD) is a common, chronic neuropsychiatric disorder that causes significant psychosocial impairment (Fineberg et al., 2015). It is characterized by recurrent and persistent obsessions and/or compulsions that the individual feels driven to perform (American Psychiatric Association, 2013). OCD equally affects males and females and has a lifetime prevalence of 1.6% worldwide (Stein et al., 2012). Seeking treatment is often delayed (Stein et al., 2012), and is associated with a poorer outcome, whereas effective pharmacological treatment improves quality of life (Fineberg et al., 2015).

[a]Department of Psychiatry, Harvard Medical School, VA Boston Healthcare System, Brockton Division, 940 Belmont Street, Brockton, MA 02301, United States
[b]Department of Psychiatry, NYS Psychiatric Institute, Columbia University College of Physicians and Surgeons, 1051 Riverside Drive, Box 111, New York, NY 10032, United States
*Corresponding author.
E-mail address: david.osser@va.gov (D.N. Osser).
https://doi.org/10.1016/j.psychres.2019.112583
Received 21 June 2019; Received in revised form 26 September 2019; Accepted 26 September 2019
Available online 27 September 2019

Treatments for OCD include cognitive-behavioral therapy (which may be first-line especially for patients with prominent compulsive behaviors), medication, and their combination (Foa et al., 2005). Selective serotonin reuptake inhibitors (SSRIs) are considered the first-line pharmacological treatment for patients with OCD, but these medications are effective in only 40–60% of patients (Stein et al., 2012). Evidence-informed psychopharmacology algorithms can guide clinicians in choosing appropriate medication options beyond the first-line options for OCD (Burchi et al., 2018). In this article, we present an updated version of a previously published OCD algorithm to which one of the authors (DNO) contributed (Stein et al., 2012).

Since 1995 the Psychopharmacology Algorithm Project at the Harvard South Shore Program (PAPHSS) has been creating evidence-informed treatment algorithms. Eight peer-reviewed PAPHSS algorithms have been published and can also be accessed through a publicly available website (www.psychopharm.mobi).

The PAPHSS algorithms focus on psychopharmacological treatment, but psychotherapeutic and other non-pharmacological treatments for OCD are important. Family counseling or cognitive behavioral therapy incorporating exposure and response prevention could be first-line or integrated with pharmacotherapy at any point (Burchi et al., 2018; Heyman et al., 2006). If and when medication is considered desirable, this algorithm is meant to suggest the best supported and safest options for the first and subsequent medication trials, taking into consideration the common psychiatric and medical comorbidities that might alter the selection process.

METHODS

The methods used in developing new and revised PAPHSS algorithms have been described previously (Abejuela and Osser, 2016; Ansari and Osser, 2010; Bajor et al., 2011; Giakoumatos and Osser, 2019; Hamoda and Osser, 2008; Mohammad and Osser, 2014; Osser and Dunlop, 2010; Osser et al., 2013).

In brief, the authors conducted literature searches using PubMed with key words obsessive-compulsive disorder, algorithm, management, and psychopharmacology, focusing on new randomized controlled trials (RCTs), reviews, meta-analyses, and other guidelines published since the last OCD algorithm to which current authors contributed (Stein et al., 2012).

The authors considered efficacy, tolerability, and safety as the main factors for determining the order of recommended pharmacological treatments. All recommendations to retain or change the previously published algorithm were based on the body of evidence reviewed and conclusions agreed upon by the three authors. The peer review process that follows submission of the article also adds validation to the recommendations in this and other PAPHSS algorithms. If the interpretations of the pertinent evidence, and subsequent recommendations, are plausible to reviewers, then they are retained. When differences of opinion occur, the authors make modifications to achieve consensus with the reviewers or examine the relevant evidence further in order to present additional support for their interpretation.

While the algorithm is intended to provide flexible decision-making guidance based on the evidence, clinicians must also consider the unique aspects of each patient's case.

RESULTS

Flow chart for the algorithm

An overview of the algorithm appears in Fig. 1. Each "node" represents a clinical scenario where a treatment choice must be made. The steps in the algorithm progress through initial treatments at the beginning to highly treatment-resistant scenarios at the end. The evidence and reasoning that support the recommendations at each node will be presented below.

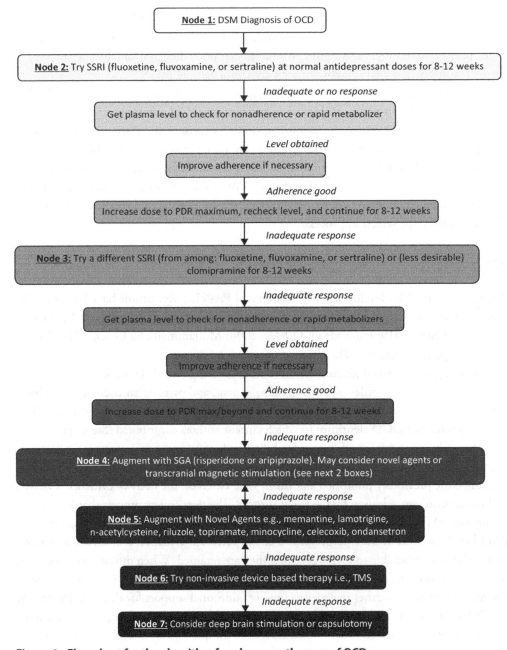

Figure 1. Flow chart for the algorithm for pharmacotherapy of OCD.

Node 1: Diagnosis of OCD

The treatment recommendations of this algorithm apply only to patients that have been diagnosed with OCD based on the American Psychiatric Association Diagnostic and Statistical Manual of Mental Disorders, edition 5 (DSM-5) criteria (American Psychiatric Association, 1994). These criteria have undergone only very minor changes since the DSM-IV criteria (American Psychiatric Association, 1994) that were in use from 1994 to 2013 when the great majority of psychopharmacology studies of OCD were conducted. The changes mostly clarify previous texts and reorganize where the disorder is found in the manual. It is reasonable to consider the results of studies utilizing the older criteria to apply to patients meeting the present criteria.

Once a diagnosis has been made based on DSM-5 criteria, it is also important to consider any co-occurring psychiatric or medical diagnoses or other circumstances that may be particularly important, such as bipolar disorder and women of childbearing potential. Table 1 provides a brief summary of how these comorbidities and other considerations would modify the basic algorithm.

Node 2: Start with an SSRI (fluoxetine, fluvoxamine, sertraline)

After making the diagnosis of OCD based on DSM-5 criteria and considering the comorbidities and conditions in Table 1 that might change the basic algorithm, the next step is to initiate a trial of an SSRI (fluoxetine, fluvoxamine, or sertraline) for 8–12 weeks. All three of these options are U.S. Food and Drug Administration (FDA) approved for OCD and are considered first-line. There have been multiple large multi-center studies of each and the details of those studies have been reviewed elsewhere and need not be repeated here (Fineberg and Gale, 2005; Fineberg et al., 2015). However, a few comments pertinent to their first-line selection follow.

Fluoxetine has been found effective in at least some studies at 20, 40, and 60 mg daily at 12–13 week end points, but with greater effectiveness with increasing dose (Tollefson et al., 1994). We will have more to say on this later.

Fluvoxamine (100–300 mg/day) is effective. In one study at a mean dose of 271 mg, 63% of the fluvoxamine CR group versus 46% of the placebo group were responders (defined as a Yale-Brown Obsessive-Compulsive Symptoms score (YBOCS) decrease of ≥ 25%). Fluvoxamine was the first SSRI approved for OCD in the United States. As a result, it is often thought of as a better medication for treating OCD than other SSRIs, but there is no evidence to suggest it is any more effective. Fluvoxamine has significant drug interactions through its inhibition of Cytochrome CYP 1A2, 2C9, C219, and 3A4 metabolizing enzymes that are important to consider (Oesterheld, 1999).

Sertraline was tested in an RCT (50 mg, 100 mg, 200 mg) and all doses were equally effective for OCD symptoms (Greist et al., 1995). In the double-blind phase of a long term 80-week trial (n = 223), sertraline was more effective than placebo in preventing: dropout due to relapse or insufficient clinical response (9% versus 24%, respectively) and acute exacerbation of symptoms (12% versus 35%) (Koran et al., 2002). Ninan et al. (2006) studied non-responders after 16 weeks of receiving sertraline 50–200 mg/day. They were randomized to receive an additional 12 weeks of high-dose sertraline (250–400 mg/day) or continue on 200 mg daily. Responder rates (defined as a decrease in YBOCS score of ≥ 25% and a Clinical Global Impression of Improvement (CGI-I) rating ≤ 3) were numerically higher for the high-dose sertraline group versus the 200 mg/day group (52% vs. 34%), although this was not statistically significant (Ninan et al., 2006).

Paroxetine is also FDA-approved for the treatment of OCD but is not recommended as a first-line treatment option due having more side effects than the others. It causes more weight gain (Fava et al., 2000; Uguz et al., 2015), sedation, and constipation (Marks et al., 2008). It also has strong drug-drug interactions due to inhibition at cytochrome P450 2D6. It is particularly prone to produce discontinuation symptoms if stopped abruptly or doses are missed (Marks et al., 2008). Paroxetine is the only SSRI with a category D rating in pregnancy (see Table 1).

Table 1	Comorbidity and Other Features in Obsessive Compulsive Disorder and How They Affect the Algorithm		
Comorbidity and other circumstances	*Considerations*	*Recommendations*
Cardiac arrhythmias	TCAs may cause cardiac arrhythmias due to their effects on cardiac sodium and potassium channels (Thanacoody and Thomas, 2005).	Try SSRIs before TCAs (clomipramine). EKG monitoring of TCA-treated patients is a more accurate way to detect cardiac toxicity than plasma level monitoring. Sertraline appears to be safe in patients at risk of arrhythmia following myocardial infarction (Glassman et al., 2002). We do not recommend citalopram or escitalopram because of concerns about QTc prolongation (Beach et al., 2013; Bird et al., 2014).
Gastrointestinal bleeding	SSRIs increase hemorrhage risk. Gastrointestinal bleeding can be increased 9-fold by SSRIs combined with NSAIDS (Anglin et al., 2014; Paton and Ferrier, 2005).	Adding proton pump inhibitors such as omeprazole decreases the risk to only slightly above controls not on SSRIs (Paton and Ferrier, 2005).
Older adults (greater than 65 years of age)	SSRIs may increase risk of bleeding; however, in a Cochrane metaanalysis of post-stroke patients, bleeding risk was non-significant (Mead et al., 2013). SSRIs are associated with higher rates of hyponatremia secondary to SIADH in older adults (De Picker et al., 2014). SSRIs, TCAs, and other antidepressant classes have been associated with increased risk of falls, particularly in frail older women (Naples et al., 2016).	Consider side effect profiles of antidepressant medications prior to initiation or titration in elderly adults. In patients with intolerable hyponatremia secondary to SSRI use, consider mirtazapine (De Picker et al., 2014). Escitalopram has fewer drug interactions than fluoxetine or fluvoxamine and less QTc prolongation than citalopram, so it might be considered but QTc should be monitored as the dose goes higher.

Table 1	Comorbidity and Other Features in Obsessive Compulsive Disorder and How They Affect the Algorithm (*continued*)		
Comorbidity and other circumstances	**Considerations**	**Recommendations**
Women of child-bearing potential and pregnant women	Severity of OCD is mostly unchanged in pregnancy and postpartum. Predictors of severity of OCD included younger age at delivery and delivery by C-section (House et al., 2016), suggesting that increased surveillance during pregnancy and postpartum may be indicated. There were no differences in neonatal outcomes including birth weight, birth length, estimated gestational age at delivery, or NICU admissions between patients with OCD and those without OCD, and severity of OCD in women who were adequately treated with pharmacotherapy, suggesting that neither disease nor treatment of OCD during pregnancy pose a direct risk to the neonate (House et al., 2016). Alternatively, late exposure to SSRIs (after 20th week of pregnancy) has been associated with increased risk of prematurity, low body weight, neonatal complications (Addis and Koren, 2000) and persistent pulmonary hypertension of the newborn in other studies (Kieler et al., 2012). Some of these could be due to confounding by indication.	The risk to the newborn of maternal treatment may be out-weighed by the impact of uncontrolled OCD symptoms on the patient (House et al., 2016). Avoid paroxetine (D rating due to atrial septal defect risk) (Reefhuis et al., 2015). If the patient is already on paroxetine, consider risks involved with switching. Consider CBT. Treatment choices are a collaborative decision with the patient.
Bipolar disorder	Antidepressants may shift euthymic patients with bipolar disorder toward a manic phase (Sahraian et al., 2017).	CBT and psychoeducation are strongly recommended as a necessary part of treatment. Among antidepressants, tricyclics (clomipramine) should particularly be avoided because of higher mania switch rates (Pacchiarotti et al., 2013). If other antidepressants such as SSRIs are used, they should be added to a mood stabilizer. Even then, their use is associated with a significant increase in [hypo]manic switches on one-year followup (McGirr et al., 2016). Of perhaps greater concern, if the bipolar disorder is rapid cycling, adding an antidepressant triples the rate of recurrent depressions compared with not starting one, according to the STEP-BD study (El-Mallakh et al., 2015). Memantine 20 mg/day showed promise as an effective adjunctive agent in reducing OCD symptoms in manic patients with bipolar I disorder (Sahraian et al., 2017).

(*continued*)

Table 1 | Comorbidity and Other Features in Obsessive Compulsive Disorder and How They Affect the Algorithm (*continued*)		
Comorbidity and other circumstances	*Considerations*	*Recommendations*
Schizophrenia	Obsessive-compulsive symptoms (OCS) occur in the course of many patients with schizophrenia (Schirmbeck et al., 2019) and also can be a new-onset side effect of second generation antipsychotics (SGAs) in these patients, most often with clozapine, due to mechanisms that are unclear (Grillault Laroche and Gaillard, 2016). In addition, some patients with OCD have psychotic symptoms (Cederlof et al., 2015) and such patients may be at risk for developing schizophrenia (Meier et al., 2014). Schizotypal personality, a condition genetically linked to schizophrenia, can present with OCS as well (De Haan, 2015).	CBT and psychoeducation are strongly recommended as a necessary part of treatment if the patient has the capacity to cognitively process and cooperate with the procedures. Use of SSRI antidepressants added to the antipsychotic for these symptoms is reasonable if there is no history of mania (as in schizoaffective disorder). If there is a mania history, review the suggestions for bipolar-related disorders. For treating OCS due to clozapine, first check a plasma level (Meyer, 2019). If it is above usual therapeutic levels, consider lowering the dose to see if the OCS are dose-related and the antipsychotic benefits can be retained. Next, consider treating with sertraline which has the least drug interactions and would be preferred over fluvoxamine (especially), fluoxetine, and paroxetine. When adding an SSRI to other SGAs, other interactions may need to be considered.

Citalopram and escitalopram are not FDA-approved but they are effective for OCD (Montgomery et al., 2001; Stein et al., 2007). Citalopram can cause QTc prolongation with doses of 40 mg and above (Beach et al., 2013), and escitalopram causes moderate dose-dependent QTc prolongation at approved doses (Bird et al., 2014) (see reference 2). Above the maximum dose of 20 mg/day, QTc was prolonged more than the control moxifloxacin. Therefore, we prefer to avoid citalopram and escitalopram because higher doses are often needed.

In summary, the first SSRI trial could be either sertraline, fluoxetine, or fluvoxamine. Unfortunately, SSRIs do have many side effects and these need to be discussed with patients. Perhaps the most disturbing are the sexual side effects and these usually do not diminish over time (Serretti and Chiesa, 2009). Some medical considerations related to these side effects are presented in Table 1.

Considering these side effects, it is recommended to carefully evaluate whether improvement on an SSRI was medication-related and not due to other reasons. As noted above, placebo response rates can be as high as 46%. This can be accomplished by trials off the medication when patients are well and have supports in place.

As noted, some evidence suggests that higher doses (and for a longer time) than usually used for depression may be necessary for maximum results (Bloch et al., 2010; Ninan et al., 2006; Pampaloni et al., 2010). However, over 20 years ago, the Expert Consensus Panel for OCD recommended that patients be treated with moderate doses at first and only increased to high doses after a period of assessment at regular doses (March, 1997). This still seems reasonable. The informative fixed-dose study by Tollefson et al. (1994) showed very little difference in benefit in the first three weeks of treatment with fluoxetine at any dose (20 mg, 40 mg, or 60 mg) or placebo in mean YBOCS total score (Tollefson et al., 1994). At 5 weeks, all the doses start separating from placebo. Then, there appears to be a decision point at about week 7, when the fluoxetine 60 mg dose begins separating slightly from the 40 mg dose. It therefore seems reasonable to recommend that, to minimize unnecessary dose escalation and associated increased side effects, clinicians wait a minimum of 7 weeks before increasing beyond the moderate dose, if the response is inadequate.

There may be three possible outcomes as one proceeds with the moderate dose of the selected SSRI; an adequate response, a partial but inadequate response, or no response. If there is an adequate response, continue with maintenance treatment for at least 1–2 years and then consider tapering to evaluate if the improvement was a placebo effect. Earlier drug discontinuation can be followed by a high likelihood of symptom recurrence (Ravizza et al., 1996). If there is a partial but inadequate response, or no response, the next step is to get a plasma SSRI level to check for nonadherence or rapid metabolizers. This adds "precision medicine" to the case, checking to see if the medication is bioavailable, and it could also help explain problematic side effects (Grunder, 2018). If the plasma level is zero, the patient is most likely non-adherent, so this should be discussed with the patient to see if the problem can be corrected. If adherence appears satisfactory but the plasma level is low, the patient may be a rapid metabolizer of that SSRI. Seven percent of Caucasians and 3% of other ethnicities can be ultrarapid metabolizers of some SSRIs (Bertilsson et al., 1993). Genetic testing could confirm this. The testing could then indicate which SSRI would be metabolized normally (Brandl et al., 2014). SSRIs do not have therapeutic levels for treating OCD (Koran et al., 1996) but the laboratory will provide the usual range of levels associated with a given dose.

Once adherence is confirmed, the next step is to increase the dose (if tolerated) to the maximum FDA-recommended dose for OCD (e.g., fluoxetine 80 mg, fluvoxamine 300 mg, or sertraline 200 mg daily) for 8–12 weeks and recheck the plasma SSRI level. A meta-analysis showed that patients obtain only a 9 or 7% greater decline in OCD symptoms on high-dose SSRI compared to low and medium dose SSRI treatment, respectively (Bloch et al., 2010). Therefore, expectations for the results of this increase should be realistic and weighed against any possible associated additional harms.

Are there other antidepressants that could be considered for initial treatment of OCD?

Bupropion, trazodone, venlafaxine, and duloxetine have received study in OCD but the evidence is not convincing for priority in the algorithm (Balachander et al., 2019; Denys et al., 2003; Phelps and Cates, 2005; Pigott et al., 1992; Sansone and Sansone, 2011; Vulink et al., 2005).

Mirtazapine is a dual neurotransmitter action agent that has the benefit of fewer sexual side effects than SSRIs and SNRIs, and its sedative effects could be useful for anxiety and insomnia. There is one small study of 30 participants who received open-label high-dose mirtazapine 60 mg daily for 12 weeks. It suggested that mirtazapine may be superior to placebo in treating OCD, but the study needs replication (Koran et al., 2005). Of perhaps greater interest regarding mirtazapine, there is a single-blind study of 49 OCD patients (never previously treated) comparing initiating them on citalopram 40–80 mg/day plus mirtazapine 15–30 mg/day versus citalopram plus placebo (Pallanti et al., 2004). Raters were not blind to the treatment group, undermining confidence in the findings, but over the first 4 weeks the results with the combined treatment were significantly better (p < 0.001) on YBOC scores. However, by 12 weeks there was no significant difference. It appeared that mirtazapine accelerated the response to the SSRI, though it did not ultimately produce a greater response. Accelerating response would be highly desirable given the discussions above about how long it takes for the SSRIs to achieve their maximum effects. However, it could come at the cost of mirtazapine side effects like weight gain – unless the mirtazapine could be removed after the acceleration and the OCD results maintained. It seems that these findings should be replicated in an appropriately-designed double-blind placebo-controlled study before it should become routine practice to add mirtazapine (Schule and Laakmann, 2005). However, it may be reasonable to explain this option to patients and the evidence behind it, and give it consideration.

Node 3: Try another SSRI (preferable) or clomipramine

If the patient fails to achieve an adequate improvement on the first SSRI trial, the next recommendation is to try another SSRI from the three first-line options, or consider the tricyclic clomipramine. Clomipramine is effective for OCD and was the first medication approved by the FDA for OCD in the United States (Thoren et al., 1980). Some meta-analyses have concluded that clomipramine has slightly greater efficacy than the SSRIs, but direct comparisons have found no differences (Fineberg and Gale, 2005; Stein et al., 2012). Moreover, early studies with clomipramine may have employed particularly medication-responsive subjects (Fineberg and Gale, 2005). Mostly in Europe, clomipramine has also been used IV to produce a faster response (Koran et al., 1994). Since clomipramine has many more side effects than SSRIs especially seizures, cardiotoxicity, weight gain, anticholinergic effects, particularly strong sexual dysfunction, and overdose lethality, the general preference is to try another SSRI for the second trial. Controlled studies, however, have not been done to evaluate whether patients who failed one adequate SSRI trial would respond to a second SSRI trial versus other medication options like augmentation strategies. The Expert Consensus group estimated a 40% likelihood of a significant response to a second SSRI trial (March, 1997). Notably, other disorders that can be treated with SSRIs such as major depression can respond to a different SSRI after failure on a first (Rush et al., 2006). SSRIs differ somewhat in their neurotransmitter-based activities. Furthermore, the side effects for patients are probably greater when adding the most-studied augmenting medications (second generation antipsychotics), compared with trying a different SSRI.

As in the first SSRI trial, there are three potential outcomes; an adequate response in which the maintenance dose would be continued, a partial but inadequate response, or no response. Again, plasma levels should be checked for nonadherence and rapid metabolizers. Once adherence is confirmed, the dose should then be increased if tolerated, to the maximum recommended dose. However, node 3 differs from node 2 in that if the response is inadequate or there is no response, and the plasma level has been adjusted to typical levels, consideration could be given for pushing the dose of the second SSRI beyond that recommended in the manufacturer's package insert. This suggestion is based on limited evidence. As described earlier, Ninan et al. (2006) found that among acute phase non-responders, continuation treatment with high-dose (250–400 mg) sertraline sometimes gave greater and more rapid improvement in OCD symptoms compared to continuing the maximal-labeled dose of sertraline (200 mg). This suggests that some patients who do not respond with doses up to 200 mg/day of sertraline may benefit from higher doses. However, these patients did not have baseline sertraline plasma levels before the dose increases. In this algorithm, this would have occurred, and dose adjustments made. It is unclear if the benefits seen in Ninan et al. (2006) could occur in patients raised to above normal plasma levels, and it is unclear if the side effect burden would be increased in such cases. However, if typical levels have been well tolerated, it seems reasonable to consider a dose increase as in Ninan et al. (2006). There were, in fact, somewhat higher rates of tremor and agitation seen on the higher doses. In the next step in the algorithm (node 4) the recommendation is to augment with SGAs, which have significant side effect profiles and, often, marginal benefits. Therefore, it may be a safer and possibly effective option for some patients to try an SSRI dose above the FDA maximum.

Other antidepressant options to consider for node 3:

Venlafaxine was mentioned earlier and has evidence of comparable effectiveness to a second SSRI. However, it has more side effects including hypertension especially at high doses, higher overdose lethality risk, and greater gastrointestinal problems (Giakoumatos and Osser, 2019).

Node 4: Augment the SSRI with a second-generation antipsychotic

If there is no or a partial but inadequate response to the second SSRI, options could include a third SSRI or clomipramine, or an augmentation strategy. The latter have received much more study and there are some positive findings. Among the augmentations, the most evidence has accumulated with SGAs, and, of those, the results favor choosing aripiprazole or risperidone. Antipsychotic augmentation has been associated with significant improvement in approximately one third of patients (Diniz et al., 2011). Other augmentations and treatment strategies are discussed in nodes 5 and 6, and prescribers should look over those options as well before making a decision at this point since they may appear better suited to the individual patient.

Risperidone (0.5 mg/day) and aripiprazole (10 mg/day or possibly lower) have the most evidence of short-term benefit (Veale et al., 2014). In this meta-analysis, there were 5 small studies involving low-dose risperidone, with a total of 77 participants receiving risperidone and 89 participants receiving placebo. The risperidone group had a 3.9-point reduction in overall mean YBOCS score, which was statistically significant compared to the placebo. The number needed to treat (NNT) for significant improvement was 4.65. There were 2 aripiprazole trials including a total of 41 participants on aripiprazole and 38 on placebo. There was a 6.3-point improvement on YBOCS outcome scores between the aripiprazole group and placebo, which was statistically and clinically significant. Of note, 50% of participants on the SGAs had a greater than 10% increase in body mass index (BMI) compared to 15.2% with an elevated BMI in the SSRI plus placebo group. The SGA group also had a higher fasting blood sugar. These risks should be taken into consideration and discussed with the patient before choosing an SGA as an augmentation strategy. Notably, the benefits from the augmentation seemed to plateau at 4 weeks and there was no further improvement after that. Therefore, if aripiprazole or risperidone are used for treatment-resistant OCD, they should be trialed for no longer than 4 weeks (and without other interventions) to determine effectiveness. If a patient is determined to be a responder at 4 weeks, then another discussion should be had regarding the possible long-term risks and need for regular monitoring of weight, blood sugar, and lipid profile.

There is also one single-blind head-to-head comparison of risperidone versus aripiprazole which found a greater response rate for risperidone. Participants were placed on high doses of either sertraline, fluoxetine, or paroxetine for 12 weeks, and those who did not achieve an improvement of $\geq$ 35% on the YBOCS were considered refractory and augmented for an additional 8 weeks with aripiprazole 15 mg/day or risperidone 3 mg/day (Selvi et al., 2011). It was found that YBOCS scores for both risperidone and aripiprazole significantly declined over the 8 weeks, but risperidone showed a significantly greater response rate of $\geq$ 35% on the YBOCS (72.2%, 13 patients) compared to aripiprazole (50%, 8 patients). However, risperidone has a more severe long-term side effect profile in terms of weight gain, sedation, extrapyramidal effects and problems associated with hyperprolactinemia including amenorrhea and sexual dysfunction (Veale et al., 2014).

Of note, most of these SGA trials only last for 8–12 weeks, but when deciding on a medication regimen, it should be taken into consideration that OCD has a chronic relapsing and remitting pattern. One long-term open-label study did not support the effectiveness of SGA augmentation of SSRIs for treatment-resistant OCD. SSRI non-responders who required atypical antipsychotic augmentation had significantly higher total YBOCS scores both at initial assessment and after one year of treatment (initial assessment = 29.3 ± 9.9, after 1 year = 19.3 ± 6.8) compared to SSRI responders (at initial assessment = 25.8 ± 11.4, after 1 year = 13.7 ± 4.6) (Matsunaga et al., 2009). Moreover, the SSRI + atypical antipsychotic group had significantly more side effects.

Veale et al. (2014) found no evidence for the effectiveness of quetiapine or olanzapine (Veale et al., 2014). In one study, quetiapine as an augmentation of an SSRI was actually less effective than placebo (Diniz et al., 2011). Notably, in the same study, clomipramine as an augmenter was not different from adding placebo. Some clinicians report from experience that combining an SSRI and clomipramine is an effective augmentation strategy, but the evidence does not support that impression. Haloperidol has some evidence of efficacy as an augmenter; however, it is not recommended due to increased risk of long-term adverse effects with the use of first-generation antipsychotics including tardive dyskinesia (Veale et al., 2014).

Node 5: Novel agents

If there is still an inadequate response, augmentation with novel agents can be considered. As noted in node 4, they might be preferred over the recommended SGAs if the side effects of the SGAs would be unacceptable.

The benefit from some of these novel agents, including memantine, riluzole, topiramate, n-acetylcysteine, lamotrigine and ketamine, theoretically occurs via modulation of glutamatergic pathways. Of these, memantine seems particularly promising based on a small amount of evidence. In one RCT, participants with a YBOCS score of 21 or higher were started on fluvoxamine 100–200 mg/day for 8 weeks, and randomly assigned to also receive memantine 20 mg/day (n = 19) or placebo (n = 19). By the end of the trial 89% of the memantine group compared to 32% of the placebo group achieved remission (YBOCS score ≤ 16) (Ghaleiha et al., 2013). Side effects were not different between the two groups. Another RCT (n = 29) demonstrated that, compare to patients with adjuvant placebo, patients who received adjuvant memantine 5–10 mg/day in addition to standard SSRI or clomipramine medication, improved significantly after 12 weeks and were more likely to achieve a full response (35% or more in Y-BOCS reduction) and show a decline in CGI severity over time. It was also found that adjuvant memantine not only affects overall response rate, but also may accelerate monotherapy response rate with a standard SSRI or clomipramine (Haghighi et al., 2013).

Riluzole is a glutamate-blocking agent approved for the treatment of symptoms of amyotrophic lateral sclerosis. An 8-week RCT (n = 50) investigated adding adjuvant riluzole 50 mg twice daily or placebo to fluvoxamine 200 mg/day in patients with moderate to severe OCD. Thirteen patients in the riluzole group achieved remission (YBOCS score ≤ 16), versus 5 patients in the placebo group, which was significantly different (Emamzadehfard et al., 2016).

Topiramate 50–400 mg/day (mean dose 177.8 mg/day) is another inhibitor of glutamatergic function that has been studied in OCD. When added as an adjuvant to participants' stable SSRI doses, it was shown to significantly reduce compulsion scores on the YBOCS by 5.38 points (versus 0.6 points in the placebo group), but not obsessions or total YBOCS scores (Berlin et al., 2011). However, 28% of 18 subjects receiving topiramate discontinued due to adverse effects.

N-acetylcysteine (NAC) 2000 mg/day is also a glutamate-inhibiting agent that has been studied as an augmenter. NAC or placebo were added to fluvoxamine 200 mg/day in a 10-week double-blind RCT (n = 22 participants in each group). NAC significantly reduced YBOCS total scores and the obsession subscale compared to the control group (Paydary et al., 2016).

Another trial investigated augmentation with lamotrigine 100 mg/ day or placebo in 33 subjects with persistent OCD symptoms despite an adequate trial on an SSRI for at least 12 weeks. In this 16-week double-blind placebo-controlled trial, significant improvement was achieved on the YBOCS obsession, compulsion, total scores, as well as CGI scores of the lamotrigine group in comparison to the placebo group at the end of the study (Bruno et al., 2012). Thirty-five percent of the lamotrigine group had a reduction of 35% or greater in YBOCS total score, corresponding to a full response, while none of the patients in the placebo group met response criteria of even 25% improvement in YBOCS total score. Lamotrigine was well-tolerated in this trial. Another 12-week study of lamotrigine by Khalkhali et al. (2016) found that SSRI-resistant patients who received adjuvant lamotrigine 100 mg/day to their SSRI (n = 26) had a significant reduction in obsessive and compulsive symptoms on the YBOCS total score and subscores compared to SSRI + placebo (n = 27) (Khalkhali et al., 2016).

Ketamine infusions (0.5 mg/kg over 40 min) were compared with saline infusions in 15 patients with OCD (Rodriguez et al., 2013). In further support of the proposed importance of glutamate mechanisms in OCD, the ketamine subjects had a significant rapid reduction in obsessions mid-infusion, 230 min post-infusion, and 1-week post-infusion. Fifty percent of the ketamine group (n = 8) met treatment response criteria (≥ 35% reduction in YBOCS score) at 1-week post-infusion versus 0% of the placebo group (n = 7), suggesting ketamine's effects on OCD symptoms can last at least a week (Rodriguez et al., 2013). The most common side effects included increases in blood pressure and pulse, and dissociative symptoms during the ketamine infusion. We mention ketamine because of current interest in this product, but much more research is needed before it should be used routinely for OCD.

Other novel agents may reduce OCD symptoms by different mechanisms. Ondansetron is a serotonin-3 receptor antagonist used to treat nausea. Patients with OCD symptoms receiving fluoxetine 20 mg/day were augmented with ondansetron 4 mg/day or placebo in an 8-week trial. Patients treated with ondansetron had significantly lower YBOCS scores at weeks 2 and 8 compared to placebo (Soltani et al., 2010). Another 8-week trial (n = 44) involved augmentation of fluvoxamine 100–200 mg/day with either ondansetron 4 mg twice daily or placebo over 8 weeks. It was found that the ondansetron group showed a significant reduction in YBOCS total score from week 4 and thereafter compared to the placebo, such that at the end of the trial, 14 (64%) patients in the ondansetron group versus 6 (27%) patients in the placebo group achieved remission (YBOCS score ≤ 16) (Heidari et al., 2014).

Agents that reduce neuroinflammation may also serve as effective augmenters for patients with OCD. In one 10-week trial of augmentation of fluvoxamine 100–200 mg/day with minocycline 100 mg twice daily versus augmentation with placebo (n = 47 in each group), it was found that the minocycline group had a significantly lower YBOCS total scores compared to the placebo group at the end of the trial. The minocycline group also achieved higher remission, partial, and complete response rates compared to placebo at the end of the trial. Furthermore, there was a significantly shorter period of time needed in the minocycline group than the placebo group for a partial response to be achieved (Esalatmanesh et al., 2016).

In an 8-week trial investigating the anti-inflammatory agent celecoxib as an adjunctive treatment of OCD, 27 patients were placed on fluoxetine 20 mg/day plus celecoxib 200 mg twice daily, and 25 patients were placed on fluoxetine 20 mg/day plus placebo. It was found that patients in the celecoxib group had significantly lower YBOCS scores at the end of the study compared to placebo. Both groups showed a decline in mean YBOCS scores during the trial, but the celecoxib group started to decline sooner (by week 2) versus the placebo group (week 4) (Sayyah et al., 2011).

These experimental agents are placed after the SGAs in this algorithm due to the limited amount of evidence on each agent. However, they do show some positive benefit and one could debate whether they should be offered as a group at node 4. It is reasonable to present these options at the same time as antipsychotics, as most of the novel agents, except for ketamine and maybe topiramate, have fewer side effects compared to SGAs.

Node 6: Non-invasive device based therapy

If SGAs and any novel agents selected are not effective, the next step to consider is transcranial magnetic stimulation (rTMS). It is also reasonable to offer this treatment option at the same time as the novel agents to patients who might prefer this somatic therapy compared to taking another medication. rTMS has received many studies. A recent meta-analysis evaluated 15 RCTs with sham control as adjunctive treatment for OCD. Most of the trials targeted the dorsolateral prefrontal cortex. Active TMS was found to be significantly more effective than sham, but had questionable clinical meaningfulness due to the small effect size (2.94-point difference on YBOCS between groups) (Trevizol et al., 2016). However, media reports of interesting new data submitted to the FDA by the Brainsway "Deep" TMS System involving a study of 100 patients suggested that 38% responded with 30% reduction of YBOCS scores compared to an 11% response rate on sham. The FDA approved the device in 2018. The procedure is to apply the magnet for 25 min, 5 days a week for 6 weeks. The procedure costs over $10,000. An important additional aspect of the treatment in this study was the provision of a brief session just before each procedure in which patients were asked to think about their obsessions and compulsions. Hence, it was really a study of combined cognitive processing and magnetic stimulation. None of the other 15 RCTs employed this method and it may account for the (as yet unpublished) better results. It is unclear where this costly procedure belongs in the algorithm at this time. More study is needed. Also, nothing is known about what maintenance procedures would be needed to sustain the benefit.

Traditional electroconvulsive therapy could be considered for OCD patients who have severe comorbid depression that has not responded to the antidepressant trials (Hanisch et al., 2009).

Node 7: Neurosurgery

Finally, deep brain stimulation (DBS) and ablative surgery have been shown to be beneficial for severe and intractable OCD, but remain experimental. A meta-analysis of 31 DBS trials showed that YBOCS scores improved 45.1% in patients treated with DBS (Alonso et al., 2015). It was also found that 60% of patients treated with DBS met criteria for response to treatment (defined as a reduction of $\geq$ 35% on YBOCS). DBS responders had a significantly older age at onset of OCD than nonresponding patients (responders 17.1 years $\pm$ 7.9 vs non-responders 13.7 years $\pm$ 6.9) and more frequently reported obsessions and compulsions of sexual/religious content than non-responders (33% of responders compared to 0% of non-responders) (Alonso et al., 2015). Most responding patients also reported significant improvement in quality of life. Severe adverse events were less common with DBS than lesional neurosurgery (Alonso et al., 2015). Of note, the optimal brain region is still being established.

There is one double-blind RCT of radiosurgery (gamma ventral capsulotomy - GVC) of the anterior limb of the internal capsule, for patients with intractable OCD, which showed that 2 out of 8 patients (25%) in the active treatment group reached a response at 12 months (defined as a 35% or greater reduction in YBOCS and "improved" or "much improved" on the CGI-I) compared to 0 out of 8 patients in the sham group. This finding suggests that patients who underwent GVC may have benefited more than those who underwent sham surgery, although the difference was not statistically significant. However, in the open long-term follow-up phase, 3 additional patients in the active treatment group responded at post-GVC month 24, raising the response rate to 62.5% (Lopes et al., 2014). Furthermore, 2 out of 4 patients who received active treatment, after having been in the sham group initially, became responders at post-GVC months 12 and 24. In sum, of the 12 patients who ultimately received GVC, 7 (58.3%) became responders. Review of open-label gamma capsulotomy trials showed response rates of at least 55% in patients with severe refractory OCD (Leveque et al., 2013; Ruck et al., 2008). Capsulotomy is also effective in reducing OCD symptoms at long-term follow-up (mean of 10.9 years after surgery), but has a substantial risk of adverse effects, including problems with executive function, apathy, and disinhibition, particularly in patients who received high doses of radiation or underwent multiple surgical procedures (Ruck et al., 2008).

DISCUSSION

This algorithm organizes the evidence systematically for practical clinical application and can serve as a guide for clinicians in the management of OCD. It stresses the importance of adequate trials of SSRIs including adding the benefits of measuring plasma levels at times before going on to less established or more side-effect-prone augmentations or somatic procedures. Nevertheless, the treatment of OCD still has many challenges. There is much to be learned about the pathophysiology, genetics, and neurobiology of OCD that could improve future treatment and algorithms.

Declaration of Competing Interest

The authors declare that they have no known competing financial interests or personal relationships that could have appeared to influence the work reported in this paper.

Funding

This research did not receive any specific grant from funding agencies in the public, commercial, or not-for-profit sectors.

REFERENCES

Abejuela, H.R., Osser, D.N., 2016. The psychopharmacology algorithm project at the Harvard South Shore Program: an algorithm for generalized anxiety disorder. Harv. Rev. Psychiatry 24 (4), 243–256.

Addis, A., Koren, G., 2000. Safety of fluoxetine during the first trimester of pregnancy: a meta-analytical review of epidemiological studies. Psychol. Med. 30 (1), 89–94.

Alonso, P., Cuadras, D., Gabriels, L., Denys, D., Goodman, W., Greenberg, B.D., Jimenez-Ponce, F., Kuhn, J., Lenartz, D., Mallet, L., Nuttin, B., Real, E., Segalas, C., Schuurman, R., du Montcel, S.T., Menchon, J.M., 2015. Deep brain stimulation for obsessive-compulsive disorder: a meta-analysis of treatment outcome and predictors of response. PLoS ONE 10 (7), e0133591.

American Psychiatric Association, 1994. Diagnostic and Statistical Manual of Mental Disorders, IV ed. American Psychiatric Association, Washington, D.C.

American Psychiatric Association, 2013. Diagnostic and Statistical Manual of Mental Disorders, 5th ed. American Psychiatric Publishing, Washington, D.C.

Anglin, R., Yuan, Y., Moayyedi, P., Tse, F., Armstrong, D., Leontiadis, G.I., 2014. Risk of upper gastrointestinal bleeding with selective serotonin reuptake inhibitors with or without concurrent nonsteroidal anti-inflammatory use: a systematic review and meta-analysis. Am. J. Gastroenterol. 109 (6), 811–819.

Ansari, A., Osser, D.N., 2010. The psychopharmacology algorithm project at the Harvard South Shore Program: an update on bipolar depression. Harv. Rev. Psychiatry 18 (1), 36–55.

Bajor, L.A., Ticlea, A.N., Osser, D.N., 2011. The psychopharmacology algorithm project at the Harvard South Shore Program: an update on posttraumatic stress disorder. Harv. Rev. Psychiatry 19 (5), 240–258.

Balachander, S., Kodancha, P.G., Arumugham, S.S., Sekharan, J.T., Narayanaswamy, J.C., Reddy, Y.C.J., 2019. Effectiveness of venlafaxine in selective serotonin reuptake inhibitor-resistant obsessive-compulsive disorder: experience from a specialty clinic in India. J. Clin. Psychopharmacol. 39 (1), 82–85.

Beach, S.R., Celano, C.M., Noseworthy, P.A., Januzzi, J.L., Huffman, J.C., 2013. QTc prolongation, torsades de pointes, and psychotropic medications. Psychosomatics 54 (1), 1–13.

Berlin, H.A., Koran, L.M., Jenike, M.A., Shapira, N.A., Chaplin, W., Pallanti, S., Hollander, E., 2011. Double-blind, placebo-controlled trial of topiramate augmentation in treatment-resistant obsessive-compulsive disorder. J. Clin. Psychiatry 72 (5), 716–721.

Bertilsson, L., Dahl, M.L., Sjoqvist, F., Aberg-Wistedt, A., Humble, M., Johansson, I., Lundqvist, E., Ingelman-Sundberg, M., 1993. Molecular basis for rational mega-prescribing in ultrarapid hydroxylators of debrisoquine. Lancet 341 (8836), 63.

Bird, S.T., Crentsil, V., Temple, R., Pinheiro, S., Demczar, D., Stone, M., 2014. Cardiac safety concerns remain for citalopram at dosages above 40 mg/day. Am. J. Psychiatry 171 (1), 17–19.

Bloch, M.H., McGuire, J., Landeros-Weisenberger, A., Leckman, J.F., Pittenger, C., 2010. Meta-analysis of the dose-response relationship of SSRI in obsessive-compulsive disorder. Mol. Psychiatry 15 (8), 850–855.

Brandl, E.J., Tiwari, A.K., Zhou, X., Deluce, J., Kennedy, J.L., Muller, D.J., Richter, M.A., 2014. Influence of CYP2D6 and CYP2C19 gene variants on antidepressant response in obsessive-compulsive disorder. Pharmacogen. J. 14 (2), 176–181.

Bruno, A., Mico, U., Pandolfo, G., Mallamace, D., Abenavoli, E., Di Nardo, F., D'Arrigo, C., Spina, E., Zoccali, R.A., Muscatello, M.R., 2012. Lamotrigine augmentation of serotonin reuptake inhibitors in treatment-resistant obsessive-compulsive disorder: a double-blind, placebo-controlled study. J. Psychopharmacol. 26 (11), 1456–1462.

Burchi, E., Hollander, E., Pallanti, S., 2018. From treatment response to recovery: a realistic goal in OCD. Int. J. Neuropsychopharmacol. 21 (11), 1007–1013.

Cederlof, M., Lichtenstein, P., Larsson, H., Boman, M., Ruck, C., Landen, M., Mataix-Cols, D., 2015. Obsessive-Compulsive disorder, psychosis, and bipolarity: a longitudinal cohort and multigenerational family study. Schizophr. Bull. 41 (5), 1076–1083.

De Haan, L., Schirmbeck, F., Zink, M., 2015. Obsessive-compulsive Symptoms in Schizophrenia. Springer.

De Picker, L., Van Den Eede, F., Dumont, G., Moorkens, G., Sabbe, B.G., 2014. Antidepressants and the risk of hyponatremia: a class-by-class review of literature. Psychosomatics 55 (6), 536–547.

Denys, D., van der Wee, N., van Megen, H.J., Westenberg, H.G., 2003. A double blind comparison of venlafaxine and paroxetine in obsessive-compulsive disorder. J. Clin. Psychopharmacol. 23 (6), 568–575.

Diniz, J.B., Shavitt, R.G., Fossaluza, V., Koran, L., Pereira, C.A., Miguel, E.C., 2011. A double-blind, randomized, controlled trial of fluoxetine plus quetiapine or clomipramine versus fluoxetine plus placebo for obsessive-compulsive disorder. J. Clin. Psychopharmacol. 31 (6), 763–768.

El-Mallakh, R.S., Vohringer, P.A., Ostacher, M.M., Baldassano, C.F., Holtzman, N.S., Whitham, E.A., Thommi, S.B., Goodwin, F.K., Ghaemi, S.N., 2015. Antidepressants worsen rapid-cycling course in bipolar depression: a step-BD randomized clinical trial. J. Affect. Disord. 184, 318–321.

Emamzadehfard, S., Kamaloo, A., Paydary, K., Ahmadipour, A., Zeinoddini, A., Ghaleiha, A., Mohammadinejad, P., Zeinoddini, A., Akhondzadeh, S., 2016. Riluzole in augmentation of fluvoxamine for moderate to severe obsessive-compulsive disorder: randomized, double-blind, placebo-controlled study. Psychiatry Clin. Neurosci. 70 (8), 332–341.

Esalatmanesh, S., Abrishami, Z., Zeinoddini, A., Rahiminejad, F., Sadeghi, M., Najarzadegan, M.R., Shalbafan, M.R., Akhondzadeh, S., 2016. Minocycline combination therapy with fluvoxamine in moderate-to-severe obsessive-compulsive disorder: a placebo-controlled, double-blind, randomized trial. Psychiatry Clin. Neurosci. 70 (11), 517–526.

Fava, M., Judge, R., Hoog, S.L., Nilsson, M.E., Koke, S.C., 2000. Fluoxetine versus sertraline and paroxetine in major depressive disorder: changes in weight with longterm treatment. J. Clin. Psychiatry 61 (11), 863–867.

Fineberg, N.A., Gale, T.M., 2005. Evidence-based pharmacotherapy of obsessive-compulsive disorder. Int. J. Neuropsychopharmacol. 8 (1), 107–129.

Fineberg, N.A., Reghunandanan, S., Simpson, H.B., Phillips, K.A., Richter, M.A., Matthews, K., Stein, D.J., Sareen, J., Brown, A., Sookman, D., 2015. Obsessive-compulsive disorder (OCD): practical strategies for pharmacological and somatic treatment in adults. Psychiatry Res. 227 (1), 114–125.

Foa, E.B., Liebowitz, M.R., Kozak, M.J., Davies, S., Campeas, R., Franklin, M.E., Huppert, J.D., Kjernisted, K., Rowan, V., Schmidt, A.B., Simpson, H.B., Tu, X., 2005. Randomized, placebo-controlled trial of exposure and ritual prevention, clomipramine, and their combination in the treatment of obsessive-compulsive disorder. Am. J. Psychiatry 162 (1), 151–161.

Ghaleiha, A., Entezari, N., Modabbernia, A., Najand, B., Askari, N., Tabrizi, M., Ashrafi, M., Hajiaghaee, R., Akhondzadeh, S., 2013. Memantine add-on in moderate to severe obsessive-compulsive disorder: randomized double-blind placebo-controlled study. J. Psychiatr. Res. 47 (2), 175–180.

Giakoumatos, C.I., Osser, D., 2019. The psychopharmacology algorithm project at the Harvard South Shore Program: an update on unipolar nonpsychotic depression. Harv. Rev. Psychiatry 27 (1), 33–52.

Glassman, A.H., O'Connor, C.M., Califf, R.M., Swedberg, K., Schwartz, P., Bigger Jr., J.T., Krishnan, K.R., van Zyl, L.T., Swenson, J.R., Finkel, M.S., Landau, C., Shapiro, P.A., Pepine, C.J., Mardekian, J., Harrison, W.M., Barton, D., McLvor, M., 2002. Sertraline treatment of major depression in patients with acute MI or unstable angina. JAMA 288 (6), 701–709.

Greist, J.H., Jefferson, J.W., Kobak, K.A., Chouinard, G., DuBoff, E., Halaris, A., Kim, S.W., Koran, L., Liebowtiz, M.R., Lydiard, B., et al., 1995. A 1 year double-blind placebo-controlled fixed dose study of sertraline in the treatment of obsessive-compulsive disorder. Int. Clin. Psychopharmacol. 10 (2), 57–65.

Grillault Laroche, D., Gaillard, A., 2016. Induced Obsessive Compulsive Symptoms (OCS) in schizophrenia patients under atypical 2 antipsychotics (AAPs): review and hypotheses. Psychiatry Res. 246, 119–128.

Grunder, G., 2018. Editorial to consensus guidelines for therapeutic drug monitoring in neuropsychopharmacology. Pharmacopsychiatry 51 (1-02), 5–6.

Haghighi, M., Jahangard, L., Mohammad-Beigi, H., Bajoghli, H., Hafezian, H., Rahimi, A., Afshar, H., Holsboer-Trachsler, E., Brand, S., 2013. In a double-blind, randomized and placebo-controlled trial, adjuvant memantine improved symptoms in inpatients suffering from refractory obsessive-compulsive disorders (OCD). Psychopharmacology (Berl) 228 (4), 633–640.

Hamoda, H.M., Osser, D.N., 2008. The psychopharmacology algorithm project at the Harvard South Shore Program: an update on psychotic depression. Harv. Rev. Psychiatry 16 (4), 235–247.

Hanisch, F., Friedemann, J., Piro, J., Gutmann, P., 2009. Maintenance electroconvulsive therapy for comorbid pharmacotherapy-refractory obsessive-compulsive and schizoaffective disorder. Eur. J. Med. Res. 14 (8), 367–368.

Heidari, M., Zarei, M., Hosseini, S.M., Taghvaei, R., Maleki, H., Tabrizi, M., Fallah, J., Akhondzadeh, S., 2014. Ondansetron or placebo in the augmentation of fluvoxamine response over 8 weeks in obsessive-compulsive disorder. Int. Clin. Psychopharmacol. 29 (6), 344–350.

Heyman, I., Mataix-Cols, D., Fineberg, N.A., 2006. Obsessive-compulsive disorder. BMJ 333 (7565), 424–429.

House, S.J., Tripathi, S.P., Knight, B.T., Morris, N., Newport, D.J., Stowe, Z.N., 2016. Obsessive-compulsive disorder in pregnancy and the postpartum period: course of illness and obstetrical outcome. Arch. Womens Ment. Health 19 (1), 3–10.

Khalkhali, M., Aram, S., Zarrabi, H., Kafie, M., Heidarzadeh, A., 2016. Lamotrigine augmentation versus placebo in serotonin reuptake inhibitors-resistant obsessive-compulsive disorder: a randomized controlled trial. Iran J. Psychiatry 11 (2), 104–114.

Kieler, H., Artama, M., Engeland, A., Ericsson, O., Furu, K., Gissler, M., Nielsen, R.B., Norgaard, M., Stephansson, O., Valdimarsdottir, U., Zoega, H., Haglund, B., 2012. Selective serotonin reuptake inhibitors during pregnancy and risk of persistent pulmonary hypertension in the newborn: population based cohort study from the five Nordic countries. BMJ 344, d8012.

Koran, L.M., Cain, J.W., Dominguez, R.A., Rush, A.J., Thiemann, S., 1996. Are fluoxetine plasma levels related to outcome in obsessive-compulsive disorder? Am. J. Psychiatry 153 (11), 1450–1454.

Koran, L.M., Faravelli, C., Pallanti, S., 1994. Intravenous clomipramine for obsessive-compulsive disorder. J. Clin. Psychopharmacol. 14 (3), 216–218.

Koran, L.M., Gamel, N.N., Choung, H.W., Smith, E.H., Aboujaoude, E.N., 2005. Mirtazapine for obsessive-compulsive disorder: an open trial followed by doubleblind discontinuation. J. Clin. Psychiatry 66 (4), 515–520.

Koran, L.M., Hackett, E., Rubin, A., Wolkow, R., Robinson, D., 2002. Efficacy of sertraline in the long-term treatment of obsessive-compulsive disorder. Am. J. Psychiatry 159 (1), 88–95.

Leveque, M., Carron, R., Regis, J., 2013. Radiosurgery for the treatment of psychiatric disorders: a review. World Neurosurg. 80 (3–4), e31–e39 S32.

Lopes, A.C., Greenberg, B.D., Canteras, M.M., Batistuzzo, M.C., Hoexter, M.Q., Gentil, A.F., Pereira, C.A., Joaquim, M.A., de Mathis, M.E., D'Alcante, C.C., Taub, A., de Castro, D.G., Tokeshi, L., Sampaio, L.A., Leite, C.C., Shavitt, R.G., Diniz, J.B., Busatto, G., Noren, G., Rasmussen, S.A., Miguel, E.C., 2014. Gamma ventral capsulotomy for obsessive-compulsive disorder: a randomized clinical trial. JAMA Psychiatry 71 (9), 1066–1076.

March, J.S., 1997. The expert consensus guideline series: treatment of obsessive-compulsive disorder. J. Clin. Psychiatry 58 (Suppl), 1–72.

Marks, D.M., Park, M.H., Ham, B.J., Han, C., Patkar, A.A., Masand, P.S., Pae, C.U., 2008. Paroxetine: safety and tolerability issues. Expert Opin. Drug Saf. 7 (6), 783–794.

Matsunaga, H., Nagata, T., Hayashida, K., Ohya, K., Kiriike, N., Stein, D.J., 2009. A longterm trial of the effectiveness and safety of atypical antipsychotic agents in augmenting SSRI-refractory obsessive-compulsive disorder. J. Clin. Psychiatry 70 (6), 863–868.

McGirr, A., Vohringer, P.A., Ghaemi, S.N., Lam, R.W., Yatham, L.N., 2016. Safety and efficacy of adjunctive second-generation antidepressant therapy with a mood stabiliser or an atypical antipsychotic in acute bipolar depression: a systematic review and meta-analysis of randomised placebo-controlled trials. Lancet Psychiatry 3 (12), 1138–1146.

Mead, G.E., Hsieh, C.F., Hackett, M., 2013. Selective serotonin reuptake inhibitors for stroke recovery. JAMA 310 (10), 1066–1067.

Meier, S.M., Petersen, L., Pedersen, M.G., Arendt, M.C., Nielsen, P.R., Mattheisen, M., Mors, O., Mortensen, P.B., 2014. Obsessive-compulsive disorder as a risk factor for schizophrenia: a nationwide study. JAMA Psychiatry 71 (11), 1215–1221.

Meyer, J.M., Stahl, S.M., 2019. The Clozapine Handbook. Cambridge University Press, New York, NY.

Mohammad, O., Osser, D.N., 2014. The psychopharmacology algorithm project at the Harvard South Shore Program: an algorithm for acute mania. Harv. Rev. Psychiatry 22 (5), 274–294.

Montgomery, S.A., Kasper, S., Stein, D.J., Bang Hedegaard, K., Lemming, O.M., 2001. Citalopram 20 mg, 40 mg and 60 mg are all effective and well tolerated compared with placebo in obsessive-compulsive disorder. Int. Clin. Psychopharmacol. 16 (2), 75–86.

Naples, J.G., Kotlarczyk, M.P., Perera, S., Greenspan, S.L., Hanlon, J.T., 2016. Non-tricyclic and non-selective serotonin reuptake inhibitor antidepressants and recurrent falls in frail older women. Am. J. Geriatr. Psychiatry 24 (12), 1221–1227.

Ninan, P.T., Koran, L.M., Kiev, A., Davidson, J.R.T., Rasmussen, S.A., Zajecka, J.M., Robinson, D.G., Crits-Christoph, P., Mandel, F.S., Austin, C., 2006. High-Dose sertraline strategy for nonresponders to acute treatment for obsessive-compulsive disorder: a multicenter double-blind trial. J. Clin. Psychiatry 67 (1), 15–22.

Oesterheld, J., Osser, D.N., 1999. Drug interactions in augmentation strategies for pharmacotherapy of OCD. J. Pract. Psychiatry Behav. Health 5 (3), 179–183.

Osser, D.N., Dunlop, L.R., 2010. The psychopharmacology algorithm project at the Harvard South Shore Program an update on generalized social anxiety disorder. Psychopharm. Rev. 45 (12), 91–98.

Osser, D.N., Roudsari, M.J., Manschreck, T., 2013. The psychopharmacology algorithm project at the Harvard South Shore Program: an update on schizophrenia. Harv. Rev. Psychiatry 21 (1), 18–40.

Pacchiarotti, I., Bond, D.J., Baldessarini, R.J., Nolen, W.A., Grunze, H., Licht, R.W., Post, R.M., Berk, M., Goodwin, G.M., Sachs, G.S., Tondo, L., Findling, R.L., Youngstrom, E.A., Tohen, M., Undurraga, J., Gonzalez-Pinto, A., Goldberg, J.F., Yildiz, A., Altshuler, L.L., Calabrese, J.R., Mitchell, P.B., Thase, M.E., Koukopoulos, A., Colom, F., Frye, M.A., Malhi, G.S., Fountoulakis, K.N., Vazquez, G., Perlis, R.H., Ketter, T.A., Cassidy, F., Akiskal, H., Azorin, J.M., Valenti, M., Mazzei, D.H., Lafer, B., Kato, T., Mazzarini, L., Martinez-Aran, A., Parker, G., Souery, D., Ozerdem, A., McElroy, S.L., Girardi, P., Bauer, M., Yatham, L.N., Zarate, C.A., Nierenberg, A.A., Birmaher, B., Kanba, S., El-Mallakh, R.S., Serretti, A., Rihmer, Z., Young, A.H., Kotzalidis, G.D., MacQueen, G.M., Bowden, C.L., Ghaemi, S.N., Lopez-Jaramillo, C., Rybakowski, J., Ha, K., Perugi, G., Kasper, S., Amsterdam, J.D., Hirschfeld, R.M., Kapczinski, F., Vieta, E., 2013. The International Society for Bipolar Disorders (ISBD) task force report on antidepressant use in bipolar disorders. Am. J. Psychiatry 170 (11), 1249–1262.

Pallanti, S., Quercioli, L., Bruscoli, M., 2004. Response acceleration with mirtazapine augmentation of citalopram in obsessive-compulsive disorder patients without comorbid depression: a pilot study. J. Clin. Psychiatry 65 (10), 1394–1399.

Pampaloni, I., Sivakumaran, T., Hawley, C.J., Al Allaq, A., Farrow, J., Nelson, S., Fineberg, N.A., 2010. High-dose selective serotonin reuptake inhibitors in OCD: a systematic retrospective case notes survey. J. Psychopharmacol. 24 (10), 1439–1445.

Paton, C., Ferrier, I.N., 2005. SSRIs and gastrointestinal bleeding. BMJ 331 (7516), 529–530.

Paydary, K., Akamaloo, A., Ahmadipour, A., Pishgar, F., Emamzadehfard, S., Akhondzadeh, S., 2016. N-acetylcysteine augmentation therapy for moderate-to-severe obsessive-compulsive disorder: randomized, double-blind, placebo-controlled trial. J. Clin. Pharm. Ther. 41 (2), 214–219.

Phelps, N.J., Cates, M.E., 2005. The role of venlafaxine in the treatment of obsessive-compulsive disorder. Ann. Pharmacother. 39 (1), 136–140.

Pigott, T.A., L'Heureux, F., Rubenstein, C.S., Bernstein, S.E., Hill, J.L., Murphy, D.L., 1992. A double-blind, placebo controlled study of trazodone in patients with obsessive-compulsive disorder. J. Clin. Psychopharmacol. 12 (3), 156–162.

Ravizza, L., Barzega, G., Bellino, S., Bogetto, F., Maina, G., 1996. Drug treatment of obsessive-compulsive disorder (OCD): long-term trial with clomipramine and selective serotonin reuptake inhibitors (SSRIs). Psychopharmacol. Bull. 32 (1), 167–173.

Reefhuis, J., Devine, O., Friedman, J.M., Louik, C., Honein, M.A., 2015. Specific SSRIs and birth defects: bayesian analysis to interpret new data in the context of previous reports. BMJ 351, h3190.

Rodriguez, C.I., Kegeles, L.S., Levinson, A., Feng, T., Marcus, S.M., Vermes, D., Flood, P., Simpson, H.B., 2013. Randomized controlled crossover trial of ketamine in obsessive-compulsive disorder: proof-of-concept. Neuropsychopharmacology 38 (12), 2475–2483.

Ruck, C., Karlsson, A., Steele, J.D., Edman, G., Meyerson, B.A., Ericson, K., Nyman, H., Asberg, M., Svanborg, P., 2008. Capsulotomy for obsessive-compulsive disorder: long-term follow-up of 25 patients. Arch. Gen. Psychiatry 65 (8), 914–921.

Rush, A.J., Trivedi, M.H., Wisniewski, S.R., Nierenberg, A.A., Stewart, J.W., Warden, D., Niederehe, G., Thase, M.E., Lavori, P.W., Lebowitz, B.D., McGrath, P.J., Rosenbaum, J.F., Sackeim, H.A., Kupfer, D.J., Luther, J., Fava, M., 2006. Acute and longer-term outcomes in depressed outpatients requiring one or several treatment steps: a STAR*D report. Am. J. Psychiatry 163 (11), 1905-1917.

Sahraian, A., Jahromi, L.R., Ghanizadeh, A., Mowla, A., 2017. Memantine as an adjuvant treatment for obsessive compulsive symptoms in manic phase of bipolar disorder: a randomized, double-blind, placebo-controlled clinical trial. J. Clin. Psychopharmacol. 37 (2), 246–249.

Sansone, R.A., Sansone, L.A., 2011. SNRIs pharmacological alternatives for the treatment of obsessive compulsive disorder? Innov. Clin. Neurosci. 8 (6), 10–14.

Sayyah, M., Boostani, H., Pakseresht, S., Malayeri, A., 2011. A preliminary randomized double-blind clinical trial on the efficacy of celecoxib as an adjunct in the treatment of obsessive-compulsive disorder. Psychiatry Res. 189 (3), 403–406.

Schirmbeck, F., Konijn, M., Hoetjes, V., Zink, M., de Haan, L., For Genetic, R., 2019. Obsessive-compulsive symptoms in psychotic disorders: longitudinal associations of symptom clusters on between-and within-subject levels. Eur. Arch. Psychiatry Clin. Neurosci. 269 (2), 245–255.

Schule, C., Laakmann, G., 2005. Mirtazapine plus citalopram has short term but not longer term benefits over citalopram alone for the symptoms of obsessive compulsive disorder. Evid. Based Ment. Health 8 (2), 42.

Selvi, Y., Atli, A., Aydin, A., Besiroglu, L., Ozdemir, P., Ozdemir, O., 2011. The comparison of aripiprazole and risperidone augmentation in selective serotonin reuptake inhibitor-refractory obsessive-compulsive disorder: a single-blind, randomised study. Hum. Psychopharmacol. 26 (1), 51–57.

Serretti, A., Chiesa, A., 2009. Treatment-emergent sexual dysfunction related to antidepressants: a meta-analysis. J. Clin. Psychopharmacol. 29 (3), 259–266.

Soltani, F., Sayyah, M., Feizy, F., Malayeri, A., Siahpoosh, A., Motlagh, I., 2010. A doubleblind, placebo-controlled pilot study of ondansetron for patients with obsessive-compulsive disorder. Hum. Psychopharmacol. 25 (6), 509–513.

Stein, D.J., Andersen, E.W., Tonnoir, B., Fineberg, N., 2007. Escitalopram in obsessive-compulsive disorder: a randomized, placebo-controlled, paroxetine-referenced, fixed-dose, 24-week study. Curr. Med. Res. Opin. 23 (4), 701–711.

Stein, D.J., Koen, N., Fineberg, N., Fontenelle, L.F., Matsunaga, H., Osser, D., Simpson, H. B., 2012. A 2012 evidence-based algorithm for the pharmacotherapy for obsessive-compulsive disorder. Curr. Psychiatry Rep. 14 (3), 211–219.

Thanacoody, H.K., Thomas, S.H., 2005. Tricyclic antidepressant poisoning : cardiovascular toxicity. Toxicol. Rev. 24 (3), 205–214.

Thoren, P., Asberg, M., Cronholm, B., Jornestedt, L., Traskman, L., 1980. Clomipramine treatment of obsessive-compulsive disorder. I. A controlled clinical trial. Arch. Gen. Psychiatry 37 (11), 1281–1285.

Tollefson, G.D., Rampey Jr., A.H., Potvin, J.H., Jenike, M.A., Rush, A.J., kominguez, R.A., Koran, L.M., Shear, M.K., Goodman, W., Genduso, L.A., 1994. A multicenter investigation of fixed-dose fluoxetine in the treatment of obsessive-compulsive disorder. Arch. Gen. Psychiatry 51 (7), 559–567.

Trevizol, A.P., Shiozawa, P., Cook, I.A., Sato, I.A., Kaku, C.B., Guimaraes, F.B., Sachdev, P., Sarkhel, S., Cordeiro, Q., 2016. Transcranial magnetic stimulation for obsessive-compulsive disorder: an updated systematic review and meta-analysis. J. ect 32 (4), 262–266.

Uguz, F., Sahingoz, M., Gungor, B., Aksoy, F., Askin, R., 2015. Weight gain and associated factors in patients using newer antidepressant drugs. Gen. Hosp. Psychiatry 37 (1), 46–48.

Veale, D., Miles, S., Smallcombe, N., Ghezai, H., Goldacre, B., Hodsoll, J., 2014. Atypical antipsychotic augmentation in SSRI treatment refractory obsessive-compulsive disorder: a systematic review and meta-analysis. BMC Psychiatry 14, 317.

Vulink, N.C., Denys, D., Westenberg, H.G., 2005. Bupropion for patients with obsessive-compulsive disorder: an open-label, fixed-dose study. J. Clin. Psychiatry 66 (2), 228–230.

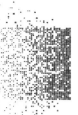

Pharmacologic Approach to the Psychiatric Inpatient*

Arash Ansari, MD, David N. Osser, MD, Leonard S. Lai, MD, Paul M. Schoenfeld, MD, and Kenneth C. Potts, MD

CHARACTERISTICS OF INPATIENT TREATMENT

The role of inpatient psychiatric treatment has evolved in recent decades. Psychopharmacologic advances have enabled more successful treatment of major mental illnesses. The movement to deinstitutionalize psychiatric patients and shift care to community-based agencies and the economic realities of the health care marketplace have had major impact to reduce the length of stay. Nevertheless, a recent study by the U.S. Health and Human Services Agency for Healthcare Research and Quality[1] found that in 2004, 1.9 million out of 32 million admissions (6%) to US community hospitals were primarily for a mental health or substance abuse diagnosis, while an additional 5.7 million admissions (18%) also involved depression, bipolar disorder, schizophrenia, or other mental health diagnoses or substance abuse-related disorders as a secondary diagnosis. The top five diagnoses reported were mood disorders, substance abuse-related disorders, delirium/dementia, anxiety disorders, and schizophrenia. The average length of stay for a patient with a primary mental health or substance abuse diagnosis was 8 days compared to 5 days for nonmental health-related diagnoses.

Because of time limitations, the goals of inpatient psychiatry have shifted from striving to achieve full remission to symptom alleviation through the judicious use of psychotropic medication so that the stay can be brief. Patients may therefore be discharged as long as they are evaluated to be unlikely to harm themselves or others, even though only some of the most distressing symptoms have improved, for example, agitation, anxiety, or insomnia. Medication treatment plans focus on these symptoms with the understanding that the full effect and benefit may not occur for several weeks. Psychosocial treatments such as intensive short-term individual psychotherapy, group therapy, and milieu interventions that apply the principles of psychodynamic, cognitive, behavioral, and dialectic behavioral techniques are vital in helping patients reduce problematic thoughts, behavior, feelings, and other responses to their stressors and symptoms in the inpatient setting. As no patient exists in a vacuum, outreach to families, significant others, and social supports to address possible acute psychosocial precipitants will contribute to helping reduce the likelihood of a relapse or a recurrence. Consultations with outpatient providers can be of critical importance. The inpatient stay can often provide an opportunity to clarify how the community treatment network can be made more efficient and responsive to the patient's needs.

---

*From Principles of Inpatient Psychiatry. Ovsiew F and Munich RI, Eds. Wolters Kluwer Health/Lippincott Williams & Wilkins. New York, 2009: 43-69.

FACTORS INFLUENCING PHARMACOTHERAPY ON AN INPATIENT UNIT

Publicly and privately funded inpatient psychiatric treatment is usually authorized for patients who present a danger to themselves or to others or who have demonstrated that they are unable to care for themselves. Inpatient treatment is monitored closely by mental health review agencies hired to ensure that this most expensive level of psychiatric care is used effectively and minimally in order to contain costs. Inpatient treatment teams must be vigilant about the time limitations imposed on each admission. This is made more difficult by the fact that the safety concerns that open the door to an inpatient admission generally are often found to be complicated by a myriad of additional reasons for which the patient has come to the attention of health care providers. Thorough assessment and formulation of why the patient is in a crisis must be done quickly and with a careful evaluation of which symptoms and contributing factors are the most important to address. These factors can range from noncompliance with treatment because of poor insight to limited treatment access and to destabilizing forces such as homelessness and family or relationship conflicts. Patients have comorbid medical illnesses or substance abuse-related factors that confound and prevent successful outpatient interventions. Therefore, the challenge for the inpatient multidisciplinary treatment team is to be able to evaluate and stabilize the sickest patients in the psychiatric care continuum in the shortest time possible.

In some cases, keeping the inpatient stay brief may be therapeutic, especially in the more character-disordered where the inpatient treatment milieu may encourage regressive behaviors.

GOAL OF INPATIENT TREATMENT AS RELATED TO PHARMACOTHERAPY

The task of the psychiatrist is to alleviate some of the presenting symptoms. This may mean the commencement of a new medicine or the resumption or adjustment of a medication regimen that has been effective in the past. The choices made have to enable prompt and effective symptom relief while the patient is in the hospital and to be feasible for the outpatient treatment team to continue in the community. Some medicines will be effective in the short run, for example, benzodiazepines for anxiety, whereas other medicines such as antidepressants are initiated with the expectation that in time a more definitive effect will occur. In other situations, it may be preferable to withhold initiation of pharmacologic treatment, such as when the presenting picture is complicated by significant substance abuse that obscures determination of whether Axis I pathology is primary or secondary. The opportunity to observe the initial response to medication will also allow evaluation of side effects, such as excess sedation or akathisia, which may preclude the use of that particular drug.

Close observations by the treatment team facilitate psychopharmacology decisions dependent on symptoms rather than syndromal diagnoses. For example, medicine may be given to target anxiety symptoms while it is determined if the symptoms are part of a mood disorder or an independent anxiety disorder.

It is important to explain to the patient and his or her family that the short length of stay allowed does not commonly result in full remission. They need to understand that the goal is to reduce troubling symptoms and to enable the patient to feel safer, be in better behavioral control, and to be able to function better with or without the assistance of others in the community. Often the suicidal or homicidal ideation that prompted the admission will resolve soon after admission because of the containment and structure of the supportive inpatient milieu. The focus will then quickly shift to the crucial question of whether the patient still requires inpatient level of care.

SELECTING TREATMENT

Selecting initial psychopharmacologic treatment for a newly admitted patient can be a complicated process and is based on multiple considerations and variables. Often the prescribing physician must weigh many of these variables simultaneously and rapidly given the complicated psychiatric, medical, and psychosocial presentations of most hospitalized patients. Ten factors that influence choice of initial agent will be reviewed.

SYMPTOM CONTROL—THE AGITATED PATIENT AND THE USE OF P.R.N. MEDICATION

The inpatient psychiatrist is faced with the challenge of making a provisional diagnosis and an initial treatment plan for the patient. Sometimes this diagnosis is based on very limited or even contradictory clinical and historical data. The clinician must be aware that new information may come to light, and the diagnoses may need to be modified. Recalling the guiding principles of "safety first" and "do no harm" is frequently helpful.

It is important to identify and treat the most serious symptoms regardless of diagnosis—these include violence, aggression, assault, self-harm, suicide, disorganizing psychosis, agitation, and risk of dying from inanition or other complications of poor oral intake and immobility (e.g., deep venous thrombosis [DVT], aspiration pneumonia, and skin breakdown). A symptom-based approach to psychopharmacologic treatment in an inpatient setting is therefore often necessary. This section will focus on the treatment of the agitated patient and the use of p.r.n. medication.

The Agitated Patient

A patient may become agitated at any time during the admission. Upon entry to the hospital, factors include the effects of being confined, the change in environment, and the loss of autonomy. A patient may become agitated later in the admission, such as if too rapidly allowed out of a contained situation or denied privileges. Nicotine-dependent patients can become extremely agitated if not permitted to smoke when they want. Interestingly, a recent study found that when units become smoke-free, incidents of agitation and restraint are markedly reduced.[2]

The violent, aggressive, or out-of-control patient can be very difficult to manage. The risk of assault or of self-harm must be assessed and reassessed. Prevention is the best approach, of course, with active treatment of any patient who may be at risk.

Certainly, the intensive use of the structure of the inpatient milieu can be instrumental in minimizing the need for medication. The containment of quiet rooms and destimulation can reduce potentially stressful situations for the patient, allowing time for a treatment plan to help an agitated patient.

However, there are situations where all the best efforts fail. Safety of the patient or staff is at risk, and sometimes urgent medication is necessary. When a rapid response is required, parenteral medication is indicated (although in less acute situations oral medication should be considered). A combination of an intramuscular typical antipsychotic and a benzodiazepine has been shown to be more effective than either one used alone.[3] This combination can avoid the need for an adjunctive dose of an anticholinergic; extrapyramidal symptoms (EPS) are infrequent. The advantages are avoiding both additional injections and anticholinergic toxicity. A common combination includes haloperidol 2 to 5 mg along with lorazepam 1 to 2 mg intramuscularly (in the same syringe) given every 30 to 60 minutes, up to three doses. Haloperidol is often considered first-line because of its relative safety profile, the lack of an established ceiling dose, and years of clinical experience. Other typical antipsychotics are less often used in this situation and have become less available. Intramuscular chlorpromazine is not recommended because of its high risk of hypotension. Intramuscular droperidol should not be used in the emergency treatment of agitation because of the increased risk of QTc prolongation with this agent.

The role of intramuscular atypical antipsychotics (i.e., ziprasidone, olanzapine, aripiprazole) is less clear. The upper limit of dosing and risks of drug interactions (e.g., QTc prolongation issues) may preclude ongoing use in an agitated patient. Although these drugs are heavily promoted by their manufacturers and many clinicians use them, the evidence base is unsatisfactory. All have been compared with haloperidol alone, without lorazepam or concomitant anticholinergic agents.[4-6] This gave the atypicals an unfair advantage.

One alternative to consider is monotherapy with parenteral lorazepam. This can be a valuable option when exposure to a typical antipsychotic is undesirable. A usual dose may be 1 to 3 mg intramuscularly hourly up to three doses. Some clinicians may be hesitant to use benzodiazepines with a substance-using patient. However, its efficacy in treating agitation in an emergency may well outweigh these concerns. Some clinicians are also concerned about the risk of "disinhibition" or a paradoxical reaction. There are no clear risk factors for this, and it appears to be rare. The risk of respiratory depression with repeated doses of benzodiazepines should be taken into account, especially if the patient has other sedating drugs on board, or has pulmonary insufficiency. As with all medication, an elderly agitated patient may require significant dose reduction and greater intervals between dosing.

Use of p.r.n. Medication

The use of so-called p.r.n. medication (*pro re nata*—"as the thing is born") is common in inpatient psychiatry to treat a variety of symptoms, including agitation (see preceding text), anxiety, breakthrough psychotic symptoms, and insomnia. Judicious use of p.r.n. medication can be very helpful in evaluating the need to change the standing medication plan. For example, the psychotic patient who is not "held" by his standing medication and needs "extra" doses may need a reevaluation of the standing medication dose.

However, there are also potential pitfalls. There is the risk of forming an association, on the part of the patient, between an undesirable behavior and taking an extra pill, thereby reinforcing drug-seeking behavior and externalization of responsibility. On many units, the culture is to actively encourage patients, if in distress, to ask for a p.r.n. medication. The astute clinician then helps the patient identify the precipitating factor and solve the problem, thereby fostering more of a sense of self-control on the part of the patient.

The milieu effect of p.r.n. medication is important to consider. Asking for extra medicine may be a patient's way of communicating the need for more contact, especially in a busy inpatient unit. The patient may then feel heard, attended to, and held, even if medicine is not offered. The interaction allows for more patient-staff contact. In addition, nursing staff often feel safer if p.r.n. medication is "on the books" for a challenging patient. The placebo effect of p.r.n. medication must not be overlooked.

The choice of a p.r.n. agent should take into account the relevant symptom and the current medication list. Attention should be paid to the total daily dose (standing plus p.r.n. available) so as to avoid exceeding maximum recommended doses. When treating psychosis or mania, p.r.n. medication should ideally be the same as the standing medication, so as to avoid the risks of polypharmacy, including the risks of adverse (e.g., cardiac) effects. Adjunctive use of benzodiazepines can be very helpful in psychotic patients.[3]

In patients with anxiety, short-acting or intermediate acting benzodiazepines are often used. Although not approved by the U.S. Food and Drug Administration (FDA), many clinicians use low-dose antipsychotics in these patients, especially if substance abuse is an issue. Low-dose antipsychotics may be particularly helpful in patients with anxiety or agitation associated with personality disorders[7,8] (see subsequent text). Trazodone is a cost-effective alternative that needs further study. Prazosin can be useful as a p.r.n. during the day for patients with post-traumatic stress disorder (PTSD) as well as at night for sleep.[9,10]

Insomnia is probably the single symptom for which p.r.n. medication is most frequently requested. Insomnia may be due to the environment, a side effect of medication, a complication of a general medical condition (such as restless legs syndrome [RLS] or obstructive sleep apnea), a consequence of excessive intake of caffeine or nicotine, a symptom of withdrawal, and so on. Although sleep hygiene should be addressed, often medication is required. Choices include antihistamines, benzodiazepines, trazodone, low-dose sedating tricyclic antidepressants, prazosin, and newer hypnotics.

Psychotropic medicines, both p.r.n. and standing, also play a crucial role in the treatment of patients with borderline personality disorder (BPD). Often patients with BPD are admitted to inpatient units when they are emotionally overwhelmed, regressed, and in poor behavioral control. Heightened emotional lability, irritability, anger, impulsivity, transient psychosis, and agitation can all be present. Frequently p.r.n. medicines are used to decrease the intensity of these symptoms, and, if helpful, may be continued as standing treatment. When the patient with BPD exhibits dangerous agitation that places the patient or others directly at risk of harm, then, as is the case in the schizophrenic or manic patient, intramuscular or oral antipsychotics are likely to be needed. Overall total doses needed are usually less than those employed in manic or psychotically agitated patients. Even when immediate dangerousness is not an issue, antipsychotics can be used to decrease patient hostility and transient psychosis.[11] Although there is no reason to believe that any one antipsychotic is more effective than any other, in acute situations many clinicians prefer to use an antipsychotic that can have immediate and observable effect (e.g., perphenazine, haloperidol, or risperidone). Quetiapine is also frequently used for p.r.n. treatment of anxiety in patients with BPD. Disinhibition from benzodiazepines (which as previously noted is of limited concern when treating violent behavior in general) is of particular concern in patients with BPD and may lead to further behavioral dyscontrol;[12] benzodiazepines, therefore, should not be used to treat anxiety in these patients. Once acuity has decreased and transient psychotic phenomena have subsided, continuing an antipsychotic as a standing medication may help reduce impulsivity and aggression, and improve overall functioning.[13] Again, total doses needed are usually lower than those needed for the ongoing treatment of a primary psychotic disorder.[14,15] Quetiapine and aripiprazole may also be helpful for ongoing mood and anxiety symptoms in these patients.[8,16] Serotonergic antidepressants and mood stabilizers may help primarily with affective lability and anger.[11,13] One controlled study of 30 patients suggested that omega-3 fatty acids may reduce depression and aggression in patients with moderate BPD.[17] On the other extreme with respect to toxicity, clozapine has been reported in several uncontrolled studies to be helpful in reducing morbidity in some treatment refractory patients.[18,19]

PATIENT'S PSYCHOPHARMACOLOGIC HISTORY

An advantage the inpatient psychiatrist has is extended time to obtain a history of the psychopharmacologic treatment the patient has received. It is time well spent. The psychiatrist should have several interviews with the patient over a few days to ascertain as much detail as possible about what the patient remembers about his medication history. Information about dose, efficacy, side effects, duration of treatment, and use of different medication combinations is necessary to formulate an approach and apply relevant treatment algorithms. The level of functional recovery with previous treatment interventions is critical to assess. An understanding of the factors that contribute to compliance or noncompliance is essential for establishing the ongoing medication treatment alliance. Repeating treatment trials that have failed in the past is to be avoided if possible. It is important to obtain a comprehensive list of all prescribed and over-the-counter medicines used by the patient for general medical ailments to evaluate for possible drug interactions.

Careful medication reconciliation on admission is required. The physician must accurately determine what the patient was taking immediately before admission. For each identified item, there should be clear documentation of the plan to continue, change, or stop the medication. This practice promotes the accurate administration of medication.

Because the patient may be an unreliable informant, collateral information from out-patient clinicians and family members should be actively sought as soon as possible. They often have critical insights and observations about how effective different psychopharma-cologic interventions have been.

When medical records are available to supplement the data collected from patients and significant others, history gathering is easier. Fortunately, more and more health care organizations are switching to electronic information systems that enable all clinicians to have fast, convenient, and accurate access to psychiatric and general medical histories at the touch of a keyboard. However, when the patient is treated in multiple unrelated health care systems, it can still be extremely difficult to obtain accurate, sequenced historical in-formation in a timely manner for a short inpatient stay. Error-prone educated guesswork can often not be avoided especially in the early days of an admission.

PREEXISTING GENERAL MEDICAL CONDITIONS

There are certain common general medical concerns that influence the selection of phar-macologic agents. Very early in the decision-making process, many physicians first glance at the patient's past medical history to clarify the "medical milieu" in which they will be prescribing. Rapid access to laboratory data as well as other testing (e.g., electrocardiogram [ECG]), and review of general medical history especially in an electronic medical record, when available, are extremely helpful.

Cardiac

Many psychotropics can affect cardiac conduction, with the potential to delay conduction enough to lead to fatal arrhythmias. There is an association between sudden death and the use of antipsychotics[20] and tricyclic antidepressants at high doses[21] (but not selective sero-tonin reuptake inhibitors [SSRIs]), although causality has not been completely established, and there may be multiple etiologies. The cardiovascular effects of psychotropics should therefore be taken into account before beginning treatment.

Prolonged QT interval (reported as QTc when corrected for heart rate) is believed to be associated with *torsades de pointes*, a potentially fatal ventricular arrhythmia. The QT interval includes both the QRS interval as well as the ST segment. Whereas QRS (depolarization phase) lengthening is primarily associated with the use of tricyclic antide-pressants (or low-potency typical antipsychotics with tricyclic structure) and their effect on sodium channels, atypical antipsychotics may potentially prolong the ST segment (repolarization phase) through their effect on potassium channels.[22] Although there is some question whether QT prolongation is a reliable indicator for the risk of *torsades de pointes*,[23] measuring this interval is the simplest way to estimate this risk.

Antipsychotics are not equal in their potential to affect the QT interval. Thioridazine, mesoridazine, pimozide, and droperidol[24] have shown significant potential to prolong QT and should generally be avoided. Among the newer antipsychotics, ziprasidone is considered to have the greatest potential to lengthen QT.[22] Some postmarketing studies such as the Clinical Antipsychotic Trials of Intervention Effectiveness (CATIE) have not confirmed this.[25,26] Premarketing data with aripiprazole indicate little risk.[27] Clozapine may contribute to QT prolongation primarily in patients with other risk factors.[28] The other cardiac risks of clozapine, that is risk of developing myocarditis or cardiomyopathy, are etiologically independent of its effect on cardiac conduction.

Tricyclic antidepressants, especially at high doses (particularly in the setting of overdose), have long been known for their potential to interfere with cardiac conduction and have traditionally been used with caution in patients with cardiac disease. Lithium may worsen sick sinus syndrome, produce blockade of the sinoatrial node, and also prolong QT.[29] SSRIs do not appear to significantly prolong QT, although there has been concern regarding their potential to induce bradycardia .[30-32]

Patients at higher cardiac risk should be identified before starting treatment with antipsychotics, tricyclic antidepressants, and lithium. Caution should be used in the care of the elderly, those with preexisting cardiac disease or preexisting QT prolongation, bradycardia, hypokalemia, or hypomagnesemia, and in those taking concomitant medication with proarrhythmic potential. A baseline ECG should be obtained in these patients; if the QTc is >440 to 450 msec, the patient should be monitored more carefully, and a QTc >500 msec should greatly increase concern for arrhythmias. Ziprasidone is contraindicated if the QTc is >500 msec. Magnesium and potassium abnormalities should be corrected early on. In high-risk patients, medicines with lower potential for cardiac toxicity should be used, and an effort should be made to use the lowest effective dose. Additionally, the clinician should be aware of medication interactions that may increase the serum level of the selected agent (see section on Medication Interactions). The clinician should also consider obtaining repeat ECGs on any patient who is being treated with two or more psychotropics with high risks of QT prolongation as the doses of these medications are titrated.

Blood Pressure

Many commonly used psychotropics have a-adrenergic blocking effects and can therefore lower blood pressure. Some of the observed cases of sudden death in patients taking antipsychotics or tricyclic antidepressants may be primarily due to severe hypotension rather than to cardiac arrhythmias. Vital signs, commonly checked on admission and daily thereafter, can identify those with preexisting hypotension. Patients at risk for orthostatic hypotension include the elderly, those with cardiac disease, and those taking other medicines that can lower blood pressure. Medicines whose propensity to lower blood pressure mandates caution are clozapine, chlorpromazine, risperidone, quetiapine, tricyclic antidepressants, and trazodone. Clozapine, which carries the highest risk of causing orthostasis, requires a very gradual and careful titration (i.e., starting at 12.5 mg once or twice a day with increases starting with 25 mg increments daily). In the patient who has been noncompliant it should not be restarted at prior doses if treatment has been interrupted for 2 or more days. Chlorpromazine administered intramuscularly or at sudden high oral doses carries a similar risk. Although tolerance to this side effect usually develops, care should be exercised when starting these medicines (or restarting them at previously prescribed high doses in patients who may have been recently nonadherent to their regimen). Increased fluid intake should be encouraged as tolerated and orthostatic blood pressure should be monitored in symptomatic patients until the appropriate dose is reached.

In regard to the risk of increasing blood pressure, there has been concern regarding the use of serotonin and norepinephrine reuptake inhibitors (SNRIs) in patients at risk for hypertension. Venlafaxine used at high doses can increase blood pressure.[33,34] This effect may be less pronounced with duloxetine and may not be clinically significant.[35,36] Patients with stable, effectively treated hypertension have not been found to show an increase in blood pressure from venlafaxine.[37]

Hepatic

There are two considerations regarding choice of psychiatric drug in a patient with compromised hepatic function. The first is the issue of hepatotoxicity with certain medicines, and the second is the use of hepatically metabolized agents in patients with preexisting liver disease. Baseline liver function tests should be measured, and if high, should influence care when using certain psychotropics.

Valproate, olanzapine, and quetiapine can cause hepatotoxicity. Although in the vast majority of cases any elevation in transaminases is mild and transient, these medicines should be used cautiously. The presence of clinically active liver disease or cirrhosis would suggest use of other agents (e.g., lithium rather than valproate for mania). If, during early inpatient treatment, transaminase levels increase to more than three times the upper end of the normal range, discontinuing or decreasing the dose of the offending agent should be considered. Patients with previous exposure to hepatitis B or C virus who are not acutely ill can still be treated with these medicines, although transaminases should be carefully monitored.[38,39] Given the concern that one would be exposing these patients with potentially worsening liver disease to yet another toxic insult, alternative nonhepatotoxic agents (e.g., lithium) should be considered when appropriate. Valproate may also rarely cause hyperammonemic encephalopathy without causing transaminase elevation,[40] although this is controversial.[41]

In the case of a patient admitted with preexisting liver disease, medicines which are primarily hepatically metabolized should be started at lower doses and increased slowly and agents with shorter half-lives should be used preferentially.

Renal

Measurement of kidney function, that is serum creatinine, is routinely done upon admission to an inpatient unit. Lithium, topiramate, and gabapentin are cleared by the kidneys, and any decrease in renal function warrants dose reduction of these medicines.

A common scenario is the admission to the inpatient unit of a patient whose lithium has been discontinued as an outpatient, because of concerns regarding worsening renal function (as can occur in up to 20% of patients on long-term lithium treatment).[42] Often the patient had been previously well maintained for many years on lithium. Once lithium is discontinued, however, the patient may decompensate and require multiple alternative medication trials and multiple hospitalizations for recurrent manic or depressive episodes. In these patients, the overall risks of morbidity and mortality may be less with rechallenge with lithium than if lithium treatment is withheld. After a clear risk and benefit assessment, and in close consultation with a nephrologist, it may be clinically appropriate for these patients to resume taking lithium. Close monitoring from then on, while avoiding further episodes of lithium toxicity, and administration of lithium once a day at bedtime, may decrease the risk of worsening renal effects.[43]

Metabolic Syndrome

Metabolic syndrome is characterized by dyslipidemia, hyperglycemia, and weight gain and is a major risk associated with some second-generation antipsychotics.

Hyperglycemia/Diabetes

The prevalence of diabetes is higher in patients with schizophrenia (in part because of unhealthy lifestyles) independent of treatment with antipsychotics.[44] Clozapine and olanzapine have clearly been implicated in increased risk of onset of hyperglycemia and diabetes, and in the exacerbation of preexisting diabetes, even leading to diabetic ketoacidosis. The propensity of quetiapine to cause hyperglycemia is numerically greater than that of other second-generation antipsychotics but less than that of the two agents mentioned earlier.[25] The data regarding risperidone are mixed.[45] One putative mechanism is that some of these agents rapidly induce insulin resistance, with or without causing weight gain.

Measuring fasting plasma glucose and inquiring about a patient's personal and family history of hyperglycemia and/or diabetes can help identify those at risk for developing diabetes, and determining hemoglobin A_{1c} can provide a measure of recent glycemic control. In patients at high risk of developing diabetes, aripiprazole or ziprasidone should be considered.[46] If fasting glucose is elevated, a glucose tolerance test has excellent predictive value regarding who is going to develop overt diabetes.[47]

Weight Gain

The risk of significant weight gain, particularly in the first few months of treatment, should be considered when prescribing atypical antipsychotics. A 2- to 3-kg weight gain early in the course of treatment (i.e., within the first 3 weeks) often predicts the risk of substantial weight gain over the long term.[48] However, different antipsychotics are not equal in their propensity to cause obesity. Clozapine and olanzapine are generally considered to be more likely to cause weight gain than quetiapine and risperidone, and in turn aripiprazole and ziprasidone are the least likely to contribute to weight gain.[49] Measuring baseline body mass index (BMI) and waist circumference are recommended by recent guidelines.[46] A patient's admission weight must be measured to establish a pretreatment baseline.

Hyperlipidemia

Antipsychotics that have the highest propensity to cause weight gain also carry the highest risk of worsening lipid profile. Risperidone may be more neutral in this regard, and ziprasidone may actually improve lipid profile.[25] Triglycerides are the lipids most affected by the use of atypical antipsychotics.[50] A fasting lipid profile can identify those patients already at higher cardiac risk and again serve as a pretreatment baseline. Pharmacotherapy of hyperlipidemia may be necessary. Also education on diet and lifestyle changes necessary to manage these side effects is essential, although compliance with these changes over time can be more unsatisfactory than compliance with the antipsychotic treatment itself.[51]

Leukopenia, Thrombocytopenia

Although many psychotropics (e.g., antipsychotics) can cause leukopenia, clozapine and carbamazepine are the primary medicines that need to be avoided in leukopenic patients. Of the antidepressants, mirtazapine may be associated with leukopenia, although causality has not been established and this has been rarely observed in clinical practice.[52] Gabapentin can also infrequently have a mild leukopenic effect.[27] Lithium, on the other hand, has been suggested for treatment of leukopenia and may be beneficial in this regard;[53] the mechanisms for increased white blood count may include demarginalization of neutrophils as well as possible release of colony-stimulating factors.[54-56]

The use of mood stabilizers such as carbamazepine, oxcarbazepine,[57] and valproate[58,59] is problematic in patients with preexisting thrombocytopenia because of their potential for lowering platelet count. Even when platelet count is normal, valproate may cause platelet dysfunction and prolong bleeding time.[60,61] Therefore, patients taking valproate should be assessed for bleeding risk before any invasive surgical procedures.

Hyponatremia

The syndrome of inappropriate antidiuretic hormone secretion (SIADH), resulting in hyponatremia, has been documented in patients, especially the elderly, who have been taking antidepressants. In addition to SSRIs, mirtazapine, duloxetine, and bupropion have all been implicated.[62-64] Among mood stabilizers, carbamazepine and oxcarbazepine can both cause hyponatremia,[65] although the mechanism is not secondary to SIADH and is not well understood.[66]

Neurologic Disease
Seizures

Patients with seizure disorders provide challenges in the choice of medication. Antidepressants and antipsychotics are thought to lower seizure threshold and this effect is generally dose dependent.[67] The most likely to do so are clozapine, chlorpromazine, olanzapine, quetiapine, tricyclic antidepressants, and bupropion (contraindicated in patients with seizure disorders). The risk with monoamine oxidase inhibitors (MAOIs) and SSRIs and other new antidepressants are considered to be low.[68] This is controversial, however. Depression itself appears to increase seizure risk and a review of FDA clinical trial data for antidepressants has shown a possible anticonvulsant effect of newer antidepressants at therapeutic doses[69] (although in overdoses antidepressants are still considered to increase seizure risk). Among antipsychotics, haloperidol and risperidone are less likely to affect seizure threshold.[70] All psychotropics should be used cautiously in patients with seizure disorders or when patients are seizure-prone (e.g., during alcohol or benzodiazepine withdrawal).

Stroke

Antipsychotics increase the incidence of stroke in patients with dementia.[71-73] First- and second-generation antipsychotics likely pose equal risk.[74] Possible etiologies for stroke may be related to cardiovascular effects or changes secondary to excessive sedation. In patients with dementia and significant behavioral dyscontrol or assaultiveness, SSRIs,[75] trazodone, or mood stabilizers should be considered.[76] However given their more rapid onset of action, antipsychotics should not be withheld if there is imminent risk of harm secondary to behavioral dyscontrol. The clinician should be aware that the use of both typical and atypical antipsychotics may be associated with an increased risk of death in patients with dementia.[71]

Extrapyramidal Symptoms

Patients with a prior history of dystonic reactions or substance abuse, and young, male patients are at higher risk for developing acute dystonias. Dystonias are primarily caused by typical antipsychotics but can occur with any antipsychotic with higher D_2 receptor occupancy (e.g., risperidone). Olanzapine, especially in high doses, can also cause EPS, although at lower rates than typical antipsychotics, possibly because of its own anticholinergic effects.[45] Quetiapine and clozapine are least likely to cause dystonias and parkinsonism.

Clozapine should also be considered in a patient presenting with tardive dyskinesia (TD), although all antipsychotics may mask, and therefore appear to improve, symptoms with treatment. Clinicians should attempt to avoid using typical antipsychotics in patients with preexisting abnormal movements. If abnormal movements again develop during treatment, clinicians should be aware that withdrawing the offending agent (especially if done too rapidly) could unmask and thereby worsen symptoms of TD. Patients at higher risk for TD are the elderly, women, those with prolonged treatment or past treatment with high doses of neuroleptics, those who developed significant parkinsonian side effects initially, and those with a history of affective disorders.

In contrast to other EPS, akathisia rates are generally similar among atypical antipsychotics, although there are lower overall rates with atypicals when compared with typical antipsychotics (10% to 20% vs. 20% to 50%, respectively).[45] Identifying akathisia as the cause of agitation, restlessness, or even worsening psychosis or suicidality is crucial because treatment would include decreasing rather than increasing antipsychotic dose.

Restless Legs Syndrome

RLS has been reported with the use of antidepressants such as SSRIs,[77] venlafaxine,[78] and mirtazapine[79] (as well as with several antipsychotics). Preliminary case reports suggest that bupropion, through modulation of dopaminergic effect, may be a better alternative antidepressant in patients with either preexisting or antidepressant-induced RLS.[80]

Women of Childbearing Age

Careful attention should be given to the choice of medication in young women. The general areas of concern are (a) the possibility of unplanned pregnancy while taking psychotropics and subsequent potential harm to the fetus and (b) the hormonal effects of medications on nonpregnant women.

Valproate may play a role in the development of polycystic ovary syndrome in women of reproductive age,[81] thereby affecting fertility (although there is a lack of clarity regarding rates given a higher-than-baseline occurrence of polycystic ovaries in bipolar patients not taking valproate).[82] In general, the use of mood stabilizers in young women can be very problematic given the possibility of interfering with fertility (e.g., valproate), interacting to decrease effectiveness of oral contraceptives (e.g., carbamazepine), and then increasing the chances of congenital malformations (e.g., valproate, carbamazepine, and to a lesser extent lithium) should pregnancy ensue. Considering alternatives to treatment with mood stabilizers and providing patient education are particularly important when treating women of childbearing age.

Another endocrine risk in women is the propensity of many antipsychotics to increase prolactin. Of the newer antipsychotics risperidone is the most problematic. Olanzapine, which is generally unlikely to increase prolactin, may do so at higher than usual doses (e.g., 30 mg per day).[83]

MEDICATION INTERACTIONS

The potential for interactions among psychotropics, or interactions between psychotropics and other classes of medication, often influences the inpatient clinician's choice of therapeutic agent. Although occasionally the likelihood of interactions clearly precludes the use of certain agents, more commonly the concern about interactions necessitates caution when introducing a new medicine. A complete list of interactions is beyond the scope of this chapter. The inpatient psychiatrist is well advised to consult the several available databases (web-based [e.g., www.genemedrx.com],[84] print,[85] etc.) when using multiple medicines. Nevertheless, there are commonly encountered types of interactions, both pharmacokinetic and pharmacodynamic, that should be kept in mind when choosing treatment for the hospitalized psychiatric patient. Patients at particularly high risk for dangerous medication interactions include those with impaired drug metabolism (including the elderly and those with organ insufficiencies) and those with chronic conditions (e.g., chronic psychiatric conditions, human immunodeficiency virus [HIV], cardiac patients) who require long-term complex pharmacotherapy.

Antidepressants

SSRIs are well known for their ability to interact with other medicines by affecting the hepatic cytochrome P-450 system. A primary concern is the potential for an SSRI to inhibit the enzymatic activity of specific P-450 isoenzymes, thereby increasing the serum levels of other hepatically metabolized medications (i.e., substrates), such as tricyclic antidepressants, antipsychotics, and warfarin.[86] Potentially harmful dose-dependent side effects (e.g., effects on cardiac conduction secondary to increased plasma concentrations of tricyclic antidepressants and antipsychotics, or increased bleeding secondary to increased warfarin levels) could develop. Not all SSRIs are equal in their potential for dangerous interactions. Fluoxetine, paroxetine, and fluvoxamine are more likely to inhibit hepatic enzymes; fluoxetine's inhibition of CYP2C9 and CYP2D6, paroxetine's inhibition of CYP2D6, and fluvoxamine's inhibition of CYP1A2, CYP2C9, CYP2C19, and CYP3A4 are of particular concern. Additionally, these three SSRIs exhibit nonlinear dose-concentration kinetics and small changes in dose may result in greater than expected enzyme inhibition and serum concentrations of substrates. These SSRIs should be used with caution when combined with other medication.[87]

Among SSRIs, citalopram and escitalopram have the least potential to affect serum levels of other medicines through enzymatic inhibition and should be selected preferentially in patients taking multiple medicines (however, citalopram can markedly increase clozapine levels through a mechanism that has not yet been elucidated).[88,89] Sertraline also generally causes less enzymatic inhibition than fluoxetine, paroxetine, and fluvoxamine. Other non-SSRI antidepressants that also should be favorably considered in the setting of medication combinations are venlafaxine and mirtazapine, both of which have a very low risk of medication interactions. However, although citalopram, venlafaxine, and mirtazapine are not likely to clinically affect the activity of hepatic enzymes, they themselves are substrates of these enzymes and their plasma concentrations can increase if used in combination with other enzyme-inhibiting SSRIs, thereby increasing the chances of unexpected or unwanted serotonergic effects.

Other antidepressants can also inhibit cytochrome P-450 enzymes. Duloxetine and bupropion can both moderately inhibit CYP2D6. Nefazodone is a potent CYP3A4 inhibitor and this can affect the metabolism of many common substrates such as macrolide antibiotics, statins, calcium channel blockers, and many HIV protease inhibitors, as well as many antipsychotics including ziprasidone (see subsequent text).[87,90]

The concomitant use of MAOIs and serotonergic antidepressants is contraindicated because of the potential to cause serotonin syndrome. A washout period of 2 weeks (5 weeks after discontinuation of fluoxetine) should be allowed before starting an MAOI. Two weeks should be allowed before switching from MAOIs to other antidepressants.[91] SSRIs also should not be used with linezolid, an antibiotic used for the treatment of infections caused by gram-positive bacteria, because of this drug's weak MAOI properties.[92]

Antipsychotics

Although newer antipsychotics do have weak cytochrome enzyme-inhibiting activity (and first- generation antipsychotics, such as phenothiazines, are stronger enzyme inhibitors), they are themselves substrates of P-450 enzymes and as such can be affected by enzyme-inducing and enzyme-inhibiting agents. As noted earlier, certain SSRIs, as well as other medicines (such as valproate and the frequently used antibiotic ciprofloxacin), can inhibit the metabolism of many old and new antipsychotics, thereby increasing their plasma concentrations. Specifically, clozapine and olanzapine are substrates for CYP1A2; haloperidol, risperidone, clozapine, and olanzapine are substrates for CYP2D6; and haloperidol, clozapine, risperidone, quetiapine, and ziprasidone are substrates for CYP3A4.[90] When metabolism of these antipsychotics is inhibited, there is a higher potential for side effects such as EPS or cardiac toxicity.

Using two or more antipsychotics or combining antipsychotics with other medicines that prolong the QT interval could be problematic and would require close monitoring. The addition of ziprasidone, which some studies find to have a higher propensity to cause QT prolongation, to other QT-prolonging drugs such as pentamidine, or class Ia (e.g., procainamide, quinidine) or class III (e.g., amiodarone) antiarrhythmics, should be avoided.[24]

Clozapine should not be combined with other medicines, such as carbamazepine, which can cause leukopenia. The combination of clozapine and benzodiazepines may rarely cause fatal respiratory suppression and therefore should generally be used cautiously.[93]

Clozapine and olanzapine are metabolized by CYP1A2, and cigarette smoking can decrease their levels through induction of this isoenzyme. Consequently, a newly admitted inpatient who is restricted from smoking may experience an increased plasma clozapine concentration and therefore should be monitored for increased risk of adverse effects.[90] Enzyme induction by cigarette smoke is primarily a function of polycyclic aromatic hydrocarbons found in tobacco smoke rather than of nicotine—the use of nicotine replacement therapy would not therefore cause similar induction.[94] Although paroxetine and fluoxetine can increase clozapine levels through enzyme inhibition, the use of fluvoxamine is of particular concern. Fluvoxamine can increase clozapine concentrations 5- to 10-fold through CYP1A2 inhibition[87,90] and this combination should usually be avoided or used very cautiously. Interestingly, however, the addition of fluvoxamine has been used as a strategy to boost low clozapine levels and possibly minimize adverse effects of the metabolite norclozapine, including weight gain.[95]

Mood Stabilizers

Carbamazepine is an inducer of many hepatic enzymes (CYP1A2, CYP2C9, CYP2C19, CYP3A4) and as such can lower the concentration of other medicines including many tricyclic antidepressants, antipsychotics, benzodiazepines, and other mood stabilizers, including lamotrigine, as well as nonpsychotropic medications such as warfarin.[90] In the manic patient who requires rapid behavioral control, and who may be receiving carbamazepine in addition to an antipsychotic and/or a benzodiazepine, the clinician should be aware that these adjunctive or other medicines may not be providing full clinical effect because of decreased plasma levels. This effect seriously limits the utility of carbamazepine in these situations. (In this regard the clinician should also be aware that in addition to carbamazepine, the antiepileptic drugs phenobarbital, phenytoin, and primidone also have similarly strong enzyme-inducing properties.)[96]

Along with carbamazepine, oxcarbazepine, high-dose topiramate,[97] and possibly lamotrigine may also stimulate the metabolism of oral contraceptives, and if used would require patients to undertake additional precautions to avoid pregnancy and/or a change to a stronger contraceptive dose.[98] In women relying on oral contraceptives, alternative treatments should be considered. Valproate and gabapentin are less likely to affect oral contraceptive levels.[96]

Valproate can inhibit the glucuronidation of lamotrigine, and this combination requires very slow titration of lamotrigine to decrease the risk of dangerous rash.[96,99] Sertraline, possibly also through inhibition of glucuronidation, may also significantly increase lamotrigine levels.[100] Valproate can also increase the plasma levels of substrates of CYP2C9 and CYP2C19 such as phenobarbital, phenytoin, many tricyclic antidepressants, and warfarin. Valproate is also highly protein bound and competition in protein binding with warfarin can cause a significant increase in the free fraction of warfarin and the prothrombin time.[27,101]

Lithium and gabapentin are renally excreted and are not likely to interact with other mood stabilizers.[102] Lithium levels, however, can increase with concomitant use of nonsteroidal anti-inflammatory drugs (NSAIDs), thiazide diuretics, angiotensin-converting enzyme (ACE) inhibitors, metronidazole, and tetracyclines.[103]

SPEED OF RESPONSE

In the acute inpatient setting, speed of pharmacotherapy response is critical. Unfortunately, there has been little study focused on speed as the primary outcome measure. Clinicians have been forced to rely on their clinical experience or that of trusted colleagues and form their own opinion. The present authors will survey the applicable or possibly applicable literature on strategies for maximizing speed of response to treatment of schizophrenia, mania, and depression.

Antipsychotics in Schizophrenia and Schizoaffective Disorder
Osser and Sigadel in 2001[3] published a comprehensive review of antipsychotic response speed in schizophrenia. This review concluded that risperidone may work faster than other antipsychotics, and that olanzapine worked fastest when started at relatively higher doses (e.g.,15 mg daily) compared with lower doses (e.g., 5 or 10 mg daily). Risperidone was the only second-generation antipsychotic that appeared to work faster than the control first-generation antipsychotic. However, that difference was not statistically significant, and it was of questionable clinical significance because the data on which it was based were not primary outcome data in the studies from which it was derived. Notably, quetiapine and ziprasidone numerically trailed the control first-generation antipsychotic in the first week or two of treatment. However, the authors of these studies did not note this in their discussions, although the implications for antipsychotic therapy in the acute inpatient setting might be important. This could be because the studies were not designed to focus on the outcome at 1 or 2 weeks.

Recent studies have suggested that rapid, as opposed to conventional, dosing of quetiapine speeds response in acute schizophrenia during the first week of treatment.[104] The starting dose of rapid treatment was 200 mg on the first day, followed by 400 mg on the second day, 600 mg on the third day, and 800 mg on day 4. However, the conventional dosing was to begin with 50 mg on day 1, 100 mg on day 2, 200 on day 3, 300 on day 4, and 400 mg on day 5. This is slower than most clinicians would go, but the side effects of dizziness, restlessness, and excess sedation on the faster titration were significant.

The possibility of early onset of therapeutic response to risperidone versus conventional antipsychotics was confirmed in a more recent review.[105] In this *post hoc* analysis of four studies involving 757 patients, a significantly greater proportion of patients at weeks 1 or 2 achieved a 20% reduction in Positive and Negative Syndrome Scale (PANSS) total scores with risperidone, compared with perphenazine (mean dose 28 mg daily) or haloperidol 10 to 20 mg daily. This may be clinically important because a meta-analysis has shown that failure to achieve a 25% reduction of symptoms on an antipsychotic in the first 2 weeks predicts poor outcome at 4 weeks (positive predictive value of 63%).[106]

The large National Institute of Mental Health (NIMH)-sponsored CATIE study could have been an opportunity to collect prospective data on early response, but the investigators did not design the study to shed light on this. The first evaluation point was 1 month after starting randomized antipsychotic therapy.

The short-term comparative effectiveness of antipsychotics was tested in another recent randomized trial that was not supported by pharmaceutical companies.[107] Three hundred and twenty seven acute schizophrenia and schizoaffective patients who were newly admitted to a public sector hospital were randomized in a 3-week open-label study to haloperidol (mean maximum dose 16 mg), aripiprazole (22 mg), olanzapine (19 mg), quetiapine (650 mg), risperidone (5.2 mg), or ziprasidone (150 mg). Effectiveness was defined, controversially, as whether the patient was well enough for discharge. By this criterion, haloperidol (89%), olanzapine (92%), and risperidone (88%) were significantly more effective than aripiprazole (64%), quetiapine (63%), and ziprasidone (64%) over the 3-week period of the study

Secondary outcome measures involving various rating scales did not show significant differences. This "pragmatic" outcome measure of dischargeability could have been subject to a variety of biases, but the study is interesting in that it supports the suggestion that not all antipsychotics are equal in rapidity of response and finds olanzapine, the conventional antipsychotic, and (again) risperidone to work faster.

When antipsychotics do work, they work fairly quickly. Leucht et al. pooled data from seven randomized trials of one antipsychotic (amisulpride, not available in the United States) and found that more reduction of positive and total symptoms occurred in the first 2 weeks than in the second 2 weeks ($p < 0.0001$).[108] By the end of 4 weeks, 68% of the improvement that will be found at 1 year was already achieved.

Speed of Response in Mania

Rapid response is highly desirable in the management of the acutely manic patient, especially when there is extreme hyperactivity or serious medical illness that may be exacerbated by the manic state. For this reason, many clinicians combine mood stabilizers and antipsychotics early, for example, in the first week of admission. Some evidence supports this, but the relevant studies did not compare untreated patients assigned to either cotherapy or monotherapy. Rather, the patients studied had already been treated with mood stabilizers and had failed on them (or received inadequate doses) after which they had an antipsychotic or placebo added.[109] Often, newly admitted patients will have been tried on monotherapy with a mood stabilizer or antipsychotic in the community before needing admission; therefore, it is certainly reasonable for them to get early combination treatment once hospitalized.

Regarding the choice of which antipsychotic to add, typical or atypical, naturalistic data seem to favor the atypicals at least with respect to extrapyramidal side effects,[110] but head-to-head comparisons (e.g., olanzapine vs. haloperidol) have found no efficacy differences in mania.[111]

If monotherapy is to be initiated in a first-onset or untreated, newly admitted patient, it is difficult to discern what choice would work most rapidly. There is no clear evidence to favor a mood stabilizer or an antipsychotic as monotherapy. However, oral-loaded divalproex seems to work faster than standard-titration methods.[112] With rapid oral loading, the patient is given (in one method) 30 mg/kg/day on days 1 and 2, followed by 20 mg/kg/day on subsequent days. In a pooled analysis of three studies involving 348 patients, this approach worked faster than lithium (300 mg three times daily for 2 days followed by titration to levels 0.4 to 1.5 mEq per L), and it worked equally rapidly to olanzapine 10 mg for 2 days followed by increase to a maximum of 20 mg daily.[112]

All five atypical antipsychotics have been approved by the FDA for the treatment of acute mania based on placebo-controlled studies. However, it must be kept in mind that the ethical requirements of placebo-controlled studies mandated that the sicker patients were not included.[113] Therefore, the effectiveness of monotherapy with atypicals in real-world patients is unclear.

Although there have been claims that the evidence suggests some atypicals work faster than others in mania, this seems to be an artifact of design variations in the registration trials.[114] Risperidone and ziprasidone patients were first rated at 1 and 2 days, aripiprazole at 4 days, and olanzapine at 7 days in these trials. Doses used were risperidone 1 mg every 6 to 8 hours, with maximum 6 to 10 mg daily; aripiprazole 30 mg daily (although a recent study used 15 mg and it worked well[115]); ziprasidone 40 mg twice daily with food, increased to 60 to 80 mg twice daily on the second day; olanzapine 15 mg daily to start and then adjusted to 5 to 20 mg daily. As is the case in schizophrenia treatment, quetiapine may work most rapidly in mania with an oral-loading schedule of 200 mg on day 1 with daily increases of 200 mg until 800 mg is reached by day 4, given in two divided doses.[116]

Patients who have new-onset bipolar mania who do not need urgent behavioral control are best treated with monotherapy with lithium. Although slower in treating the acute episode, no other treatment has performed as well in preventing recurrences of mania and depression and in reducing risk of suicidal behavior.[117] Observational data indicate that monotherapy with lithium, if initiated, is more likely to be sustained as a monotherapy, compared with anticonvulsants and antipsychotics which lead more often to polytherapy.[118]

Speed of Response in Depression

There has been a long-standing interest in finding ways to increase the response rate to antidepressants because of the clinical impression that they require many weeks to work. However, is this impression based on fact? According to a meta-analysis of 47 double-blind, placebo-controlled trials that evaluated the progression of improvement weekly or biweekly, >60% of the improvement that was going to occur on medication occurred in the first 2 weeks.[119] Also, the biggest differences between drug and placebo were seen during this initial period, suggesting that this initial improvement was a true antidepressant effect. This analysis also failed to support another long-standing impression, that rapid early response is a predictor of placebo response.

Are there any differences in the speed of response of different individual antidepressants? In a recent meta-analysis of all antidepressant controlled trials by the U.S. Agency for Healthcare Research and Quality,[120] one antidepressant had sufficient evidence to deserve mention as possibly having a faster onset of action. Mirtazapine, in seven studies, all sponsored by the manufacturer, consistently had faster effect in comparison with four different SSRIs. The effect size was moderate; the number needed to treat to yield one additional responder after 1 to 2 weeks of treatment was 7. Also, one antidepressant seemed to work consistently slower than at least four other antidepressants—fluoxetine. This is presumed to be due to the long half-life of fluoxetine and its metabolite norfluoxetine, which results in a long period (which can be months) until development of steady-state levels when the patient is started on the lowest effective dose of 20 mg daily.[121]

Augmentation strategies to speed response have been the subject of interest for decades. Prospects that have had periods of popularity include combining SSRIs and tricyclic antidepressants and adding pindolol to SSRIs (which seems to speed response in Europe but not in the United States).[122] More recently, studies in which atypical antipsychotics are added to SSRIs have been financed by the atypical antipsychotic drug companies.[123] This costly approach can augment a partial response to an SSRI, but there have been no studies evaluating whether initial cotherapy would speed response.

There is a possibility that antidepressants will be developed that have a much more rapid onset, even within hours, based on recent studies with intravenous infusions of the *N*-methyl-D-aspartate receptor agonist ketamine.[124] More research is needed to find a way of sustaining the benefits and dealing with toxicity, but the findings are of great interest.

Suicidal depressed patients present a particular challenge. There is an urgent need to see rapid improvement in suicidal thinking. With effective treatment, most patients will become less suicidal, but for a few, suicidal ideation and activity may increase, or occur *de novo*, in the early weeks of treatment. This has been observed since the beginning of the antidepressant era. It was thought to be due to a progression of response to antidepressants. Patients might initially show improvement in psychomotor retardation, with a lag in improvement in mood, leading to increased risk of suicidal actions. Possibly, this might be the mechanism with antidepressants like tricyclics with their primarily noradrenergically mediated pharmacodynamics. Other causes of increased suicidality have been proposed with the SSRIs and other second-generation antidepressants, including an activation or akathisia-like effect associated with dysphoria. All antidepressants could cause the emergence of a mixed state in a latent bipolar patient. The FDA has recently, though controversially, determined that the risk for antidepressant-emergent suicidality is higher in children, adolescents, and young adults, and required package insert alerts to watch for this adverse effect.[125] In any case, it is reasonable to monitor all patients closely when they are started on antidepressants.

MATCHING SIDE EFFECT PROFILES TO PRESENTING SYMPTOMS

A simple, yet common, consideration when choosing among treatment options concerns the issue of attempting to match the immediate effects (or side effects) of medication to patients' presenting symptoms. For example, while waiting for the effect of an antidepressant on the primary depressive disorder, the patient may have prominent neurovegetative symptoms that cause much distress. Choosing an antidepressant that could ameliorate, or at least not worsen, these symptoms may decrease the need to use multiple drugs and increase the likelihood of continued treatment adherence.

Sleep Changes

When choosing an antidepressant, mirtazapine or nefazodone given at bedtime may be more helpful than other serotonergic antidepressants for a patient with insomnia. On the other hand, patients prescribed paroxetine may subjectively feel more tired but are just as likely to have continued insomnia.[126] Bupropion or fluoxetine given during the day may be better suited for a depressed patient with somnolence. Among antipsychotics, quetiapine and olanzapine would probably help more with sleep, whereas aripiprazole or ziprasidone might be better suited for the already somnolent or anergic psychotic patient.

Appetite Changes

If the depressed patient is cachectic, mirtazapine can increase appetite and oral intake earlier than the time required for the antidepressant effect to occur. In contrast, bupropion, nefazodone, or venlafaxine would be good choices for an overweight patient. In a bipolar patient, lithium and valproate can be helpful if weight loss is a presenting symptom. Among antipsychotics, olanzapine and quetiapine could be chosen if weight gain would actually be desirable. However, the risks would include increased triglycerides, hyperglycemia, and insulin resistance. For the already overweight psychotic patient, aripiprazole or ziprasidone may be more appropriate.

POLYPHARMACY

Polypharmacy—or more appropriately "polytherapy"—may be defined as the concomitant use of two or more agents within the same class (e.g., two antipsychotics). The addition of medication from other classes, possibly for amelioration of side effects or improved control of symptoms (e.g., an antipsychotic plus a mood stabilizer for acute mania), is not always considered to be polytherapy. However, these combinations may still constitute "relative" polytherapy if the use of an available alternative single agent would have worked equally well.

Most practice guidelines and evidence-based algorithms recommend the use of sequential trials of monotherapy for treatment of acute episodes of psychiatric illness and may suggest polytherapy only as a last resort. There continues to be a dearth of controlled trials studying the use of polytherapy in hospitalized patients. Still, if one considers the use of combination psychotropics across different classes of medication, then clearly the use of polytherapy is the norm rather than the exception in the hospitalized patient.[127]

However, the concomitant use of multiple drugs within the same class (e.g., two or more antipsychotics) is also highly prevalent—40% to 50% for antipsychotics in schizophrenic and schizoaffective patients[128,129]—and this use has increased over time.[130] Probable reasons for both types of increase likely include the availability of a greater number of pharmacotherapeutic agents and the presumed increase in safety of many of the newer available agents. Furthermore, psychiatric units provide treatment for patients with (a) severe mental illness, (b) histories of multiple past hospitalizations and medication trials, (c) treatment resistance, and/or (d) dangerous behavioral problems, indicating the likelihood of an even greater perceived need for polytherapy for symptom control. The pressure from managed care for more rapid control of symptoms during briefer inpatient stays has also contributed to the use of polytherapy in this population. Understandably, in the absence of evidence, factors such as personal preference, historical patterns of practice, and pressures from milieu and nursing staff to treat patients more aggressively[131] have further contributed to the continued prevalence of polytherapy in inpatient clinical practice.

Although it is frequently unclear if there is any added benefit from the use of multiple medicines, the downsides and risks of polytherapy are clear. These include the risks of increased (a) medication-related adverse effects,[132] (b) dangerous drug-drug interactions, (c) medication errors, (d) mortality rates,[133] (e) medication nonadherence after discharge, and (f) cost.[134] Inpatient polytherapy has also been associated with longer hospital stays, although this may be because the most ill patients may be the most likely to be treated with multiple medicines.[132] It is reasonable then that generally polytherapy should be avoided when possible. To this end the use of treatment algorithms, periodic reviews of inpatient practice, and raising awareness regarding the risks of polytherapy can decrease its use in the inpatient setting.[135] However, there are certain circumstances in which, after a clear review of risks and benefits, polytherapy may be appropriate in hospitalized patients.

Cross-Titration

Clinicians commonly use cross-titration when adding a new medicine while discontinuing a previously ineffective one. The first agent is not discontinued abruptly in an effort to decrease the risks of withdrawal or discontinuation-related phenomena or worsening due to loss of an occult partial response. In the case of antipsychotics, for example, a 3-week taper can significantly reduce crossover exacerbations.[136] Frequently, however, as the patient improves with the addition of the second drug, the clinician is tempted to believe that the combination therapy (rather than the second drug alone) is responsible for this improvement and hence both medicines are continued. However, if one assumes that the response to the first drug was unsatisfactory despite an appropriate trial (i.e., dosing was appropriate and duration of treatment was adequate), it is not likely that it would have new-found effectiveness at a subsequently lower dose. In most cases it is recommended that the cross-titration continue until a clear switch is made to the second drug.[137] Completing the cross-titration switch need not occur in the hospital and may continue on an outpatient basis after the patient is well enough to be discharged. In these circumstances, clear communication with outpatient providers is necessary to convey the inpatient team's treatment plan in order to decrease the chance of continued polytherapy.

The Agitated Manic and/or Psychotic Patient

In manic patients, mood stabilizers may not be immediately effective in the treatment of mania and a 1- to 2-week time period or longer may be needed to achieve significant therapeutic effect. Preliminary studies comparing olanzapine, risperidone, or quetiapine in combination with lithium or valproate versus the use of either mood stabilizer alone suggest that the combination treatments may be more effective—although the addition of an antipsychotic increased the rate of adverse effects.[138-142] It is not clear, however, whether polytherapy results in earlier response. Also, as noted earlier, in these studies patients had a second agent added because they were not satisfactorily responding to monotherapy; the studies did not evaluate whether it is more desirable to commence treatment with the two agents simultaneously.

In schizophrenic patients there can be variable response time with the use of different antipsychotics.[3] In both the agitated manic patient and the agitated psychotic patient, there can be a real need early on for adjunctive medications such as benzodiazepines. Clinical experience suggests that adjunctive first-generation antipsychotics may acutely decrease the risk of harm secondary to behavioral dyscontrol. They may also be needed for severe insomnia. The rationale for adding typical antipsychotics should not be to hasten overall recovery—a prospect for which there is no good evidence—but in the hope of decreasing dangerous behavior in the short term. Clinicians should take into account the risks of medication interactions and the increase in risk of antipsychotic-related adverse effects and carefully balance these against the potential benefits when considering adding neuroleptics. Once the patient's behavior improves and remains stable, adjunctive drugs such as benzodiazepines and typical antipsychotics can be withdrawn. If the patient has required high doses of these agents, it is recommended that they be tapered and not abruptly discontinued, and again, clear communication with the outpatient psychiatrist is essential to ensure that the taper continues following discharge.

In the nonagitated psychotic patient there is less justification for adjunctive polytherapy. If there is no response to the first antipsychotic drug within the first week, increasing to more optimal dosing or switching to a new antipsychotic (to clozapine if appropriate) should be considered.[3] The temptation to use polytherapy within the first week (or to change to another antipsychotic prematurely) occurs if there is little response in terms of targeted psychotic symptoms. With partial response, deciding on the next step is complicated by the possibilities that (a) the patient may respond better given enough time and that (b) the observed improvement may be due to placebo effect or to other therapeutic effects of hospitalization.[3] The clinician should ensure that optimum dosing is being used and despite the uncertainty the best course of action may be to allow for gradual response. If after 2 to 3 weeks of optimal dosing—by which time most of the improvement that one is likely to see will have occurred[143]—there is still insufficient response, the antipsychotic agent should be changed. (This would constitute a briefer trial and more rapid switch than recommended by algorithms based on outpatient treatment.[144]) Again if appropriate the change should be to clozapine. A lengthy taper of the first agent is usually not needed under these circumstances.

The Depressed Patient

In depressed patients, unless multiple monotherapies have failed, the use of combination antidepressant therapy is usually not needed and a relatively rapid taper can precede the use of a new antidepressant. The concomitant use of two SSRIs should be avoided due to the risk of serotonergic side effects. If a combination of antidepressants is considered, then agents with different mechanisms of action should be used,[145] although dose increase to the optimal or maximal dose of the first agent should be tried before adding a second antidepressant. In addition, clinicians should not underestimate the effectiveness of psychotherapy when combined with antidepressant therapy and its ability to reduce the need for antidepressant polytherapy.[146-148]

Adding an antidepressant to an acutely psychotic schizophrenic patient's antipsychotic regimen is generally not helpful and may cause symptom exacerbations or drug interactions. Mood symptoms generally improve as the patient responds to the prescribed antipsychotic.[149]

In the patient with bipolar depression, lithium[150] or quetiapine[151] and possibly lamotrigine[152] may be used as monotherapies, although there are three unpublished negative or failed studies with lamotrigine monotherapy.[103] However, if these agents cannot be used, then antidepressants may need to be considered, despite disappointing data on the efficacy of antidepressants over the long term.[153] In these cases, it may be prudent to treat the patient with another mood stabilizer (and to reach therapeutic serum levels if applicable) before carefully introducing an antidepressant, thereby reducing the risk of inducing mania.

TREATMENT RESISTANCE

Patients who are admitted to acute psychiatric units have frequently had a number of medication trials with unsatisfactory results, leading to their need for admission. Therefore, treatment resistance is a typical challenge encountered in this setting. There are also more severe levels of treatment resistance. Exhaustive trials may have already occurred in recidivistic patients, and it will be difficult to determine what to do next. Or the patient may have had more than one significant trial during the present admission, without success, and the length of stay to that point may require that the patient be transferred to a tertiary-care facility.

Although detailed algorithms for the approach to treatment-resistant problems would require going beyond the scope of this chapter, a list of sometimes overlooked or avoided options that are especially worthy of consideration will be offered. As a general principle, making one medication change at a time, and giving it adequate time to be dosed properly, produces better and faster results than "treatment as usual" that lacks this organized and consistent approach.[154]

Schizophrenia and Schizoaffective Disorder

In the treatment of schizophrenia and schizoaffective disorder, one must first rule out the perhaps most frequent cause of poor response—noncompliance (e.g., cheeking, self-induced vomiting, purging). The most evidence-supported pharmacotherapy option after there have been a minimum of two adequate monotherapy trials of anti-psychotics is clozapine.[155,156] The two trials should include one first-generation anti-psychotic and either risperidone or olanzapine. The resistance to using clozapine comes from fear of side effects and concern about the amount of time it takes to start a rea-sonable trial. Also, a very common conceptual obstacle on the part of the physician is the assumption that a previously noncompliant patient would not be willing or able to adhere to the monitoring regime (i.e., blood draws) that would be needed with clozap-ine treatment. This concern is usually misplaced, however, given that if the patient re-sponds well to clozapine, outpatient compliance could be much better than expected. The physician has to be prepared to make an appropriately positive and convincing description of the potential benefits versus the risks of this option during the consent process. This is the true "art" of medicine—the ability to persuade the patient (and the managed care reviewer) to agree to an effective, highly evidence-based, but arduous treatment course. The improvisational throwing together of unproven combinations of multiple classes of disparate psychotropic agents is closer to alchemy than to art. (Clozapine is also an important option for treatment-resistant cases of bipolar disorder and BPD.)[18,19]

If clozapine cannot be used, many patients have never had an adequate trial of a rea-sonably well-tolerated first-generation antipsychotic such as perphenazine, and may bene-fit substantially even if the more esteemed second-generation drugs have been ineffective. Fully a quarter of well-defined treatment-resistant patients with schizophrenia had a sub-stantial response (>30% improvement in PANSS score) with perphenazine in a controlled study at a dose of approximately 40 mg daily.[157]

Surprisingly, aripiprazole at a dose of 30 mg did equally well in this trial, although there were somewhat more dropouts due to side effects.

Finally, in thinking about treatment resistance in the pharmacotherapy of schizo-phrenia, it is useful to recall the original observations of Dr. Heinz Lehmann from the 1950s regarding the phases of response to chlorpromazine.[158] He observed three phases, as follows:

1. Medicated cooperation. The patient is no longer assaultive or uncooperative but does not interact socially and still has persistent delusions, hallucinations, or formal thought disorder. This phase is usually achieved within the first week of treatment.
2. Socialization. The patient is able to interact reasonably well but still has persistent psy-chotic symptoms on questioning. It may take 4 to 6 weeks to achieve this phase.
3. Elimination of thought disorder. The patient is in substantial remission, with refine-ment of social and occupational capacities. It may take several months to reach this phase, if it occurs at all.

If the patient's improvement seems to have plateaued at level (1) or (2), further med-ication trials including clozapine are indicated. One may then have the opportunity to observe the patient progressing further on this continuum of response.

Mania

In the treatment of mania, lithium may be the most overlooked option in the United States currently.[159] Marketing influences may have led American physicians to routinely overlook the significant benefits of lithium over the long term, particularly for suicidal patients and others with resistant depression, and underestimate the risks of alternative agents (e.g., the greater weight gain and teratogenicity associated with valproate).

Depression

Inpatients with psychotic depression are often not given the most evidence-supported pharmacotherapy,[160] which is to use full doses of antipsychotics and antidepressants in combination.

In the approach to pharmacotherapy-resistant nonpsychotic depression, it is important to delineate and intervene to ameliorate stress-related and personality style-mediated contributions to the depressed state.[161] Beyond that, Sequenced Treatment Alternatives to Relieve Depression (STAR*D) has suggested that thyroid hormone augmentation of an SSRI, and the quadruple-action combination of venlafaxine and mirtazapine may deserve more consideration than previously thought.[162,163] ECT, with its high remission rates,[164] deserves consideration as an alternative to either of these options.[165] Unfortunately, the likelihood of use of ECT is strongly dependent on its availability in the hospital to which the patient is admitted.

PHARMACOGENETICS

Pharmacogenetics, the study of genetically determined drug response, can guide treatment selection by helping to predict how an individual patient would respond to specific agents. A brief discussion of promising developments can shed light on the ways in which better understanding of genetically determined factors can affect clinical treatment. Pharmacogenetic understanding holds significant potential to decrease morbidity by decreasing the risk of adverse drug effects and decreasing overall treatment time—time that would otherwise be spent trying ineffective treatments. At a minimum, it is important to obtain the family history of drug response in patients admitted to the psychiatric unit. It may also be of value to think about how psychopharmacologic choices may be influenced by ethnic and population-based considerations.[166]

A primary area has been the improved understanding of genetic polymorphisms in CYP450 enzymes, especially the CYP2D6 and CYP2C19 variants, and their impact on the pharmacokinetics of drug response and tolerance.[167] Laboratory testing for 19 genes is now available[168] but not yet part of mainstream clinical practice, in part because it is not covered by any insurance programs. Individual genotypes can be identified based on the function of the enzymatic phenotype (e.g., poor, intermediate, extensive, or ultrarapid metabolizers). For example, "ultrarapid" metabolizers may carry three or more active CYP2D6 alleles, whereas "poor metabolizers" may lack enzymatic activity. Poor metabolizers may therefore be at higher risk of adverse effects if treated with medicines that are substrates of this isoenzyme, whereas ultrarapid metabolizers may not show clinical response.

Ultrarapid metabolism, for example, may be one reason for treatment refractoriness to antipsychotics, many of which are metabolized by CYP2D6. What is additionally important is that relevant genotypes are represented differently in different populations. For example, approximately 30% of patients from North Africa and the Middle East may be ultrarapid metabolizers of CYP2D6 substrates;[167] up to 50% of Asians may have a partially deficient form of the CYP2D6 allele.[169]

Pharmacodynamic implications of genetically determined response could also have direct influence on choice of treatment. A major area of study is that of the genetic variants of the serotonin transporter gene (*SLC6A4*). The "short" form of the serotonin transporter gene promoter has a polymorphism that has been associated with decreased response to SSRIs, whereas the presence of the long allele is associated with positive drug response.[170] Also interestingly the short allele variant may be associated with increased risk of antidepressant-induced mania.[171] This correlation of long versus short forms of the alleles with treatment response, however, may apply only to SSRIs and not to antidepressants with other mechanisms of action (e.g., mirtazapine).[172]

For antipsychotics, polymorphisms in receptor genes have been associated with both effectiveness and with the risk of adverse effects. Examples particularly relevant to inpatient psychiatry are studies showing the possibility of an association between variations in D2-receptor genes and the speed of response to antipsychotics[173] and effects of variations in D3-receptor genes on the development of TD.[170] There also could be important economic ramifications—the potential to predict those who can benefit from more affordable first-generation antipsychotics without being genetically predisposed to TD would significantly influence treatment decisions.[174]

In regard to mood stabilizers, the study of lithium responders and genetic inheritance of bipolar disorder may eventually guide treatment. Positive response to lithium may be associated with bipolar disorder that is more genetically based.[175] A known clear family history of bipolar disorder therefore may argue for the selection of lithium for these patients.

MANAGED CARE AND FINANCIAL CONSIDERATIONS

Although physicians would like to feel that they have the autonomy, right, and responsibility to prescribe whatever they think is best, the reality is that health care resources are limited and it is impossible to avoid oversight by managed care. Questions will be raised about the high costs of certain medicines. At the same time, the primary interest of managed care review teams is to keep the length of stay as short as possible and their criteria mainly focus on safety issues and ensuring that "active treatment" is occurring. Often this means to them that there have to be frequent medication changes. They see this as concrete evidence of active interventions, whereas the other no less important and effective inpatient interventions such as intensive individual or group psychotherapy are less appreciated in justifying ongoing inpatient stay. There is often scant acknowledgment that most psychotropic medicines have latency periods before their onset of action and often it is the therapeutic milieu that is responsible for the rapid initial improvement in the patient's distress.

Nevertheless, difficult as it is, psychiatrists should avoid the temptation, fanned by the impatience of managed care reviewers, to increase doses too rapidly or to add additional medicines before current ones have had a reasonable chance to take effect. Evidence-supported approaches should influence treatment decisions and not the usually unseen managed care criteria for allowing additional days of inpatient care that usually have little scientific basis.

Drug formularies inform physicians of the availability of more economical choices when selecting medication. The hope and expectation is that these lists are guided not only by economic concerns but also by the realities of clinical practice. Requests by physicians for exceptions based on these realities should follow from thoughtful, cost-effective, stepwise sequences of choices that can be justified to the cost managers in terms that they will understand.

With a significant proportion of the population in the United States lacking health benefits, the psychiatrist may have to opt for alternative medication to accommodate a patient's ability to pay for it.

Sometimes, this may expose the patient to the risk of more side effects compared with a newer drug. For example, the atypical antipsychotics have fewer motor side effects but they are not currently available in a generic formulation and therefore none may be affordable without health benefits. Even if the health plan allows the use of newer medicines, they may still be unaffordable because of the high copayments or limited allowable yearly coverage. Psychiatrists in many parts of the world confront this problem routinely. As the costs of health care continue to escalate and fewer financial resources are available for patient care, physicians can expect to be required to factor economics more and more into their clinical decisions.

IMPROVING OUTCOME AFTER DISCHARGE

Up to 50% of discharged psychiatric inpatients may be readmitted within 1 year of discharge.[176] Many factors can help prevent readmission but the two most important ones are compliance with treatment appointments and medication. Studies have shown that up to half of discharged patients with schizophrenia or related disorders miss their first follow-up appointment after their hospital release.[177] Boyer et al.[178] reported that aftercare appointment compliance can be enhanced by three clinical "bridging strategies." These are (a) communication between inpatient and outpatient providers about discharge plans, (b) starting outpatient programs before discharge, and (c) family involvement during the hospitalization.

Disease-management programs promoted by managed care companies for medical diagnoses are beginning to be developed for psychiatric illnesses. Kopelowicz et al.[179] demonstrated that patients and their families who received skills training had better outcomes in the first 9 months in regard to relapse, functioning, and rehospitalization.

Psychoeducation of patients, especially when their families are involved, has produced reduction of relapse and readmission rates of up to 50%. Inpatient teams should therefore take advantage of the ability to involve family members in meetings during the hospital stay.

Finally, compliance is negatively associated with the complexity of a medication regimen. The inpatient psychiatrist has the opportunity to examine closely whether poly-therapy regimens that require multiple daily doses of various therapeutic agents are really necessary. Simplification of a patient's pharmacotherapeutic regimen can significantly con-tribute to continued improvement and stability after discharge from the inpatient setting.

SUMMARY

The pharmacologic approach to the psychiatric inpatient is influenced by multiple consid-erations. Treatment needs to be provided for the most severely psychiatrically ill patients within a short period of time and it needs to be safe and effective and also to increase the likelihood that patients remain well after discharge.

1. The provision of safe treatment means that any dangerous or assaultive behavior has to be treated urgently, often before a definitive diagnosis is reached. Typical antipsychot-ics and benzodiazepines remain the mainstay for rapid parenteral treatment.
2. In decreasing patient distress, p.r.n. medication does play a role in decreasing patient distress, although the request for such medication by patients and staff may suggest a need to consider psychological methods of managing this distress.
3. Efforts should be made to clarify patients' past pharmacotherapeutic treatments. Collateral information is often necessary. Data regarding past medication trials, both successful and otherwise, as well as information regarding reasons for past medication nonadherence, can be invaluable.
4. In all patients, but particularly in those with concomitant medical illness, the choice of agent should be guided by an effort to decrease overall medical risk and to avoid worsening the patient's medical comorbidities. The effect of psychiatric medication on all major systems, including cardiovascular, neurologic, hematologic, hepatic, renal, metabolic, and reproductive should be considered, and adequate steps should be taken to identify high-risk patients and monitor them when appropriate.
5. Antipsychotics, antidepressants, and mood stabilizers carry the risk of dangerous med-ication interactions. In the patient being treated with multiple medicines, psychiatric or otherwise, an effort should be made to decrease the risk of these interactions.
6. Although some agents may bring about response quicker than others (e.g., risperidone for psychosis, mirtazapine for depression), dose and speed of titration also likely affect speed of response for antipsychotics (e.g., olanzapine and quetiapine) and for mood stabilizers (e.g., valproate).
7. Psychiatric medicines should be used that would preferentially improve, rather than worsen, patients' associated neurovegetative symptoms, such as sleep and appetite changes, by matching side effect profiles to these symptoms.

8. Polytherapy should be minimized when there is a lack of evidence for its effectiveness and risk of increased overall side effects. However, in certain contexts (e.g., during cross titrations, or while treating agitated manic or psychotic patients) polytherapy may be temporarily necessary.

9. Treatment resistance constitutes a significant problem in the inpatient population. Clozapine use should not be avoided when there is clear treatment resistance to multiple other antipsychotics. In patients with bipolar disorder, lithium should not be overlooked. In refractory depressed patients, ECT and evidence-supported antidepressant combinations (e.g., venlafaxine and mirtazapine) should be considered.

10. Pharmacogenetic factors may explain lack of response to, or lack of tolerability of, certain medications in specific patients. Laboratory testing for genetic polymorphisms will increasingly aid in the identification of patients who would be likely to respond to certain therapies earlier during inpatient treatment.

11. Efforts should be made to resist managed care reviewers who push for aggressive psychopharmacologic interventions when psychotherapy is more appropriately indicated. On the other hand, outpatient insurance formularies, and patients' lack of ability to afford expensive prescribed medications after discharge cannot be ignored when deciding the inpatient choice of treatment.

12. The inpatient psychiatrist should keep in mind that for any pharmacotherapeutic regimen to be successful it should be tied to psychosocial interventions. Individual and group psychotherapy, family involvement in patient treatment, communication with outpatient systems of care, and strategies to increase likelihood of treatment adherence are all critical for a successful outcome. Comprehensive treatment of the whole patient is necessary for the ongoing provision of safe and effective treatment.

REFERENCES

1. Agency for Health Care Research and Quality. *Care of adults with mental health and substance abuse disorder in U.S. community hospitals: Health and Human Services Agency for Health Care Research and Quality,* 2004.

2. Woodward SA, Zeiss RA, Wheeler R, et al. Smoking Cessation and Decreased Behavioral Restraints in Inpatient Psychiatry. *American Psychiatric Association Annual Meeting,* New Research Poster NR 579. San Diego, 2007.

3. Osser DN, Sigadel R. Short-term inpatient pharmacotherapy of schizophrenia. *Harv Rev Psychiatry.* 2001;9(3):89-104.

4. Brook S, Walden J, Benattia I, et al. Ziprasidone and haloperidol in the treatment of acute exacerbation of schizophrenia and schizoaffective disorder: Comparison of intramuscular and oral formulations in a 6-week, randomized, blinded- assessment study. *Psychopharmacology (Berl).* 2005;178(4):514-523.

5. Breier A, Meehan K, Birkett M, et al. A double-blind, placebo-controlled dose-response comparison of intramuscular olanzapine and haloperidol in the treatment of acute agitation in schizophrenia. *Arch Gen Psychiatry.* 2002;59(5):441-448.

6. Tran-Johnson TK, Sack DA, Marcus RN, et al. Efficacy and safety of intramuscular aripiprazole in patients with acute agitation: A randomized, double-blind, placebo-controlled trial. *J Clin Psychiatry.* 2007;68(1):111-119.

7. Raj YP. Psychopharmacology of borderline personality disorder. *Curr Psychiatry Rep.* 2004;6(3):225-231.

8. Villeneuve E, Lemelin S. Open-label study of atypical neuroleptic quetiapine for treatment of borderline personality disorder: Impulsivity as main target. *J Clin Psychiatry*. 2005;66(10):1298-1303.

9. Taylor FB, Lowe K, Thompson C, et al. Daytime prazosin reduces psychological distress to trauma specific cues in civilian trauma posttraumatic stress disorder. *Biol Psychiatry*. 2006;59(7):577-581.

10. Raskind MA, Peskind ER, Hoff DJ, et al. A parallel group placebo controlled study of prazosin for trauma nightmares and sleep disturbance in combat veterans with post-traumatic stress disorder. *Biol Psychiatry*. 2007;61(8):928-934.

11. Binks CA, Fenton M, McCarthy L, Lee T, et al. Pharmacological interventions for people with borderline personality disorder. *Cochrane Database Syst Rev*. 2006(1):CD005653.

12. Cowdry RW, Gardner DL. Pharmacotherapy of borderline personality disorder. Alprazolam, carbamazepine, trifluoperazine, and tranylcypromine. *Arch Gen Psychiatry*. 1988;45(2):111-119.

13. Nose M, Cipriani A, Biancosino B, et al. Efficacy of pharmacotherapy against core traits of borderline personality disorder: Meta-analysis of randomized controlled trials. *Int Clin Psychopharmacol*. 2006;21(6):345-353.

14. Bellino S, Paradiso E, Bogetto F. Efficacy and tolerability of quetiapine in the treatment of borderline personality disorder: A pilot study. *J Clin Psychiatry*. 2006;67(7):1042-1046.

15. Soler J, Pascual JC, Campins J, et al. Double-blind, placebo-controlled study of dialectical behavior therapy plus olanzapine for borderline personality disorder. *Am J Psychiatry*. 2005; 162(6):1221-1224.

16. Nickel MK, Loew TH, Gil FP. Aripiprazole in treatment of borderline patients, part II: An 18-month follow-up. Psychopharmacology (Berl). 2007;191(4):1023-1026.

17. Zanarini MC, Frankenburg FR. Omega-3 fatty acid treatment of women with borderline personality disorder: A double-blind, placebo-controlled pilot study. *Am J Psychiatry*. 2003;160(1):167-169.

18. Chengappa KN, Ebeling T, Kang JS, et al. Clozapine reduces severe self-mutilation and aggression in psychotic patients with borderline personality disorder. *J Clin Psychiatry*. 1999;60(7):477-484.

19. Benedetti F, Sforzini L, Colombo C, et al. Low- dose clozapine in acute and continuation treatment of severe borderline personality disorder. *J Clin Psychiatry*. 1998;59(3):103-107.

20. Straus SM, Bleumink GS, Dieleman JP, et al. Antipsychotics and the risk of sudden cardiac death. *Arch Intern Med*. 2004;164(12): 1293-1297.

21. Ray WA, Meredith S, Thapa PB, et al. Cyclic antidepressants and the risk of sudden cardiac death. *Clin Pharmacol Ther*. 2004;75(3): 234-241.

22. Glassman AH, Bigger JT Jr. Antipsychotic drugs: Prolonged QTc interval, torsade de pointes, and sudden death. *Am J Psychiatry*. 2001;158(11): 1774-1782.

23. Shah RR. Drug-induced QT dispersion: Does it predict the risk of torsade de pointes? *J Electrocardiol*. 2005;38(1):10-18.

24. Fayek M, Kingsbury SJ, Zada J, et al. Cardiac effects of antipsychotic medications. *Psychiatr Serv*. 2001;52(5):607-609.

25. Lieberman JA, Stroup TS, McEvoy JP, et al. Effectiveness of antipsychotic drugs in patients with chronic schizophrenia. *N Engl J Med*. 2005; 353(12):1209-1223.

26. Breier A, Berg PH, Thakore JH, et al. Olanzapine versus ziprasidone: Results of a 28-week double-blind study in patients with schizophrenia. *Am J Psychiatry*. 2005;162(10):1879-1887.

27. *Physician's desk reference*. Montvale: Thomson PDR; 2007.

28. Merrill DB, Dec GW, Goff DC. Adverse cardiac effects associated with clozapine. *J Clin Psychopharmacol*. 2005;25(1):32-41.

29. Mamiya K, Sadanaga T, Sekita A, et al. Lithium concentration correlates with QTc in patients with psychosis. *J Electrocardiol*. 2005;38(2): 148-151.

30. Brucculeri M, Kaplan J, Lande L. Reversal of citalopram-induced junctional bradycardia with intravenous sodium bicarbonate. *Pharmacotherapy*. 2005;25(1):119-122.

31. Isbister GK, Prior FH, Foy A. Citalopram- induced bradycardia and presyncope. *Ann Pharmacother*. 2001;35(12):1552-1555.

32. Pae CU, Kim JJ, Lee CU, et al. Provoked bradycardia after paroxetine administration. *Gen Hosp Psychiatry*. 2003;25(2):142-144.

33. Mbaya P, Alam F, Ashim S, et al. Cardiovascular effects of high dose venlafaxine XL in patients with major depressive disorder. *Hum Psychopharmacol.* 2007;22(3):129-133.

34. Johnson EM, Whyte E, Mulsant BH, et al. Cardiovascular changes associated with venlafaxine in the treatment of late-life depression. *Am J Geriatr Psychiatry.* 2006;14(9):796-802.

35. Raskin J, Goldstein DJ, Mallinckrodt CH, et al. Duloxetine in the long-term treatment of major depressive disorder. *J Clin Psychiatry.* 2003;64(10):1237-1244.

36. Wohlreich MM, Mallinckrodt CH, Prakash A, et al. Duloxetine for the treatment of major depressive disorder: Safety and tolerability associated with dose escalation. *Depress Anxiety.* 2007;24(1):41-52.

37. Feighner JP. Cardiovascular safety in depressed patients: Focus on venlafaxine. *J Clin Psychiatry.* 1995;56(12):574-579.

38. Felker BL, Sloan KL, Dominitz JA, et al. The safety of valproic acid use for patients with hepatitis C infection. *Am J Psychiatry.* 2003;160(1): 174-178.

39. Lott RS, Helmboldt KM, Madaras-Kelly KJ. Retrospective evaluation of the effect of valproate therapy on transaminase elevations in patients with hepatitis C. *Pharmacotherapy.* 2001; 21(11):1345-1351.

40. Mallet L, Babin S, Morais JA. Valproic acid- induced hyperammonemia and thrombocytopenia in an elderly woman. *Ann Pharmacother.* 2004;38(10):1643-1647.

41. Carr RB, Shrewsbury K. Hyperammonemia due to valproic acid in the psychiatric setting. *Am J Psychiatry.* 2007;164(7):1020-1027.

42. Lepkifker E, Sverdlik A, Iancu I, et al. Renal insufficiency in long-term lithium treatment. *J Clin Psychiatry.* 2004;65(6):850-856.

43. *Gitlin M. Lithium and the kidney: An updated* review. *Drug Saf.* 1999;20(3):231-243.

44. Dixon L, Weiden P, Delahanty J, et al. Prevalence and correlates of diabetes in national schizophrenia samples. *Schizophr Bull.* 2000;26(4): 903-912.

45. Shirzadi AA, Ghaemi SN. Side effects of atypical antipsychotics: Extrapyramidal symptoms and the metabolic syndrome. *Harv Rev Psychiatry.* 2006;14(3):152-164.

46. Clark NG. Consensus development conference on antipsychotic drugs and obesity and diabetes. *Diabetes Care.* 2004;27(2):596-601.

47. van Winkel R, De Hert M, Van Eyck D, et al. Screening for diabetes and other metabolic abnormalities in patients with schizophrenia and schizoaffective disorder: Evaluation of incidence and screening methods. *J Clin Psychiatry.* 2006;67(10):1493-1500.

48. Lipkovich I, Citrome L, Perlis R, et al. Early predictors of substantial weight gain in bipolar patients treated with olanzapine. *J Clin Psychopharmacol.* 2006;26(3):316-320.

49. Gentile S. Long-term treatment with atypical antipsychotics and the risk of weight gain: A literature analysis. *Drug Saf.* 2006;29(4): 303-319.

50. Osser DN, Najarian DM, Dufresne RL. Olanzapine increases weight and serum triglyceride levels. *J Clin Psychiatry.* 1999;60(11):767-770.

51. Piette JD, Heisler M, Ganoczy D, et al. Differential medication adherence among patients with schizophrenia and comorbid diabetes and hypertension. *Psychiatr Serv.* 2007;58(2): 207-212.

52. Anghelescu I, Klawe C, Dahmen N. Venlafaxine in a patient with idiopathic leukopenia and mirtazapine-induced severe neutropenia. *J Clin Psychiatry.* 2002;63(9):838.

53. Sedky K, Lippmann S. Psychotropic medications and leukopenia. *Curr Drug Targets.* 2006;7(9):1191-1194.

54. Hager ED, Dziambor H, Hohmann D, et al. Effects of lithium on thrombopoiesis in patients with low platelet cell counts following chemotherapy or radiotherapy. *Biol Trace Elem Res.* 2001;83(2):139-148.

55. Hager ED, Dziambor H, Winkler P, et al. Effects of lithium carbonate on hematopoietic cells in patients with persistent neutropenia following chemotherapy or radiotherapy. *J Trace Elem Med Biol.* 2002;16(2):91-97.

56. Gallicchio VS, Messino MJ, Hulette BC, et al. Lithium and hematopoiesis: Effective experimental use of lithium as an agent to improve bone marrow transplantation. *J Med.* 1992;23(3-4):195-216.

57. Mahmud J, Mathews M, Verma S, et al. Oxcarbazepine-induced thrombocytopenia. *Psychosomatics.* 2006;47(1):73-74.

58. Conley EL, Coley KC, Pollock BG, et al. Prevalence and risk of thrombocytopenia with valproic acid: Experience at a psychiatric teaching hospital. *Pharmacotherapy.* 2001;21(11):1325-1330.

59. Trannel TJ, Ahmed I, Goebert D. Occurrence of thrombocytopenia in psychiatric patients taking valproate. *Am J Psychiatry.* 2001;158(1):128-130.

60. Gerstner T, Teich M, Bell N, et al. Valproate-associated coagulopathies are frequent and variable in children. *Epilepsia.* 2006;47(7):1136-1143.

61. De Berardis D, Campanella D, Matera V, et al. Thrombocytopenia during valproic acid treatment in young patients with new-onset bipolar disorder. *J Clin Psychopharmacol.* 2003;23(5):451-458.

62. Kruger S, Lindstaedt M. Duloxetine and hyponatremia: A report of 5 cases. *J Clin Psychopharmacol.* 2007;27(1):101-104.

63. Ladino M, Guardiola VD, Paniagua M. Mirtazapine-induced hyponatremia in an elderly hospice patient. *J Palliat Med.* 2006;9(2):258-260.

64. Bagley SC, Yaeger D. Hyponatremia associated with bupropion, a case verified by rechallenge. *J Clin Psychopharmacol.* 2005;25(1):98-99.

65. Dong X, Leppik IE, White J, et al. Hyponatremia from oxcarbazepine and carbamazepine. *Neurology.* 2005;65(12):1976-1978.

66. Sachdeo RC, Wasserstein A, Mesenbrink PJ, et al. Effects of oxcarbazepine on sodium concentration and water handling. *Ann Neurol.* 2002;51(5):613-620.

67. Alldredge BK. Seizure risk associated with psychotropic drugs: Clinical and pharmacokinetic considerations. *Neurology.* 1999;53(5 Suppl 2):S68-S75.

68. Montgomery SA. Antidepressants and seizures: Emphasis on newer agents and clinical implications. *Int J Clin Pract.* 2005;59(12):1435-1440.

69. Alper K, Schwartz KA, Kolts RL, et al. Seizure incidence in psychopharmacological clinical trials: An analysis of Food and Drug Administration (FDA) summary basis of approval reports. *Biol Psychiatry.* 2007;62(4):345-354.

70. Pisani F, Oteri G, Costa C, et al. Effects of psychotropic drugs on seizure threshold. *Drug Saf.* 2002;25(2):91-110.

71. Schneider LS, Dagerman KS, Insel P. Risk of death with atypical antipsychotic drug treatment for dementia: Meta-analysis of randomized placebo-controlled trials. *JAMA.* 2005;294(15):1934-1943.

72. Schneider LS, Dagerman K, Insel PS. Efficacy and adverse effects of atypical antipsychotics for dementia: Meta-analysis of randomized, placebo-controlled trials. *Am J Geriatr Psychiatry.* 2006;14(3):191-210.

73. Herrmann N, Lanctot KL. Do atypical antipsychotics cause stroke? *CNS drugs.* 2005;19(2): 91-103.

74. Gill SS, Rochon PA, Herrmann N, et al. Atypical antipsychotic drugs and risk of ischaemic stroke: Population based retrospective cohort study. *Br Med J.* 2005;330(7489):445.

75. Pollock BG, Mulsant BH, Rosen J, et al. Comparison of citalopram, perphenazine, and placebo for the acute treatment of psychosis and behavioral disturbances in hospitalized, demented patients. *Am J Psychiatry.* 2002;159(3):460-465.

76. Salzman C. Treatment of the agitation of late-life psychosis and Alzheimer's disease. *Eur Psychiatry.* 2001;16(Suppl 1):25s-28s.

77. Yang C, White DP, Winkelman JW. Antidepressants and periodic leg movements of sleep. *Biol Psychiatry.* 2005;58(6):510-514.

78. Salin-Pascual RJ, Galicia-Polo L, Drucker-Colin R. Sleep changes after 4 consecutive days of venlafaxine administration in normal volunteers. *J Clin Psychiatry.* 1997;58(8):348-350.

79. Agargun MY, Kara H, Ozbek H, et al. Restless legs syndrome induced by mirtazapine. *J Clin Psychiatry.* 2002;63(12):1179.

80. Kim SW, Shin IS, Kim JM, et al. Bupropion may improve restless legs syndrome: A report of three cases. *Clin Neuropharmacol.* 2005;28(6): 298-301.

81. Bilo L, Meo R. Epilepsy and polycystic ovary syndrome: Where is the link? *Neurol Sci.* 2006; 27(4):221-230.

82. Klipstein KG, Goldberg JF. Screening for bipolar disorder in women with polycystic ovary syndrome: A pilot study. *J Affect Disord.* 2006;91(2-3):205-209.

83. Wilson DR. High dose olanzapine and prolactin levels. *Presented at the 51st American Psychiatric Association Institute on Psychiatric Services.* New Orleans, 1999. www.genemedrx.com.

84. Ciraulo DA, ed. *Drug interactions in psychiatry,* 3rd ed. Philadelphia: Lippincott Williams & Wilkins; 2006.

85. Sayal KS, Duncan-McConnell DA, McConnell HW, et al. Psychotropic interactions with warfarin. *Acta Psychiatr Scand.* 2000;102(4): 250-255.

86. Ereshefsky L, Jhee S, Grothe D. Antidepressant drug-drug interaction profile update. *Drugs R D.* 2005;6(6):323-336.

87. Borba CP, Henderson DC. Citalopram and clozapine: Potential drug interaction. *J Clin Psychiatry.* 2000;61(4):301-302.

88. Novartis. Product Information: Drug Warning and New Information, Clozaril(R), clozapine. 2005.

89. Spina E, Scordo MG, D'Arrigo C. Metabolic drug interactions with new psychotropic agents. *Fundam Clin Pharmacol.* 2003;17(5): 517-538.

90. Boyer EW, Shannon M. The serotonin syndrome. *N Engl J Med.* 2005;352(11):1112-1120.

91. Huang V, Gortney JS. Risk of serotonin syndrome with concomitant administration of linezolid and serotonin agonists. *Pharmacotherapy.* 2006;26(12):1784-1793.

92. Grohmann R, Ruther E, Sassim N, et al. Adverse effects of clozapine. *Psychopharmacology (Berl).* 1989;99(Suppl):S101-S104.

93. Kroon LA. Drug interactions with smoking. *Am J Health Syst Pharm.* 2007;64(18):1917-1921.

94. Lu ML, Lane HY, Lin SK, et al. Adjunctive fluvoxamine inhibits clozapine-related weight gain and metabolic disturbances. *J Clin Psychiatry.* 2004;65(6):766-771.

95. Perucca E. Clinically relevant drug interactions with antiepileptic drugs. *Br J Clin Pharmacol.* 2006;61(3):246-255.

96. Bialer M, Doose DR, Murthy B, et al. Pharmacokinetic interactions of topiramate. *Clin Pharmacokinet.* 2004;43(12):763-780.

97. Crawford P. Interactions between antiepileptic drugs and hormonal contraception. *CNS Drugs.* 2002;16(4):263-272.

98. Yuen AW, Land G, Weatherley BC, et al. Sodium valproate acutely inhibits lamotrigine metabolism. *Br J Clin Pharmacol.* 1992;33(5):511-513.

99. Kaufman KR, Gerner R. Lamotrigine toxicity secondary to sertraline. *Seizure.* 1998;7(2): 163-165.

100. Guthrie SK, Stoysich AM, Bader G, et al. Hypothesized interaction between valproic acid and warfarin. *J Clin Psychopharmacol.* 1995; 15(2):138-139.

101. Spina E, Perucca E. Clinical significance of pharmacokinetic interactions between antiepileptic and psychotropic drugs. *Epilepsia.* 2002;43(Suppl 2):37-44.

102. Janicak PG, Davis JM, Preskorn SH, et al. *Principles and practice of psychopharmacotherapy,* 4th ed. Lippincott Williams & Wilkins; 2006.

103. Pae CU, Kim JJ, Lee CU, et al. Rapid versus conventional initiation of quetiapine in the treatment of schizophrenia: A randomized, parallel-group trial. *J Clin Psychiatry.* 2007; 68(3):399-405.

104. Glick ID, Shkedy Z, Schreiner A. Differential early onset of therapeutic response with risperidone versus conventional antipsychotics in patients with chronic schizophrenia. *Int Clin Psychopharmacol.* 2006;21(5):261-266.

105. Leucht S, Busch R, Kissling W, et al. Early prediction of antipsychotic nonresponse among patients with schizophrenia. *J Clin Psychiatry.* 2007;68(3):352-360.

106. McCue RE, Waheed R, Urcuyo L, et al. Comparative effectiveness of second-generation antipsychotics and haloperidol in acute schizophrenia. *Br J Psychiatry.* 2006;189:433-440.

107. Leucht S, Busch R, Hamann J, et al. Early- onset hypothesis of antipsychotic drug action: A hypothesis tested, confirmed, and extended. *Biol Psychiatry.* 2005;57(12):1543-1549.

108. Smith LA, Cornelius V, Warnock A, et al. Acute bipolar mania: A systematic review and metaanalysis of co-therapy versus monotherapy. *Acta Psychiatr Scand.* 2007;115:12-20.

109. Letmaier M, Schreinzer D, Reinfried L, et al. Typical neuroleptics versus atypical antipsychotics in the treatment of acute mania in a natural setting. *Int J Neuropsychopharmacol.* 2006;9(5):529-537.

110. Rendell JM, Gijsman HJ, Keck P, et al. Olanzapine alone or in combination for acute mania. *Cochrane Database Syst Rev.* 2003;CD004040.

111. Hirschfeld RMA, Baker JD, Wozniak P, et al. The safety and early efficacy of oral-loaded divalproex versus standard-titration divalproex, lithium, olanzapine, and placebo in the treatment of acute mania associated with bipolar disorder. *J Clin Psychiatry.* 2003;64(7):841-846.

112. Licht RW, Gouliaev G, Vestergaard P, et al. Generalisability of results from randomized drug trials: A trial on antimanic treatment. *Br J Psychiatry.* 1997;170:264-267.

113. Goodwin FK, Jamison KR. *Manic-depressive illness: bipolar disorders and recurrent depression,* 2nd ed. New York: Oxford University Press; 2007.

114. Keck PE, Sanchez R, Torbenys A, et al. Aripiprazole monotherapy in the treatment of acute bipolar I mania: A Randomized Placebo and Lithium Controlled Study. *American Psychiatric Association Annual Meeting,* New Research Poster NR 304. San Diego, 2007.

115. Hatim A, Habil H, Jesjeet SG, et al. Safety and efficacy of rapid dose administration of quetiapine in bipolar mania. *Hum Psychopharmacol.* 2006;21(5):313-318.

116. Baldessarini RJ, Tondo L, Hennen J, et al. Is lithium still worth using? An update of selected recent research. *Harv Rev Psychiatry.* 2002;10(2):59-75.

117. Baldessarini RJ, Leahy L, Arcona S, et al. Patterns of psychotropic drug prescription for U.S. patients with diagnoses of bipolar disorders. *Psychiatr Serv.* 2007;58(1):85-91.

118. Posternak MA, Zimmerman M. Is there a delay in the antidepressant effect? A meta-analysis. *J Clin Psychiatry.* 2005;66(2):148-158.

119. Gartlehner G, Hansen RA, Thieda P, et al. *Comparative effectiveness of second-generation antidepressants in the pharmacologic treatment of adult depression: comparative effectiveness review No. 7.* Rockville: Agency for Healthcare Research and Quality; 2007.

120. Janicak PG, Davis JM, Preskorn SH. *Principles and practice of psychopharmacotherapy,* 4th ed. New York: Lippincott Williams & Wilkins; 2006:228.

121. Ballesteros J, Callado LF. Review: Combining pindolol with an SSRI improves early outcomes in people with depression. *J Affect Disord.* 2004;79:137-147.

122. Berman RM, Marcus RN, Swanink R, et al. The efficacy and safety of aripiprazole as adjunctive therapy in major depressive disorder:

123. A multicenter, randomized, double-blind, placebo-controlled study. *J Clin Psychiatry.* 2007;68(6):843-853.

124. Zarate CA Jr, Singh JB, Carlson PJ, et al. A randomized trial of an N-methyl-D-aspartate antagonist in treatment-resistant major depression. *Arch Gen Psychiatry.* 2006;63(8):856-964.

125. Leon AC. The revised warning for antidepressants and suicidality: Unveiling the black box of statistical analyses. *Am J Psychiatry.* 2007;164(12):1786-1788.

126. Preskorn S. *Outpatient management of depression,* 2nd ed. Caldo: Professional Communications, Inc; 1999.

127. Rittmannsberger H, Meise U, Schauflinger K, et al. Polypharmacy in psychiatric treatment. Patterns of psychotropic drug use in Austrian psychiatric clinics. *Eur Psychiatry.* 1999;14(1):33-40.

128. Jaffe AB, Levine J. Antipsychotic medication coprescribing in a large state hospital system. *Pharmacoepidemiol Drug Saf.* 2003;12(1):41-48.

129. Procyshyn RM, Thompson B. Patterns of antipsychotic utilization in a tertiary care psychiatric institution. *Pharmacopsychiatry.* 2004;37(1):12-17.

130. Botts S, Hines H, Littrell R. Antipsychotic polypharmacy in the ambulatory care setting, 1993-2000. *Psychiatr Serv.* 2003;54(8):1086.

131. Ito H, Koyama A, Higuchi T. Polypharmacy and excessive dosing: Psychiatrists' perceptions of antipsychotic drug prescription. *Br J Psychiatry.* 2005;187:243-247.

132. Centorrino F, Goren JL, Hennen J, et al. Multiple versus single antipsychotic agents for hospitalized psychiatric patients: Case-control study of risks versus benefits. *Am J Psychiatry.* 2004;161(4):700-706.

133. Waddington JL, Youssef HA, Kinsella A. Mortality in schizophrenia. Antipsychotic polypharmacy and absence of adjunctive anticholinergics over the course of a 10-year prospective study. *Br J Psychiatry.* 1998;173:325-329.

134. Stahl SM, Grady MM. High-cost use of second-generation antipsychotics under California's Medicaid program. *Psychiatr Serv.* 2006;57(1):127-129.

135. Patrick V, Schleifer SJ, Nurenberg JR, et al. Best practices: An initiative to curtail the use of antipsychotic polypharmacy in a state psychiatric hospital. *Psychiatr Serv.* 2006;57(1):21-23.

136. Viguera AC, Baldessarini RJ, Hegarty JD, et al. Clinical risk following abrupt and gradual withdrawal of maintenance neuroleptic treatment. *Arch Gen Psychiatry.* 1997;54(1):49-55.

137. Stahl SM. Antipsychotic polypharmacy: Evidence based or eminence based?. *Acta Psychiatr Scand.* 2002;106(5):321-322.

138. Tohen M, Chengappa KN, Suppes T, et al. Efficacy of olanzapine in combination with valproate or lithium in the treatment of mania in patients partially nonresponsive to valproate or lithium monotherapy. *Arch Gen Psychiatry.* 2002;59(1):62-69.

139. Sachs GS, Grossman F, Ghaemi SN, et al. Combination of a mood stabilizer with risperidone or haloperidol for treatment of acute mania:

140. A double-blind, placebo-controlled comparison of efficacy and safety. *Am J Psychiatry.* 2002;159(7):1146-1154.

141. Yatham LN, Grossman F, Augustyns I, et al. Mood stabilisers plus risperidone or placebo in the treatment of acute mania. International, double-blind, randomised controlled trial. *Br J Psychiatry.* 2003;182:141-147.

142. Sachs G, Chengappa KN, Suppes T, et al. Quetiapine with lithium or divalproex for the treatment of bipolar mania: A randomized, double-blind, placebo-controlled study. *Bipolar Disord.* 2004; 6(3):213-223.

143. Yatham LN, Paulsson B, Mullen J, et al. Quetiapine versus placebo in combination with lithium or divalproex for the treatment of bipolar mania. *J Clin Psychopharmacol.* 2004;24(6):599-606.

144. Leucht S, Busch R, Hamann J, et al. Early- onset hypothesis of antipsychotic drug action: A hypothesis tested, confirmed and extended. *Biol Psychiatry.* 2005;57(12):1543-1549.

145. Miller AL, Chiles JA, Chiles JK, et al. The Texas Medication Algorithm Project (TMAP) schizophrenia algorithms. *J Clin Psychiatry.* 1999;60(10):649-657.

146. Dodd S, Horgan D, Malhi GS, et al. To combine or not to combine? A literature review of antidepressant combination therapy. *J Affect Disord.* 2005;89(1-3):1-11.

147. Simon J, Pilling S, Burbeck R, et al. Treatment options in moderate and severe depression: Decision analysis supporting a clinical guideline. *Br J Psychiatry.* 2006;189:494-501.

148. Keller MB, McCullough JP, Klein DN, et al. A comparison of nefazodone, the cognitive behavioral-analysis system of psychotherapy, and their combination for the treatment of chronic depression. *N Engl J Med.* 2000;342(20):1462-1470.

149. Schramm E, van Calker D, Dykierek P, et al. An intensive treatment program of interpersonal psychotherapy plus pharmacotherapy for depressed inpatients: Acute and long-term results. *Am J Psychiatry.* 2007;164(5):768-777.

150. Levinson DF, Umapathy C, Musthaq M. Treatment of schizoaffective disorder and schizophrenia with mood symptoms. *Am J Psychiatry.* 1999;156(8):1138-1148.

151. Goodnick PJ. Bipolar depression: A review of randomised clinical trials. *Expert Opin Pharmacother.* 2007;8(1):13-21.

152. Keating GM, Robinson DM. Quetiapine: A review of its use in the treatment of bipolar depression. *Drugs.* 2007;67(7):1077-1095.

153. Goldsmith DR, Wagstaff AJ, Ibbotson T, et al. Lamotrigine: A review of its use in bipolar disorder. *Drugs.* 2003;63(19):2029-2050.

154. Leverich G, Altshuler L, Suppes T, et al. Risk of switch in mood polarity to hypomania or mania in patients with bipolar depression during acute and continuation trials of venlafaxine, sertraline, and bupropion as adjuncts to mood stabilizers. *Am J Psychiatry.* 2006;163(2):232-239.

155. Adli M, Bauer M, Rush AJ. Algorithms and collaborative-care systems for depression: Are they effective and why? A systematic review. *Biol Psychiatry.* 2006;59:1029-1038.

156. Kane JM, Honigfeld G, Singer J, et al. Clozapine for the treatment-resistant schizophrenic: A double-blind comparison with chlorpromazine. Arch Gen Psychiatry. 1988;45(9):789-796.

157. McEvoy JP, Lieberman JA, Stroup TS, et al. Effectiveness of clozapine versus olanzapine, quetiapine, and risperidone in patients with chronic schizophrenia who did not respond to prior atypical antipsychotic treatment. *Am J Psychiatry.* 2006;163(4):600-610.

158. Kane JM, Meltzer HY, Carson WH, et al. Aripiprazole for treatment-resistant schizophrenia: Results of a multicenter, randomized, double-blind, comparison study versus perphenazine. *J Clin Psychiatry.* 2007;68(2):213-223.

159. Lehmann H. On acute schizophrenia patients. In: Lehmann H, Ban T, eds. *The butyrophenones in psychiatry.* Montreal, Canada: Quebec Psychopharmacological Research Association; 1964.

160. Baldessarini RJ, Leahy L, Arcona S, et al. Patterns of psychotropic drug prescription for U.S. patients with diagnoses of bipolar disorders. *Psychiatr Serv.* 2007;58(1):85-91.

161. Andreescu C, Mulsant MH, Peasley-Miklus C, et al. Persisting low use of antipsychotics in the treatment of major depressive disorder with psychotic features. *J Clin Psychiatry.* 2007;68(2):194-200.

162. Parker G, Manicavasagar V. *Modelling and managing the depressive disorders: a clinical guide.* New York: Cambridge University Press; 2005.

163. McGrath PJ, Stewart JW, Fava M, et al. Tranylcypromine versus venlafaxine plus mirtazapine following three failed antidepressant medication trials for depression: A STAR*D report. *Am J Psychiatry.* 2006;163:1531-1541.

164. Nierenberg AA, Fava M, Trivedi MH, et al. A comparison of lithium and T3 augmentation following two failed medication treatments for depression: A STAR*D report. *Am J Psychiatry.* 2006;163(9):1519-1530.

165. Husain MM, Rush AJ, Fink M, et al. Speed of response and remission in major depressive disorder with acute electroconvulsive therapy (ECT): A Consortium for Research in ECT (CORE) report. *J Clin Psychiatry.* 2004;65(4):485-491.

166. McCall WV. What does STAR*D tell us about ECT? *JECT.* 2007;23(1):1-2.

167. Ruiz PE. *Review of psychiatry, Ethnicity and psychopharmacology,* Vol. 19. American Psychiatric Publishing, Inc; 2000.

168. de Leon J, Armstrong SC, Cozza KL. Clinical guidelines for psychiatrists for the use of pharmacogenetic testing for CYP450 2D6 and CYP450 2C19. *Psychosomatics.* 2006;47(1):75-85.

169. De Leon J. Amplichip CYP450 test: Personalized medicine has arrived in psychiatry. *Expert Rev Mol Diagn.* 2006;6(3):277-286.

170. Bertilsson L. Geographical/interracial differences in polymorphic drug oxidation. Current state of knowledge of cytochromes P450 (CYP) 2D6 and 2C19. *Clin Pharmacokinet.* 1995; 29(3):192-209.

171. Malhotra AK, Murphy GM Jr, Kennedy JL. Pharmacogenetics of psychotropic drug response. *Am J Psychiatry.* 2004;161(5):780-796.

172. Mundo E, Walker M, Cate T, et al. The role of serotonin transporter protein gene in antidepressant-induced mania in bipolar disorder: Preliminary findings. *Arch Gen Psychiatry.* 2001;58(6):539-544.

173. Murphy GM Jr, Hollander SB, Rodrigues HE, et al. Effects of the serotonin transporter gene promoter polymorphism on mirtazapine and paroxetine efficacy and adverse events in geriatric major depression. *Arch Gen Psychiatry.* 2004;61(11):1163-1169.

174. Lencz T, Robinson DG, Xu K, et al. DRD2 promoter region variation as a predictor of sustained response to antipsychotic medication in first-episode schizophrenia patients. *Am J Psychiatry.* 2006;163(3):529-531.

175. Ozdemir V, Aklillu E, Mee S, et al. Pharmacogenetics for off-patent antipsychotics: Reframing the risk for tardive dyskinesia and access to essential medicines. *Expert Opin Pharmacother.* 2006;7(2):119-133.

176. Alda M. Pharmacogenetics of lithium response in bipolar disorder. *J Psychiatry Neurosci.* 1999;24(2): 154- 158.

177. Bridge JA, Barbe RP. Reducing hospital readmission in depression and schizophrenia: Current evidence. *Curr Opin Psychiatry.* 2004;17(6):505-511.

178. Klinkenberg WD, Calsyn RJ. Predictors of receipt of aftercare and recidivism among persons with severe mental illness: A review. *Psychiatr Serv.* 1996;47(5):487-496.

179. Boyer CA, McAlpine DD, Pottick KJ, et al. Identifying risk factors and key strategies in linkage to outpatient psychiatric care. *Am J Psychiatry.* 2000;157(10):1592-1598.

180. Kopelowicz A, Zarate R, Gonzalez SV, et al. Disease management in Latinos with schizophrenia: A family-assisted, skills training approach. *Schizophr Bull.* 2003;29(2):211-227.

UPDATE

INPATIENT PSYCHOPHARMACOLOGY

In the 11 years since the publication of this book chapter on the use of psychopharmacology with the psychiatric inpatient, the general and specific principles and advice seem to have changed very little. It is surprisingly current. Anyone working on an inpatient unit, it would seem, could profit from reading this material—there will likely be at least a few practical or informational points that will be immediately applicable. A few updates for certain sections of the chapter are provided below.

Selecting Treatment

This long section begins with advice on managing the agitated patient with oral or parenteral medication directed at symptoms that must be addressed urgently. A new and fairly large prospective randomized double-blind controlled trial evaluated four intramuscular (IM) treatments for acute agitation in an emergency room setting in Brazil.[1] A total of 100 consecutive patients (consent obtained from relatives or friends accompanying the subjects) were randomized to haloperidol 2.5 mg plus midazolam 7.5 mg, haloperidol 2.5 mg plus promethazine 25 mg, olanzapine 10 mg, or ziprasidone 10 mg. The majority of the patients had schizophrenia, with 36% having a diagnosis of mania. One hour after the treatment, the best results were with either the haloperidol plus benzodiazepine or the olanzapine. However, the odds ratio for significant side effects was 1.6 higher for olanzapine. The other two treatments were inferior in effectiveness and the odds ratio for side effects was 3.6, that is, much higher, with the haloperidol plus the sedating antiparkinsonian agent promethazine. This study further supports the recommendation in the chapter that haloperidol plus a benzodiazepine (often it is lorazepam in the United States) is still the best and safest IM treatment for acute agitation in the urgent or emergency setting.

This section continues with an extended discussion of the oral use of "prn" (abbreviation for the Latin words "pro re nata," or "as the thing is born") as-needed medication for different urgent problems in the inpatient setting. The essential point, still valid today, is that while there are times when one must resort to offering prn's, there is a downside, which is that they encourage the patient in the belief that when they are feeling mental distress there is a pill they can take to immediately feel better. Usually, we are trying to teach patients to use nonmedication coping strategies for their dysphoric states, and the use of prn's can work against those strategies. It would be better, when the patient comes to the nurse to ask for the prn that he/she has on order, to sit down with the patient and figure out what is causing the distress and develop a nonmedication coping strategy for that precipitant. Many patients may already be heavily committed to self-medications for immediate symptom relief, ranging from nicotine products, to cannabis, to alcohol, cocaine, benzodiazepines, and other abusable substances. Using prn's in those patients, in particular, can be counterproductive and foster the very habits that the clinical team is working to undermine.

This section proceeds to discuss a variety of general medical conditions that inpatients may have comorbid with their psychiatric problems and how the management is affected by these comorbidities. Most of it is still very relevant and useful. The association between the use of antipsychotics and sudden death (likely in part from arrhythmias) is mentioned and new data have been added to the evidence base confirming this risk.[2] Sudden death is particularly a problem when these medications are used for dementia symptoms in the elderly, as mentioned.[3] A black box warning regarding this risk has been added to all antipsychotics. Weight gain, metabolic syndrome, and induction of diabetes are also discussed. New data indicate that even one 10 mg dose of olanzapine significantly impairs insulin resistance and elevates inflammatory markers in healthy control volunteers 4.5 hours after administration.[4] The longer term effects of this one dose were not evaluated but this "requires elucidation" according to the authors. Quetiapine probably has similar effects,[5] and clozapine almost certainly does as well. Since the chapter was written, we do have newer second-generation antipsychotics with relatively fewer metabolic side effects, including aripiprazole, lurasidone, brexpiprazole, and cariprazine—although ziprasidone still seems to have the least.

In the treatment of agitation in patients with dementia, the recommendations in the chapter are supported by more recent studies.[6,7]

Restless leg syndrome is mentioned as a problem encountered in inpatients. Quetiapine should be added to the list of medications that often cause this as a side effect.[8] Since the review by Rittmannsberger and colleagues of 16 cases from 6 years ago, there have been at least 9 other reports of varying numbers of cases in the literature.

This section ends with some discussion of issues for women including women of childbearing age. Without doubt the most undesirable (though still often used) medication in young women with bipolar disorder is valproate.[9] It received an "X" rating (for antiepileptic treatment) from the Food and Drug Administration (FDA)—because of being associated with an 11% risk of significant congenital abnormalities including spina bifida and cardiac defects.[10] Another important problem for women, and many men, is prolactin-mediated side effects of certain antipsychotics such as risperidone, paliperidone, and most first-generation antipsychotics. It is now thought that the health consequences are more significant than once thought and prolactin levels should be routinely measured and medications changed to prolactin-sparing antipsychotics (like aripiprazole) when possible.[11]

Polypharmacy, Treatment Resistance, Pharmacogenetics, Managed Care/Financial Considerations

There are discussions of polypharmacy in the management of psychotic, manic, and depressed patients. Algorithm chapters in this book will be a more updated source for the most current thinking on sequences of medications to use for these disorders and when use of more than one medication within the same class (e.g., anticonvulsants or antipsychotics) might be justified. Treatment resistance is also addressed much more comprehensively than it is in this overview chapter and the reader is referred to the individual diagnoses and their algorithms. The discussion of pharmacogenetics still seems pertinent—which is surprising given the lapse of 11 years since this was written.

REFERENCES

1. Mantovani C, Labate CM, Sponholz A Jr, et al. Are low doses of antipsychotics effective in the management of psychomotor agitation? A randomized, rated-blind trial of 4 intramuscular interventions. *J Clin Psychopharmacol.* 2013;33:306-312.

2. Ray WA, Chung CP, Murray KT, et al. Atypical antipsychotic drugs and the risk of sudden cardiac death. *N Engl J Med.* 2009;360:225-235.

3. Chahine LM, Acar D, Chemali Z. The elderly safety imperative and antipsychotic usage. *Harv Rev Psychiatry.* 2010;18:158-172.

4. Hahn MK, Wolever TM, Arenovich T, et al. Acute effects of single-dose olanzapine on metabolic, endocrine, and inflammatory markers in healthy controls. *J Clin Psychopharmacol.* 2013;33:740-746.

5. Ngai YF, Sabatini P, Nguyen D, et al. Quetiapine treatment in youth is associated with decreased insulin secretion. *J Clin Psychopharmacol.* 2014;34:359-364.

6. Osser DN, Fischer MA. *Management of the behavioral and psychological symptoms of dementia: review of current data and best practices for health care professionals. The National Resource Center for Academic Detailing.* Boston, MA: Alosa Foundation, Inc.; December 28, 2013:1-51.

7. Walaszek A. *Behavioral and psychological symptoms of dementia.* Washington, DC: American Psychiatric Association Publishing; 2020.

8. Rittmannsberger H, Werl R. Restless legs syndrome induced by quetiapine: report of seven cases and review of the literature. *Int J Neuropsychopharmacol.* 2013;16:1427-1431.

9. Balon R, Riba M. Should women of childbearing potential be prescribed valproate? A call to action. *J Clin Psychiatry.* 2016;77:525-526.

10. Bromley RL, Weston J, Marson AG. Maternal use of antiepileptic agents during pregnancy and major congenital malformations in children. *JAMA.* 2017;318:1700-1701.

11. Osser DN. Prolactin monitoring in first-episode psychotic patients. *Schizophr Res.* 2017;189:2-3.

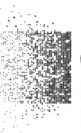

Guidelines, Algorithms, and Evidence-Based Psychopharmacology Training for Psychiatric Residents

David N. Osser, MD, Robert D. Patterson, MD, and James J. Levitt, MD

Objective: *The authors describe a course of instruction for psychiatry residents that attempts to provide the cognitive and informational tools necessary to make scientifically grounded decision making a routine part of clinical practice.*

Methods: *In weekly meetings over two academic years, the course covers the psychopharmacology of various psychiatric disorders in 32 3-hour modules. The first half of each module is a case conference, and the second is a literature review of papers related to the case. The case conference focuses on the extent to which past treatment has been consistent with evidence-supported guidelines and algorithms, and the discussants make recommendations that take the relevant scientific evidence into consideration. The second half of each module focuses on two papers: 1) a published guideline, algorithm, or review article and 2) a research study.*

Results: *Residents absorb a comprehensive overview of recommended clinical practices and acquire skills in assessing knowledge that affects decision making. Satisfaction with the course is rated highly.*

Conclusion: *The course appears useful by its face validity, but research comparing the attitudes and practice outcomes of graduates of this course compared with recipients of other training methods is needed.*

There is growing concern about how to enable physicians to use research findings in the care of their patients. Evidence-based medicine (EBM) is a way physicians can merge research with patient care (1–3). There seems to be a large gap between evidence-supported practice and typical practice (4). To narrow this gap, many practice guidelines, algorithms, and compilations of expert interpretation of evidence-based medicine have been issued in recent years. However, studies have shown that simple dissemination of these documents is generally not effective in changing practice (5, 6). Some systems designed to change behavior show promise. Examples of such systems include: computerized reminders, flowcharts posted on walls, and performance feedback and reviews. The changes in physician prescribing behavior have been modest, however (7–9). The targeted practices often return

Academic Psychiatry 2005; 29:180-186

Drs. Osser and Levitt are with the Department of Psychiatry at the Brockton Veteran's Administration Medical Center, Harvard Medical School, Brockton, Massachusetts. Dr. Patterson is with the Department of Psychiatry at the McLean Hospital, Harvard Medical School, Belmont, Massachusetts. Address correspondence to Dr. Osser, Brockton VAMC, 940 Belmont St., Brockton, MA 02301; david.osser@dmh.state.ma.us (E-mail). Copyright © 2005 Academic Psychiatry.

to preintervention levels, unless multifaceted, resource-intensive interventions are sustained (10).

This article describes a course in psychopharmacology for psychiatry residents designed to address these concerns and the problem of commercial influence in medical education. The authors wish to prepare students to be able to use valid new information and resist influences that are not evidence-based. Detailing, gifts, and sponsored educational products are highly influential, but, unfortunately, this influence is often in the direction of irrational prescribing, especially with respect to cost-effectiveness (11–13). Industry-sponsored education has been dominating residency and postgraduate training in recent years and is a concern throughout medicine (14).

The practice of EBM involves stepping back from a clinical scenario and asking questions about the scientific evidence that pertains to that situation (1). This is a rigorous approach to clinical decision making that may be unacceptably time consuming. For the psychopharmacologist, a four-step approach is required. The first step would be to make a criteria-based Diagnostic and Statistical Manual of Mental Disorders (DSM)-IV diagnostic impression, identifying subtypes and comorbidity. This is required because virtually all the evidence in the literature regarding psychopharmacological treatment involves the treatment of patients who have been identified by these criteria. Regardless of the validity of DSM criteria, their utility in the context of EBM is difficult to dispute (15). Next, a review of past treatment trials, including their adequacy and outcomes, must be completed. Then, the clinician must search for, find, read, and analyze, and apply the research evidence that pertains to the treatment situation (1). Finally, a treatment decision is made after the evidence information is integrated with the clinician's knowledge of the total patient, taking into account issues such as side effect sensitivities, patient preferences, family input, and ethnic and cultural considerations (16, 17).

This process is arduous and requires use of some cognitive disciplines that may be unfamiliar to the physician. These barriers have limited the usefulness of EBM in the day-to-day practice of medicine and psychiatry. In an effort to address this problem, high-quality, evidence-based practice guidelines and algorithms have been developed by appropriately qualified entities. The physician can consult these academic products and more quickly determine what the evidence supports for the clinical scenario at hand. However, these products will usually not address all situations, and the EBM physician must still be able to utilize the four-step process to look up particular questions or determine whether there has been important new evidence since the guideline/algorithm was published.

However, as noted, physicians often do not consult evidence-based guidelines and algorithms, much less follow them. They present many reasons for not doing so (18). The most common reasons involve lack of awareness that the guidelines exist or apply (19), belief that the recommendations will not produce a good outcome; and lack of experiences with some recommended treatments and consequent discomfort with trying them. Additionally, some physicians may not trust the guidelines/algorithms, especially if they have reason to doubt whether they were rigorously and thoughtfully constructed. Many of these products come embedded in industry sponsored educational material and contain obviously biased recommendations. Even the term "evidence-based" is losing meaning and credibility these days because of its ubiquitous presence in the titles of promotional offerings. Guidelines and algorithms may also be rejected as "cookbook medicine," even though, curiously, physicians are likely to agree with the specific recommendations in a guideline when they are presented separately from that guideline (18). Finally, some physicians assert that they do not agree with the concept of EBM in general, pointing out that much of the evidence of EBM is flawed and incomplete and thus irrelevant (20).

What is the alternative? Instead of employing EBM-informed reasoning, it is well-known that physicians often fall back on faulty processes of decision making (21–23). For example, "reflexive decisions" are impulsive judgments made without consciously considering any alternative. "Bias-driven clinical judgments" occur when the physician is overconfident and thinks that he or she knows exactly what to do based on some bias. The "availability heuristic" is the tendency to grab the first answer that comes to mind and to stick with it despite evidence to the contrary.

Use of these faulty approaches is sometimes justified by referring to them as part of the "art" of medicine. Belief in this art appears to be rooted in the apprentice/ mentor training model [eminence-based medicine (24)] and the model of placing special value on recollected clinical experience without adequately taking into account the unreliability of memories. The problem with clinical experience is that people tend to overestimate the frequency of intermittent reinforcers (25) (e.g., a gratifying positive outcome from a particular treatment). The validity of clinical experience is also limited by the small Ns of the previous experience, sample differences (i.e., the patient to be treated now is not really similar to the recollected previous patients), and investigator bias (i.e., the physician has an undue faith in the proposed treatment). At times, the art appears to be little more than treatment of symptoms without precise diagnosis and with unscientific, improvisational treatment selection. Dr. Abraham Flexner observed the same phenomena in his study of American medical practice almost 100 years ago. He urged reforms in medical education to produce a "scientific physician." Such a physician:

> . . .studies the actual situation with keener attention; he is freer of prejudiced prepossession; he is more conscious of liability to error. Whatever the patient may have to endure from a baffling disease, he is not further handicapped by reckless medication. . . (26)

Psychiatrists are committed to the principle that each patient's treatment should be uniquely crafted, in recognition of the uniqueness of each person. However, this principle may be misapplied, causing the psychiatrist to see treatment decision making as a process without significant evidence-based guideposts that should be considered. Though some of the resistance to EBM appears to come from a fear that it attacks the humanistic perspective of psychiatry, EBM should complement it.

TEACHING THE SCIENCE AND ART OF PSYCHOPHARMACOLOGY

It has been proposed that the best way to overcome these barriers is to begin training in EBM as early as possible (27, 28). This article describes a new structure for a course of classroom teaching of clinical psychopharmacology for residents at the Harvard South Shore Psychiatry Residency Training Program. It emphasizes the development of skills in practicing EBM. However, it goes beyond traditional EBM and encourages the use of rigorously constructed practice guidelines and algorithms as primary resources contributing to clinical decision making. Evidence-based guidelines and algorithms are also used as a way of organizing knowledge in psychopharmacology for the trainee (and the expert). Guidelines and algorithms provide contexts in which to place new information and compare it with previous knowledge. Using this knowledge of EBM and the contents of guidelines and algorithms, students make better decisions, and they develop the ability to identify clinical practice decisions that seem to deviate from the evidence. The course encourages them to become active consumers of many kinds of evidence (27); become skillful at detecting the biases in publications, in lectures, and in the practice of other clinicians; and learn to recognize the shortcomings of eminence-based medicine. Finally, at a time when medication costs have substantially increased, residents are encouraged to focus on evidence that pertains to making cost-effective psychopharmacology decisions (29).

THE CORE PSYCHOPHARMACOLOGY CONFERENCE: A TWO-YEAR COURSE

The Core Psychopharmacology Conference (CPC) is a 2-year program for PGY-II and III psychiatry residents that meets weekly for 1.5 hours. Each year, before the CPC begins, there is a 10-week introductory didactic lecture series in basic principles of psychopharmacology, combined with structured reading of a basic text. Topics covered in the introductory course include diagnosis, neurobiological factors in mental illness, pharmacology of the medications, kinetics, neurotransmitter issues, side effect management, and risk management strategies.

The CPC utilizes clinical case conferences coupled with practice guidelines or algorithms and research studies relevant to the cases presented, including clinical studies or papers elucidating the neurobiology of the patient's primary disorder or the mechanism of action of the medications used to treat that disorder. The CPC is organized into modules (Table 1). The first module each year focuses on basic principles of EBM and how to critically assess a paper (30, 31). Eleven psychiatric disorders are covered in the remaining 15 modules. (See Appendix 1 for specific topics.) There are a total of 64 papers read and critiqued by the resident group. Each trainee presents at least two case conferences and leads four paper discussions over 2 years.

Syllabus papers are chosen by the faculty and distributed at the beginning of the course each year. Resident-selected papers are chosen in relationship to a question raised

Table 1	Organization of Modules in Years One and Two		
	First session: Case Conference (1.5 hours)	Case presentation by resident	
		Interview of patient	
		Discussion of case	
Module (e.g., on Bipolar Mania)	Second session: Literature Study (Two papers: 45 minutes for each)	Year one, paper 1	Syllabus guideline or algorithm paper
		Year two, paper 1	Syllabus clinical research paper—related to an important recommendation from the Year one guideline or algorithm paper
		Years one and two, paper 2	Clinical or basic research paper—related to case presented in the first session, chosen by the resident

by the clinical material in the case conference: the resident (with faculty supervision) researches the question, and a relevant paper is selected for review in the meeting the following week.

Some comment is necessary about the way syllabus papers are selected. The first-year syllabus contains practice guidelines, algorithms, or review article papers, depending upon what is available for each diagnosis. Algorithms are a subset of practice guidelines that are more specific and give step-by-step elaboration of issues such as treatment sequencing, dosing, and progress assessment (32). The selections in the first year syllabus draw somewhat heavily on work by the course directors (one-third to one-half are theirs), but the course directors attempt to be rigorous in critiquing their own work during the class discussions. Algorithms can be evaluated according to several parameters (33). They should:

1. Contain a critical appraisal of the quality of supporting evidence for each recommendation, and an indication of different levels of confidence in the recommendations;
2. Be thoroughly reviewed by other experts;
3. Be free of commercial bias;
4. Consider evidence of safety as well as efficacy in determining the hierarchy of decisions;
5. Offer multiple options at each step as appropriate;
6. Cover a wide range of clinical scenarios;
7. Make special effort to explain the evidence supporting recommendations that are different from what other prominent experts have concluded in their interpretation of the literature; and
8. Be kept up-to-date. It is an advantage (34) that the algorithms and decision-support information of the Harvard South Shore Program are computerized, web-based, and frequently updated so residents can always access the most recent version.

The clinical research papers in the second-year syllabus are selected for their illustrative value on matters of contemporary clinical interest and for their usefulness to the residents in gaining experience in applying the principles of critical appraisal of papers outlined in the first module. They are not intended to comprise only the best papers. Rather, they ensure coverage of a range of problems with sampling demographics, sample size, effect size in comparison with placebo, type I or II error, and statistical analytic issues. Considerable time is spent addressing the issue of placebo effect in clinical trials, and, in general, how placebo effect confounds the interpretation of personal clinical experience in psychopharmacology practice (35). Sometimes papers are chosen that provide evidence challenging common, but questionable, practices. Other papers are selected because, although not high quality, they may be among the only studies available that pertain to important decision areas. Residents are also asked to critique the algorithm and guidelines papers according to the parameters described earlier (33). The neuroscience papers are selected by one of the course directors (JJL), who has expertise in psychiatric neuroimaging.

It should be noted that this course is not the complete curriculum in psychopharmacology at this residency program. In addition to patient-based learning through supervision in various settings, there are other courses that cover research design, epidemiology, diagnosis, biological psychiatry, integrative treatment, and a didactic lecture series in psychopharmacology. Grand rounds also cover topics in psychopharmacology.

Although increasing numbers of medical schools and residency programs are instituting courses on the principles and practice of EBM, there have been a limited number of studies of clinical outcomes of patients treated by clinicians who have adhered to evidence-based psychopharmacology guidelines or algorithms (10, 36, 37). The course directors do not encourage trainees to follow any guidelines and algorithms in a rigid way, but rather to use the structure of the algorithms for organizing or scaffolding their evidence knowledge base so that it can be readily accessed and consulted when making a clinical decision.

Course Evaluation

A survey of resident opinion about the first CPC course (1999-2001) was conducted in 2001. A questionnaire was anonymously completed by all 20 of the trainees who attended the conference, and the answers were collated. Almost all respondents indicated that the course was successful in structuring their psychopharmacological knowledge and increasing their confidence in their clinical decision making. They also approved of the emphasis placed on EBM, practice guidelines, and algorithms, and reported that they frequently considered the algorithms in their clinical decisions. Several graduates commented that having learned to practice this way, and they cannot understand how others around them do not.

Concluding Comments

Teaching methods and their impact on professional competence should not be immune from the standards that EBM educators apply to clinical treatments. In fact, there have been calls for high quality randomized trials of different methods of medical teaching (38, 39). However, there appears to be no satisfactory method of measuring the clinical performance and competence of physicians, despite numerous efforts (40). Even if there were satisfactory methods, random assignment of trainees to different training approaches would certainly be impractical. Observational studies could be done, but these would have to try to control for the many confounding covariates inherent in the baseline characteristics of the trainees and for the quality and type of teaching that occurs in other parts of the residency curriculum. Studies should also address whether trainees continue over the long term to use the thinking processes taught in this course or whether they eventually fall back upon the automatic thinking encouraged by industry-influenced education (39). Given the lack of such studies, the authors can only present this course description for its face validity, while acknowledging that the present approach should not be assumed to be efficacious. However, we are presently conducting a study to measure residents' attitudes toward EBM, guidelines, and algorithms 1 to 3 years after completion of the course. These results will be compared with the attitudes of graduates of a different psychiatry residency program in our area (41).

There is one published comprehensive model curriculum for psychopharmacology training. The American Society of Clinical Psychopharmacology (ASCP) has a 700-page volume, first published in 1997, (with a third edition published in 2004) which provides lecture outlines, reproductions of slides, and other information useful for organizing training (42). Earlier editions were discussed and reviewed (43-46). One reviewer stated that it lacked what psychiatric residents need the most: algorithms (43). One must add that residents need not just any algorithms, but rigorously evidence-based and unbiased algorithms (33).

Indeed, the ASCP's important curriculum does discuss a wide variety of evidence, but it does not teach how to assess and validate evidence for clinical application, nor does it structure the evidence into formal algorithms or guidelines. Even the authors acknowledge that the curriculum does not provide the critical thinking skills necessary for good clinical practice (47). The teaching approach described here complements and should ideally be combined with presentation of the knowledge base in curricula such as that of the ASCP. We are pleased to report that a description of this course, a citation of its web site, and the flowcharts of three algorithms reviewed in the course are included in the 2004 edition of the ASCP Model Curriculum.

In summary, the Core Psychopharmacology Conference establishes that EBM and high-quality, up-to-date psychopharmacology practice guidelines and algorithms should be routinely considered in daily clinical practice. The approach emphasizes case-centered learning, in which cases are directly associated with guidelines/algorithms and the evidence that supports them. Residents have an opportunity to absorb the knowledge that experts have filtered from the research literature and incorporated into the guidelines and algorithms. They learn how to use EBM techniques to find, filter, critically evaluate, and apply evidence and update their knowledge structures, including the knowledge summarized in the guidelines and algorithms. They also explore the cognitive, social, economic, and other factors that influence clinicians' acquisition and utilization of scientific research findings in their practice.

The authors thank Daniel Ioanitescu, M.D. for many useful discussions and for organizing the course evaluation.

APPENDIX 1: Module Topics
Evidence-based medicine and how to read a paper
Schizophrenia and related psychotic disorders (2)
Bipolar disorder (2)
Depression (2)
Anxiety disorders (4)
Dementia
Eating disorders
Attention deficit disorder
Substance abuse/dependence
Child and adolescent psychopharmacology
Overview of new developments

REFERENCES

1. Guyatt GH, Haynes RB, Jaeschke RZ, et al: Users' guides to the medical literature XXV Evidence-based medicine: principles for applying the users' guides to patient care. J the Am Med Assoc 2000; 284:1290–1296

2. Geyman JP, Deyo RA, Ramsey SD: Evidence-based clinical practice: concepts and approaches. Boston, Mass., Butterworth-Heinemann, 2000

3. Lenfant C: Clinical research to clinical practice - lost in translation? New England J Med 2003; 349:868–874

4. Jencks SF, Cuerdon T, Burwen DR, et al: Quality of medical care delivered to medicare beneficiaries: a profile at state and national levels. J the Am Med Assoc 2000; 284:1670–1676

5. Solberg LI: Guideline implementation: what the literature doesn't tell us. The Joint Commission J on Quality Improvement 2000; 26:525–537

6. Bero LA, Grilli R, Grimshaw JM, et al: Closing the gap between research and practice: an overview of systematic reviews of interventions to promote the implemetation of research findings. BMJ 1998; 317:465–468

7. Goethe JW, Schwartz HI, Szarek BL: Physician compliance with practice guidelines. Connecticut Med 1997; 61:553–558

8. Cannon DS, Allen SN: A comparison of the effects of computer and manual reminders on compliance with a mental health clinical practice guideline. J the Am Med Informatics Assoc 2000; 7:196–203

9. Shea S, DuMouchel W, Bahamonde L: A meta-analysis of 16 randomized controlled trials to evaluate computer-based clinical reminder systems for preventive care in the ambulatory setting. J the Am Med Informatics Assoc 1996; 3:399–409

10. Bauer MS: A review of quantitative studies of adherence to mental health clinical practice guidelines. Harvard Rev of Psychiatry 2002; 10:138–153

11. Wazana A: Physicians and the pharmaceutical industry: is a gift ever just a gift? J the Am Med Assoc 2000; 283:373–380

12. Goldman CR, Cutler DL: Pharmaceutical industry support of psychiatric research and education: ethical issues and remedies, in Ethics in community mental health care: commonplace concerns. Edited by Backlar P, Cutler D. New York., Kluwer Academic Press/Plenum Publishers, 2002

13. Dana J, Loewenstein G: A social science perspective on gifts to physicians from industry. J the Am Med Assoc 2003; 290:252–255

14. Relman AS: Separating continuing medical education from pharmaceutical marketing. J the Am Med Assoc 2001; 285:2009–2012

15. Kendell R, Jablensky A: Distinguishing between the validity and utility of psychiatric diagnoses. Am J Psychiatry 2003; 160:4–12

16. Goldner EM, Bilsker D: Evidence-based psychiatry. Can J Psychiatry 1995; 40:97–101

17. Sackett DL, Rosenberg WM, Gray JA, et al: Evidence-based medicine: what it is and what it isn't. It's about integrating clinical expertise and the best external evidence. BMJ 1996; 312:71–72

18. Cabana MD, Rand CS, Powe NR, et al: Why don't physicians follow clinical practice guidelines? A framework for improvement. J the Am Med Assoc 1999; 282:1458–1465

19. Azocar F, Cuffel BD, Goldman W, et al: Dissemination of guidelines for the treatment of major depression in a managed behavioral health care network. Psychiatr Services 2001; 52:1014–1016

20. Stahl SM: Does evidence from clinical trials in psychopharmacology apply in clinical practice? J Clin Psychiatry 2001; 62:6–7

21. Leape LL: Error in medicine. J the Am Med Assoc 1994; 272:1851–1857

22. Elstein AS: Cognitive processes in clinical inference and decision making, in Reasoning, inference, and judgment in clinical psychology. Edited by Turk DC, Salovey P. New York, The Free Press, 1988

23. Poses RM: One size does not fit all: questions to answer before intervening to change physician behavior. Joint Commission J on Quality Improvement 1999; 25:486–495

24. Berg AO: Dimensions of evidence. J the Am Board of Family Practice 1998; 11:216–223

25. Ferster CE, Skinner BF: Schedules of Reinforcement. New York, Appleton-Century-Crofts, 1957

26. Flexner A: Medical education in the United States and Canada: a report to the Carnegie Foundation for the Advancement of Teaching. New York, Arno Press, 1910

27. Bilsker D, Goldner EM: Teaching evidence-based practice in mental health. Evidence-Based Ment Health 1999; 2:68–69

28. Waddell C: So much research evidence, so little dissemination and uptake: mixing the useful with the pleasing. Evidence- Based Ment Health 2001; 4:3–5

29. Duckworth K, Hanson A: Using a clinical and evidence-based strategy to preserve access to psychiatric medications. Psychiatr Services 2002; 53:1231–1232

30. Miser WF: Critical appraisal of the literature. J the Am Board of Family Practice 1999; 12:315–333

31. Streiner DL: Sample size and power in psychiatric research. Can J Psychiatry 1990; 35:616–620

32. Hadorn DC, McCormick K, Diokno A: An annotated algorithm approach to clinical guideline development. J the Am Med Assoc 1992; 267:3311–3314

33. Osser DN, Patterson RD: Algorithms for psychopharmacology, in Manual of psychiatric therapeutics, third ed. Edited by Shader RI. Boston, Lippincott Williams & Wilkins, 2003

34. Trivedi MH, Kern JK, Baker SM, et al: Computerizing medication algorithms and decision support systems for major psychiatric disorders. J Psychiatr Practice 2000; 6:237–246

35. Quitkin FM: Placebos, drug effects, and study design: a clinician's guide. Am J Psychiatry 1999; 156:829–836

36. Adli M, Berghofer A, Linden M, et al: Effectiveness and feasibility of a standardized stepwise drug treatment regimen algorithm for inpatients with depressive disorders: results of a 2-year observational algorithm study. J Clin Psychiatry 2002; 63:782–790

37. Suppes T: Texas medication algorithm project, phase 3: clinical results for patients with a history of mania. J Clin Psychiatry 2003; 64:370–382

38. Epstein RM, Hundert EM: Defining and assessing professional competence. J the Am Med Assoc 2002; 287:226–235

39. Hatala R, Guyatt G: Evaluating the teaching of evidence-based medicine. J the Am Med Assoc 2002; 288:1110–1112

40. Landon BE, Normand ST, Blumenthal D, et al: Physician clinical performance assessment: prospects and barriers. J the Am Med Assoc 2003; 290:1183–1189

41. Osser DN, Patterson RD, Akhter A: Impact of a psychopharmacology course that emphasizes evidence-based medicine, practice guidelines, and algorithms, poster 290 in CINP 2004 Congress, Paris, 2004. Collegium Internationale Neuro-Psychopharmacologicum

42. American S of Clinical Psychopharmacology: Model Psychopharmacology Curriculum for Psychiatric Residency Programs, Training Directors, and Teachers of Psychopharmacology. New York, NY, American Society of Clinical Psychopharmacology, Inc., 1997

43. Rieder RO: Book review of A Model Psychopharmacology Curriculum. Acad Psychiatry 2000;24:2–3

44. Yank G: Book review of the model psychopharmacology curriculum. J Clin Psychiatry 2000; 61:952–953

45. Lomax JWI: Model curricula in psychiatric residency: evangelical failures or evocative facilitators? Acad Psychiatry 2001;25:109–111

46. Goldberg DA: Model curricula: the way we teach, the way we learn. Acad Psychiatry 2001;25:98–101

47. Glick ID, Janowsky DS, Zisook S, et al: How should we teach psychopharmacology to residents? results of the initial experiences with the ASCP model curriculum. Acad Psychiatry 2001;25:90–97

INDEX

Note: Page numbers followed by *f* and *t* indicate figures and tables, respectively.